ANNALS *of* THE NEW YORK ACADEMY OF SCIENCES

VOLUME
1285

ISBN-10: 1-57331-888-4; **ISBN-13:** 978-1-57331-888-4

ISSUE
The Year in Immunology

Basic and Clinical Research in Immunology

ISSUE EDITOR
Noel R. Rose

Johns Hopkins University

TABLE OF CONTENTS

Annals of the New York Academy of Sciences (ISSN: 0077-8923 [print]; ISSN: 1749-6632 [online]) is published 30 times a year on behalf of the New York Academy of Sciences by Wiley Subscription Services, Inc., a Wiley Company, 111 River Street, Hoboken, NJ 07030-5774.

Mailing: *Annals of the New York Academy of Sciences* is mailed standard rate.

Postmaster: Send all address changes to ANNALS OF THE NEW YORK ACADEMY OF SCIENCES, Journal Customer Services, John Wiley & Sons Inc., 350 Main Street, Malden, MA 02148-5020.

Disclaimer: The publisher, the New York Academy of Sciences, and the editors cannot be held responsible for errors or any consequences arising from the use of information contained in this publication; the views and opinions expressed do not necessarily reflect those of the publisher, the New York Academy of Sciences, and editors, neither does the publication of advertisements constitute any endorsement by the publisher, the New York Academy of Sciences and editors of the products advertised.

Copyright and Photocopying: © 2013 The New York Academy of Sciences. All rights reserved. No part of this publication may be reproduced, stored, or transmitted in any form or by any means without the prior permission in writing from the copyright holder. Authorization to photocopy items for internal and personal use is granted by the copyright holder for libraries and other users registered with their local Reproduction Rights Organization (RRO), e.g. Copyright Clearance Center (CCC), 222 Rosewood Drive, Danvers, MA 01923, USA (www.copyright.com), provided the appropriate fee is paid directly to the RRO. This consent does not extend to other kinds of copying such as copying for general distribution, for advertising or promotional purposes, for creating new collective works, or for resale. Special requests should be addressed to: permissionsUK@wiley.com.

Publisher: *Annals of the New York Academy of Sciences* is published by Wiley Periodicals, Inc., Commerce Place, 350 Main Street, Malden, MA 02148; Telephone: 781 388 8200; Fax: 781 388 8210.

Journal Customer Services: For ordering information, claims, and any inquiry concerning your subscription, please go to www.wileycustomerhelp.com/ask or contact your nearest office. *Americas:* Email: cs-journals@wiley.com; Tel:+1 781 388 8598 or 1 800 835 6770 (Toll free in the USA & Canada). *Europe, Middle East, Asia:* Email: cs-journals@wiley. com; Tel: +44 (0) 1865 778315. *Asia Pacific:* Email: cs-journals@wiley.com; Tel: +65 6511 8000. *Japan:* For Japanese speaking support, Email: cs-japan@wiley.com; Tel: +65 6511 8010 or Tel (toll-free): 005 316 50 480. Visit our Online Customer Get-Help available in 6 languages at www.wileycustomerhelp.com.

Information for Subscribers: *Annals of the New York Academy of Sciences* is published in 30 volumes per year. Subscription prices for 2013 are: Print & Online: US$6,053 (US), US$6,589 (Rest of World), €4,269 (Europe), £3,364 (UK). Prices are exclusive of tax. Australian GST, Canadian GST, and European VAT will be applied at the appropriate rates. For more information on current tax rates, please go to www.wileyonlinelibrary.com/tax-vat. The price includes online access to the current and all online back files to January 1, 2009, where available. For other pricing options, including access information and terms and conditions, please visit www.wileyonlinelibrary.com/access.

Delivery Terms and Legal Title: Where the subscription price includes print volumes and delivery is to the recipient's address, delivery terms are Delivered at Place (DAP); the recipient is responsible for paying any import duty or taxes. Title to all volumes transfers FOB our shipping point, freight prepaid. We will endeavour to fulfill claims for missing or damaged copies within six months of publication, within our reasonable discretion and subject to availability.

Back issues: Recent single volumes are available to institutions at the current single volume price from cs-journals@wiley.com. Earlier volumes may be obtained from Periodicals Service Company, 11 Main Street, Germantown, NY 12526, USA. Tel: +1 518 537 4700, Fax: +1 518 537 5899, Email: psc@periodicals.com. For submission instructions, subscription, and all other information visit: www.wileyonlinelibrary.com/journal/nyas.

Production Editors: Kelly McSweeney and Allie Struzik (email: nyas@wiley.com).

Commercial Reprints: Dan Nicholas (email: dnicholas@wiley.com).

Membership information: Members may order copies of *Annals* volumes directly from the Academy by visiting www. nyas.org/annals, emailing customerservice@nyas.org, faxing +1 212 298 3650, or calling 1 800 843 6927 (toll free in the USA), or +1 212 298 8640. For more information on becoming a member of the New York Academy of Sciences, please visit www.nyas.org/membership. Claims and inquiries on member orders should be directed to the Academy at email: membership@nyas.org or Tel: 1 800 843 6927 (toll free in the USA) or +1 212 298 8640.

Printed in the USA by The Sheridan Group.

View *Annals* online at www.wileyonlinelibrary.com/journal/nyas.

Abstracting and Indexing Services: *Annals of the New York Academy of Sciences* is indexed by MEDLINE, Science Citation Index, and SCOPUS. For a complete list of A&I services, please visit the journal homepage at www. wileyonlinelibrary.com/journal/nyas.

Access to *Annals* is available free online within institutions in the developing world through the AGORA initiative with the FAO, the HINARI initiative with the WHO, and the OARE initiative with UNEP. For information, visit www. aginternetwork.org, www.healthinternetwork.org, www.oarescience.org.

Annals of the New York Academy of Sciences accepts articles for Open Access publication. Please visit http://olabout.wiley.com/WileyCDA/Section/id-406241.html for further information about OnlineOpen.

Wiley's Corporate Citizenship initiative seeks to address the environmental, social, economic, and ethical challenges faced in our business and which are important to our diverse stakeholder groups. Since launching the initiative, we have focused on sharing our content with those in need, enhancing community philanthropy, reducing our carbon impact, creating global guidelines and best practices for paper use, establishing a vendor code of ethics, and engaging our colleagues and other stakeholders in our efforts. Follow our progress at www.wiley.com/go/citizenship.

ANNALS *of* THE NEW YORK ACADEMY OF SCIENCES

VOLUME
1285

ISSUE

The Year in Immunology

Basic and Clinical Research in Human Immunology

ISSUE EDITOR

Noel R. Rose

Johns Hopkins University

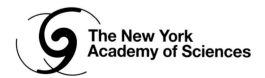
**The New York
Academy of Sciences**

Published by Blackwell Publishing
On behalf of the New York Academy of Sciences

Boston, Massachusetts
2013

Ann. N.Y. Acad. Sci. ISSN 0077-8923

ANNALS OF THE NEW YORK ACADEMY OF SCIENCES
Issue: *The Year in Immunology*

The proper study: preface to *The Year in Immunology*

Alexander Pope posited that "The proper study of mankind is man." It seems likely that the underlying motivation of most biomedical investigation is its eventual application to the betterment of humankind by the reduction of the burden of disease. This year's volume of *The Year in Immunology* emphasizes the importance of clinical and translational research to improve understanding of immune-mediated disease in humans.

Discovery in human medicine often follows a pathway leading from the clinic to the research laboratory and then back to the clinic. These steps generally begin with careful observation of individual patients, leading to larger population-based investigations, then to experimental studies in the test tube, the animal, or, in recent days, *in silico*. The ultimate outcome, after a passage of time, is improved diagnosis, treatment, and prevention.

The "proper study" of human disease, therefore, begins and ends with the patient. It is widely accepted that the patient's history of present illness provides the best starting point to gain insight into the disease process. There are numerous examples of cogent and comprehensive descriptions of illness made by patients, including physicians. Edward Trudeau's account of his tuberculosis, culminating in his self-prescribed treatment and the sanitorium movement in the United States, is a cogent example. The astute physician can frequently make a connection between a possible cause and a pathologic outcome just from careful clinical observation. Edward Jenner, noted for his later development of the vaccine for smallpox, first recorded the connection between pharyngitis and heart failure (probably due to rheumatic fever). That connection made in the 18th century waited 200 years for more data. The tools available to the clinician were greatly expanded by the widespread introduction of the autopsy, especially by Virchow and the Viennese school. William Osler, perhaps our most revered clinical observer, established his extraordinary insight into disease from the large number of autopsies he performed. On occasion, careful observation of disease in humans and a few laboratory procedures can lead to firm evidence of etiology. For example, Philip Levine clearly demonstrated the etiologic role of Rh antibody in hemolytic disease of the newborn just by skillful use of immunologic tests. The observational tools available to the clinician have expanded greatly over time with the introduction of pathologic and radiologic tests and, most recently, the increasing availability of genetic markers. The inclusion of social and environmental information, together with history of drug usage, infection, and occupational exposure, are additional examples of discovery medicine at the individual level.

After assembling the data obtainable from the individual, investigation usually proceeds to collections of individuals. Although often dismissed as anecdotes, collections of similar stories in groups of patients are frequently the first clue to the recognition of a novel disease process. The saga of John Snow and the Broad Street pump illustrates the value of epidemiologic study in providing the initial clues to the initiation and cause of disease. Yet, despite growing power based on modern bioinformatics, it is rare that epidemiology alone can establish more than an association. To develop a plausible biologic basis and define a mechanism, active intervention is needed.

doi: 10.1111/nyas.12158

Sometimes intervention takes the form of autoexperimentation, a procedure much frowned upon today. The self-transfusion of antibody by Harrington, in his effort to show that idiopathic thrombocytopenia is an antibody-mediated disease, nearly cost him his life. Because opportunities for experimental intervention in humans are limited by ethical principles and societal concerns, the search for etiology usually directs the investigator to development of a model in experimental animals.

It should be stated at the outset that a model does not necessarily reproduce all of the features of a human disease. It usually aims to replicate one aspect of the disease, in order to allow reductionist experiments leading to the demonstration of a probable mechanism. The use of animal models has been a cornerstone in the many advances of medicine during the 20th century; this tool has been spectacularly enhanced by the introduction of detailed genetic analysis and genetic engineering in rodents.

The employment of animal models can provide the first step toward translation of new knowledge back to human application. Preclinical testing of safety and efficacy are generally the first steps in introduction of a new method of treatment. Because animal models do not fully replicate the human disease, however, clinical trials must follow. Moreover, the use of animal experimentation imposes a commitment to responsible animal care. All such studies must be carefully conceived and executed. Sometimes the necessary information required for a definitive human trial can be assembled by use of *in vitro* assays or computer-based predictions.

Articles in this issue of *The Year in Immunology* represent all levels of human investigation. Mantovani *et al.* review the recent literature and their investigations concerning the long pentraxins, especially PTX3. These highly conserved molecules are important stimuli of the innate immune system, where they play a role in early resistance against pathogens, development of the inflammatory response, orientation of adaptive immunity, and, finally, in tissue repair. Although these investigations were carried out only using human specimens, the results correspond closely to results obtained in mice, suggesting that this is a fundamental step in the initiation of the immune response in infectious and immune-mediated diseases. Buerger's disease is another inflammatory disease in which there is presently no useful experimental model. Ketha and Cooper summarized the clinical, cellular, and molecular basis of this disease with special attention given to the prominent role of tobacco smoke as the environmental trigger. This is an example where the epidemiologic evidence has primarily identified tobacco as critical to the initiation and pathogenesis of the disease in the absence of an animal model. Cessation of tobacco smoking is both a primary and secondary preventative measure. Wiskott-Aldrich syndrome is a human disease that has been known for decades, but one in which there had been little understanding of the pathogenesis. It provides an example where application of genetic analysis in the human led to identification of the WAS gene located on the X-chromosome and the eventual isolation of the WAS protein. Mutations in the WAS protein are responsible for the broad array of signs of this disease. Massaad *et al.* describe how the study of this protein has led to better molecular understanding of the pathogenesis and suggest ways in which patients can be better managed.

Antiphospholipid syndrome, once regarded as a rare variant of lupus, is now known to represent a disease of increasing significance. Because of its highly variable clinical presentation involving thrombosis, unexplained pregnancy loss, and accelerated atherosclerosis, the availability of an antibody-based diagnostic test is the cornerstone of diagnosis. Unexpectedly, the major antigenic target appears to be the circulating form of the glycoprotein, beta-2 glycoprotein 1. How this antibody is generated in the course of antiphospholipid syndrome and its possible role in pathogenesis is discussed in the article by Willis and Pierangeli. Although a model of this disease has been developed in mice, the translation from animal data to human is an active area of continued investigation.

Not infrequently, new insights come from discoveries made primarily in mice and then related secondarily to humans. An example is the function of the BCL2 family. Although first discovered in human B cell lymphomas, the importance of this group of proteins has been greatly expanded by studies of their role in apoptosis of both B cells and T cells. Apoptosis is critical for regulation of inflammation, autophagy, and immune responses as well as lymphopoiesis. A comprehensive review of this growing area of investigation is provided by Renault and Chipuk.

An example of a disease where development of an animal model has opened new visions of understudied human disorders is represented in the article by Barin and Čiháková. They review the current information on inflammatory heart muscle disease as it appears in humans and how it can be reproduced in large measure by immunization of genetically susceptible mice with the requisite autoantigen, cardiac myosin. In many patients, the sequela of cardiac inflammation produced by experimental immunization or by infection with an appropriate virus is fibrotic remodeling of the heart, causing dilated cardiomyopathy. Identification of the cytokine signals leading to this often fatal outcome may provide the essential clue to recognizing this disease before it reaches its irreversible stage.

A long-standing topic of discussion in the immunologic literature is the function of B1 B cells. The cells undergo little V(D)J recombination and are believed to be involved in the production of naturally occurring, polyreactive antibodies. The presence of such a distinctive B cell population has been well established in mice, but remains controversial in humans. The relevant literature on the topic is critically summarized by Rothstein and colleagues. They describe the novel use of reverse engineering to produce a phenotype in human B cells that approximates functionally the CD5$^+$ B cell in mice. Future work will elucidate the role of B1 B cells in autoimmune and other immune system diseases in humans.

Arguably, the greatest contribution of immunology to human health and welfare during the past century was the introduction of vaccines as a public health measure. The application of vaccinology has saved millions of lives around the world. However, a medical procedure used commonly in healthy individuals requires the utmost safety as well as demonstrated efficacy. A major premium has been placed on the identification of the antigens of microorganisms that are most likely to provide protection and least likely to produce detrimental side effects. Reverse vaccinology, described by Donati and Rappuoli, is a novel approach; its safety and efficacy have been demonstrated by the development of an effective vaccine against group B *Neisseria meningitidis* infection, a worldwide cause of bacterial meningitis. The same approach can be applied to a number of other dangerous pathogens that have defied efforts to develop an effective vaccine strategy.

The final paper in this year's edition of *The Year in Immunology* describes the progress of the National Institutes of Health Center for Human Immunology, Autoimmunity, and Inflammation. As described by Dickler *et al.*, this joint effort of multiple NIH institutes is designed to overcome the fragmentation in clinical immunology, and basic immunology as applied to human diseases, by making available to individual laboratories the costly procedures for large-scale, high-throughput testing. As human immunology moves into the era of systems biology, intradisciplinary collaboration and pooled resources are of the greatest importance. Future generations of clinical immunologists will applaud the efforts of the pioneers at the NIH to create this model.

NOEL R. ROSE
Johns Hopkins University
Baltimore, Maryland

Ann. N.Y. Acad. Sci. ISSN 0077-8923

ANNALS OF THE NEW YORK ACADEMY OF SCIENCES
Issue: *The Year in Immunology*

The long pentraxin PTX3: a paradigm for humoral pattern recognition molecules

Alberto Mantovani,[1,2] Sonia Valentino,[1] Stefania Gentile,[1] Antonio Inforzato,[1] Barbara Bottazzi,[1] and Cecilia Garlanda[1]

[1]Humanitas Clinical and Research Center, Rozzano, Milan, Italy. [2]Department of Medical Biotechnology and Translational Medicine, University of Milan, Milan, Italy

Address for correspondence: Alberto Mantovani, MD, Scientific Director, Istituto Clinico Humanitas, Via Manzoni 113, 20089 Rozzano, Milano, Italy. alberto.mantovani@humanitasresearch.it

Pattern recognition molecules (PRMs) are components of the humoral arm of innate immunity; they recognize pathogen-associated molecular patterns (PAMP) and are functional ancestors of antibodies, promoting complement activation, opsonization, and agglutination. In addition, several PRMs have a regulatory function on inflammation. Pentraxins are a family of evolutionarily conserved PRMs characterized by a cyclic multimeric structure. On the basis of structure, pentraxins have been operationally divided into short and long families. C-reactive protein (CRP) and serum amyloid P component are prototypes of the short pentraxin family, while pentraxin 3 (PTX3) is a prototype of the long pentraxins. PTX3 is produced by somatic and immune cells in response to proinflammatory stimuli and Toll-like receptor engagement, and it interacts with several ligands and exerts multifunctional properties. Unlike CRP, PTX3 gene organization and regulation have been conserved in evolution, thus allowing its pathophysiological roles to be evaluated in genetically modified animals. Here we will briefly review the general properties of CRP and PTX3 as prototypes of short and long pentraxins, respectively, emphasizing in particular the functional role of PTX3 as a prototypic PRM with antibody-like properties.

Keywords: innate immunity; pentraxins; PTX3; pattern recognition molecules

Introduction

Innate immunity is a first line of resistance against pathogens, and it plays a key role in the activation and orientation of adaptive immunity and in the maintenance of tissue integrity and repair. Similar to adaptive immunity, the innate immune system consists of cellular and humoral arms, which are complementary and synergic in deciphering microbial patterns and regulating the innate response.[1,2]

Cell-associated pattern recognition molecules (PRMs) are strategically located in different cellular compartments (plasma membrane, endosomes, cytoplasm) and belong to different molecular classes, such as the Toll-like receptors (TLRs), the NOD and RIG-I–like receptors, and the scavenger receptors (Fig. 1).

Fluid phase PRMs belong to different molecular families, including collectins,[3] ficolins,[4] and pentraxins.[5] The pentraxin C-reactive protein (CRP) was the first PRM to be identified.[6,7] In spite of molecular diversity, humoral PRMs share a basic, evolutionarily conserved mode of action (complement activation; agglutination and neutralization; opsonization) (for example, see Ref. 8) and are functional ancestors of antibodies. Phagocytes serve as a source of PRMs, which are produced and released at sites of innate immune reactions: macrophages and myeloid dendritic cells (DCs) produce PRMs in a gene expression–dependent fashion, whereas neutrophils are a reservoir of ready-made PRMs that are rapidly released in minutes upon microbial encounter. In addition, epithelial tissues, the liver in particular, serve as a source of delayed, systemic mass production. Finally, some PRMs are produced constitutively to provide a ready-made line of defense in the circulation or in the lung, reminiscent of the function of natural antibodies.

doi: 10.1111/nyas.12043
Ann. N.Y. Acad. Sci. 1285 (2013) 1–14 © 2013 New York Academy of Sciences.

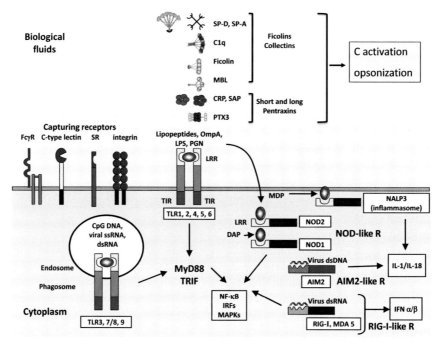

Figure 1. The humoral and the cellular arms of innate immunity: a schematic view. Fluid phase PRMs belong to different molecular families, including collectins (e.g., MBL, SP-A, SP-D), ficolins, C1q, and pentraxins (e.g., CRP, SAP, PTX3) and activate complement or facilitate opsonization of microbes. Cell-associated PRMs are located in different cellular compartments (e.g., plasma membrane, endosomes, cytoplasm) and belong to different molecular classes (e.g., TLRs; scavenger R; lectin R), some of which are shown here. The scavenger receptors (e.g., C-type lectins, integrins, and FcγR) are capturing receptors. The TLRs and NOD- and RIG-I-like receptors are signaling receptors that lead to activation of NF-κB, IRFs, and MAPKs. TLRs recognize microbial moieties. RIG-I-like receptors recognize viral double-strand RNA and induce production of type 1 IFN. AIM2-like receptors recognize viral DNA and activate the inflammasome, leading to IL-1β and IL-18 production. Muramyl dipeptide (MDP) is recognized by NOD2 and NALP3, a component of the inflammasome. Diaminopimelic acid (DAP) is recognized by NOD1. Conserved domains, such as the TIR domain, or leucin reach repeat (LRR) domain are shown (modified from Ref. 8).

Fluid phase PRMs are recognized by cellular receptors expressed on innate immunity cells. By interacting with cellular receptors directly and triggering complement activation, PRMs facilitate recognition and effector function of phagocytes and related cells.

Here we will review available information on pentraxins, with pentraxin 3, in particular, as a paradigm of humoral PRM mode of action in defense and inflammation.

CRP and short pentraxins

The presence of a highly conserved motif of primary amino acid sequence—the pentraxin signature HxCxS/TWxS, where x is any amino acid—is a distinctive feature of the members of the pentraxin family. Prototypes of the family are CRP and the closely related protein serum amyloid P (SAP) component (with 51% sequence identity to human CRP).[9] Orthologous proteins to human CRP and SAP have been described in the hemolymph of the arthropod *Limulus polyphemus*, where they are involved in the recognition and killing of pathogens.[5,10–12]

Human CRP and SAP are 25-kDa proteins produced by hepatocytes in response to IL-6.[13] They are characterized by a common structural organization that comprises, respectively, five or ten identical subunits arranged in a pentameric radial symmetry.[9,14] Each of the subunits displays a lectin-like fold composed of a two-layered β sheet with flattened jellyroll topology. Human CRP is not glycosylated, whereas human SAP has an N-linked glycosylation site occupied by sialylated glycans.[15,16]

CRP and SAP are the main acute-phase reactants in human and mouse, respectively. CRP is barely detectable in the plasma of healthy human adults ($\leq$3 mg/L), but its concentration increases by as much as 1000-fold in many pathological conditions, with a sharp rise within 6 h of induction and a maximum increase at approximately 48 hours. For this reason CRP is widely used as a marker of inflammation in several human pathological conditions, including cardiovascular diseases and infections.[7] In contrast, the level of human (but not murine) SAP does not change in pathological conditions, even during the early acute-phase response.

CRP and SAP are ancient immune molecules that share many functional properties with antibodies: they bind several molecules (Table 1), mostly in a Ca^{2+}-dependent manner, activate complement, opsonize biological particles, and bind to all three classes of Fcγ receptors (FcγR). In particular, both molecules participate in activation and regulation of the three complement pathways (i.e., classical, lectin, and alternative) by interacting with C1q,[17] ficolins,[18,19] factor H (FH),[20–22] and C4 binding protein (C4BP).[23,24] It has been suggested that complement activation by short pentraxins might favor removal of apoptotic debris, with potential implications in preventing the onset of autoimmune diseases.[25]

CRP, named after its ability to bind in a calcium-dependent fashion to the C-polysaccharide of *Streptococcus pneumonia*,[13] recognizes diverse pathogens, including fungi, yeasts, and bacteria, and promotes their removal by phagocytosis mediated through interaction with FcγR,[26–29] thus providing resistance to infection.[30] Consistent with this, CRP transgenic mice are resistant to infection with *S. pneumoniae*, displaying longer survival time and lower mortality rate than wild-type mice.[31] Similarly, SAP binds a number of bacteria (e.g., *S. pyogenes* and *Neisseria meningitides*),[32,33] influenza virus,[34] and lipopolysaccharide (LPS).[33,35] SAP has been shown to function as a β inhibitor of influenza virus by binding in a calcium-dependent fashion to mannose-rich glycans on the viral hemagglutinin (HA) and inhibiting both hemagglutination and viral infectivity.[34,36] However, the relationship between ligand binding and function of SAP and CRP is still a matter of debate.[37] For example, while CRP does not recognize *Salmonella typhimurium*, it has a protective role against this pathogen.[38] Similarly, SAP exhibits host defense functions against pathogens

Table 1. Ligand specificity of CRP, SAP, and PTX3

Ligand	CRP	SAP	PTX3
Microorganisms			
Bacteria			
Pseudomonas aeruginosa	NT[a]	NT	+
Klebsiella pneumoniae	NT	NT	+
Salmonella typhimurium	–	+	+
Fungi and yeasts			
Aspergillus fumigatus	+	NT	+
Saccharomyces cerevisiae (zymosan)	+	+	+
Paracoccidioides brasiliensis	NT	NT	+
Viruses			
Influenza virus	–	+	+
Human cytomegalovirus (HCMV)	NT	NT	+
Membrane moieties			
Phosphocholine (PC)	+	–	–
Phosphoethanolamine (PE)	–	+	–
LPS	–	+	–
Outer membrane protein A from *Klebsiella pneumoniae* (KpOmpA)	NT	NT	+
Complement components			
C1q	+	+	+
Factor H	+	NT	+
C4BP	+	+	+
M-, L-ficolin	+	–	+
MBL	–	+	+
Extracellular matrix proteins			
TNF-stimulated gene-6 (TSG-6)	NT	NT	+
Inter-α-trypsin-inhibitor (IαI)	–	NT	+
Hyaluronan	NT	NT	–
Laminin	+	+	–
Collagen IV	NT	+	–
Fibronectin	+	+	–
Growth factors			
FGF2	+/–	NT	+
FGF1 and FGF4	NT	NT	–
Adhesion molecules			
P-selectin	–	NT	+

[a]NT: not tested.

that it does not recognize.[33] In summary, pentraxins can activate both complement and FcγR pathways, which resembles the functional properties of antibodies.

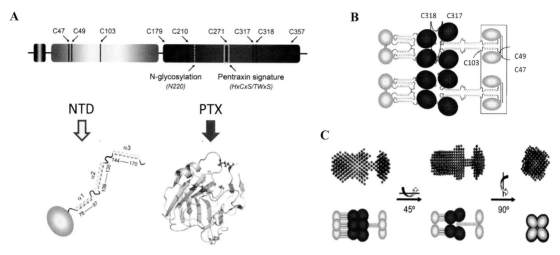

Figure 2. Model of the PTX3 protein. (A) Schematic representation of the PTX3 protomer: the N-terminal domain is in yellow and the pentraxin domain is in red. Positions of the Cys residues, the *N*-glycosylation site at Asn220, and the pentraxin signature motif are indicated. Arrows point to the model proposed for the N-terminal domain, which is believed to be composed of a globular region and three α-helical segments (α1, α2, and α3), and to a three-dimensional model of the C-terminal pentraxin domain, based on the crystal structure of C-reactive protein (Protein Data Bank ID: 1b09). (B) Disulfide bond organization of the PTX3 octamer. The α-helical regions of the N-terminal domains predicted to form coiled-coil–like structures are hypothesized to adopt two distinct structural arrangements: an extended conformation, in which four protomers associate through interchain interactions (i.e., to form tetramers), or a compact organization, where each protomer self-associates to form an antiparallel three-helix bundle (i.e., to form dimer of dimers). (C) A comparison of the small-angle X-ray scattering envelope with a schematic model for PTX3 based on the two different organizations proposed for the N-terminal domain above; the α-helical segments of the N-terminal domain are depicted as yellow rods. The C-terminal pentraxin domains are in red (adapted from Ref. 59).

The prototypic long pentraxin PTX3

General characteristics and structure

Human PTX3 is a prototype of the long pentraxin subfamily. The molecule is a multimeric glycoprotein comprising 381 amino acids, including a 17-residue signal peptide (Fig. 2A).[39] The C-terminal half containing the pentraxin signature is highly homologous to CRP and SAP,[5] with up to 57% similarity to these molecules;[39] in contrast, the N-terminal domain of PTX3 is unrelated to other known proteins. The PTX3 primary sequence is highly conserved among animal species (e.g., 92% of amino acid residues in human and murine PTX3 are conserved), suggesting a strong evolutionary pressure to maintain its structure/function relationships. The protein is rapidly and locally produced by different cells, including cells of the myeloid lineage (e.g., monocytes, macrophages, DCs, and neutrophils (PMN)), vascular and lymphatic endothelial cells, smooth muscles cells (SMCs), epithelial cells, and fibroblasts. Primary proinflammatory cytokines (namely IL-1β and TNF-α), intact microorganisms or TLR agonists

(e.g., LPS or bacterial outer membrane lipoproteins), and high-density lipoproteins (HDLs) induce PTX3.[5,40] IL-10 is a mild inducer of PTX3 in monocytes and DCs and can amplify PTX3 production induced by LPS.[41,42] Thus, PTX3 production may be part of the gene expression program activated by IL-10, an essential player of tissue injury resolution produced by anti-inflammatory M2-polarized macrophages.[43] Accordingly, PTX3 deficiency is associated with higher tissue damage in experimental models of atherosclerosis or acute heart injury, and with altered skin would healing (see Refs. 44 and 45, and A. Doni, unpublished data). Glucocorticoid hormones have divergent regulatory effects, inhibiting PTX3 production in myeloid cells or inducing and enhancing the production of the protein by fibroblasts under inflammatory conditions.[46]

The human PTX3 gene is located on chromosome 3q25 and is organized as three exons. The first and second exons code for the signal peptide and the long N-terminal domain (amino acids 18–179), while the third exon codes for the pentraxin-like C-terminal domain (amino acids 179–381). Transcription of both human and murine PTX3 gene is controlled by numerous potential enhancer binding elements, including Pu1, AP-1, NF-κB, SP1, and NF-IL6 sites.[47,48] The JNK pathway is involved in PTX3 production following TNF-α stimulation of alveolar epithelial cells,[49] while HDL induction requires activation of the PI3K/Akt pathway and the G-coupled glycosphingolipid receptor.[50] The HIF-1α and C/EBPβ pathways are involved in upregulation of PTX3 gene expression during cardiac surgery,[51] and IL-1RI or MyD88 are essential for PTX3 induction in a model of acute myocardial ischemia and reperfusion in mice.[45] The FUS/CHOP translocation involved in the pathogenesis of myxoid liposarcoma regulates PTX3 expression in liposarcoma tissues.[52,53] PTX3 production is thus controlled by several pathways, depending on the tissue compartment and inducing stimuli.

A unique N-linked glycosylation site is located in the C-terminal domain at Asn220. This glycosidic moiety includes fucosylated and sialylated biantennary sugars with a minor fraction of tri and tetraantennary glycans.[54] Despite this apparent structural conservation, we have observed a considerable heterogeneity in the relative content of bi-, tri-, and tetrantennary oligosaccharides and in the degree of sialylation among PTX3 isolates from different cellular sources, suggesting that its glycosylation status might change depending on cell type and inducing stimuli. This might have important functional implications in the modulation of PTX3 crosstalk with other molecules.

Given the high homology of PTX3 with CRP, three-dimensional models of the PTX3 C-terminal domain have been generated that are based on the crystallographic structures of CRP (PDB ID: 1b09) and SAP (PDB ID: 1sac).[54–56] Figure 2A presents a CRP-derived model showing the pentraxin-like domain of PTX3 with a β-jellyroll topology, similar to that found in legume lectins. This model contains a highly conserved disulfide bond involving Cys210 and Cys271. An additional intrachain disulfide is present that links the N- and C-terminal ends of the PTX3 C-terminal domain via Cys179 and Cys357, thus limiting the flexibility of these regions. The two remaining cysteine residues of the C-terminal fragment (i.e., Cys317 and Cys318) have been reported to form both intra- and interchain disulfide linkages that are important determinants of the complex quaternary structure of PTX3.[57] According to secondary structure prediction, the N-terminal domain is likely to form four α-helices, three of which are probably involved in the formation of coiled-coil structures (Fig. 2A).[58,59]

Mass spectrometry and site-directed mutagenesis analyses of the recombinant human protein indicate that PTX3 is an octamer made from two tetramers linked together by interchain bridges (Fig. 2B).[57] Electron microscopy (EM) and small angle X-ray scattering (SAXS) were used to generate a low-resolution model of the intact PTX3 molecule where the eight subunits of the protein fold into an elongated structure with a large and a small domain interconnected by a stalk region (Fig. 2C).[59] The association of protomers with tetramers is mediated by the PTX3 N-terminal domain via both covalent (i.e., disulfide bonds) and noncovalent (i.e., interchain coiled coils) interactions (see Fig. 2B).

Ligands and effector mechanisms

As reported for CRP and SAP, PTX3 binds a broad spectrum of cellular and molecular targets (summarized in Table 1), thus providing the basis for its multifunctional properties. A soluble pattern recognition molecule, PTX3 recognizes and binds to a wide range of microbes, including bacteria, fungi, and viruses. Specific binding has been observed to conidia of *Aspergillus fumigatus*,[60] *Paracoccidioides brasiliensis,* zymosan,[61] selected Gram-positive and Gram-negative bacteria,[1,60] and to some viruses, such as human and murine cytomegalovirus (HCMV and MCMV) and influenza virus type A (IVA).[62,63] Some microbial moieties have been identified that are specifically recognized by PTX3, including the hemagglutinin of IAV[63] and the outer membrane protein A (OMP-A) from *Klebsiella pneumonia,*[1] a member of the OMP family of Gram-negative bacteria.

As mentioned, PTX3 recognizes and modulates the activity of key components of the three complement activation cascades. It binds C1q, the main activator of the complement classical pathway, interacting with the globular head of C1q in a calcium-independent fashion.[17] Differently from CRP, no crosslinking by PTX3 is necessary for optimal *in vitro* interaction, likely because of the stable multimeric structure of PTX3. When the interaction occurs with plastic-immobilized PTX3, increased deposition of C3 and C4 is observed, demonstrating the activation of the classical complement pathway. When the interaction between PTX3 and C1q occurs in the fluid phase, in contrast, an inhibition of complement activation is observed via competitive blocking of relevant interaction sites.[25]

PTX3 interacts with members of the lectin pathway, namely ficolin-1,[64] ficolin-2[65] and mannose-binding lectin (MBL).[66] The binding occurs via the fibrinogen-binding domain (FBG) of ficolins, or via the collagen like domain of MBL, and the terminal sialic acid of the glycosidic moiety of PTX3. The physical interaction of PTX3 and ficolin-2 or MBL is accompanied by a functional cooperation that promotes recruitment of the molecules onto the surface of recognized microbes (e.g., *A. fumigatus* and *Candida albicans*) and synergistically amplifies the complement-mediated innate response.[8,65,66]

In addition to the interaction with components of the classical and lectin complement cascades, PTX3 can interact with regulators of complement activation, namely FH and C4BP.[67,68] By promoting FH deposition on PTX3-coated surfaces, PTX3 can modulate the alternative pathway and prevent exaggerated complement activation.[68] Similarly, PTX3 recruits C4BP on apoptotic cells or on the extracellular matrix (ECM), increasing the rate of C4b inactivation and reducing deposition of the lytic C5b-9 terminal complex.[67]

Several pieces of evidence indicate that PTX3 can regulate inflammatory reactions;[45,69,70] and the recent discovery that PTX3 binds the adhesion molecule P-selectin has provided a molecular mechanism for these findings.[71] The interaction with P-selectin, occuring via the N-linked glycosidic moiety of PTX3, inhibits leukocyte rolling on endothelium, as well as excessive leukocyte recruitment *in vivo*.[71] In addition, PTX3 binds the angiogenic factor fibroblast growth factor 2 (FGF2)[72] and thereby inhibits FGF2-dependent EC proliferation *in vitro* and angiogenesis *in vivo*. Also, PTX3 inhibits FGF2-dependent smooth muscle cell activation and intimal thickening after arterial injury.[73] Thus, PTX3 may contribute to the modulation of FGF2 activity in different pathological settings in which coexpression of the two proteins occurs.

Immunofluorescence data indicate that PTX3 localizes to the viscoelastic matrix of the cumulus oophorus, where it interacts with proteins of the ECM, such as TNF-α–induced protein 6 (TNFAIP6 or TSG-6) and inter-α-trypsin inhibitor (IαI).[74,75] The binding of PTX3 with TSG-6 and IαI is essential for the organization of the viscoelastic matrix

of cumuli; lack of PTX3 is associated with female subfertility as a consequence of cumulus matrix instability.[74]

While most of the ligands mentioned above required full-length PTX3 for optimal binding, for other ligands a division of labor has been observed between the C-terminal and N-terminal PTX3 domains. This is the case, for instance, of the interaction with P-selectin, mediated by the glycosidic moiety located on the C-terminal domain, or with FGF2, TSG-6, and IαI, for which the PTX3 N-terminal domain almost completely accounts for binding and for its biological effects.[71,75,76]

Functional roles

PTX3 in pathogen recognition. Genetically modified mice have enabled investigation of the *in vivo* relevance of microbe recognition by PTX3. *Ptx3*[−/−] mice are highly susceptible to invasive pulmonary aspergillosis, showing higher mortality rates.[60] In this model, PTX3-deficient neutrophils or dendritic cells and alveolar macrophages exhibit defective recognition and killing of conidia, and treatment with recombinant PTX3 or neutrophil-associated *Ptx3* expression reverses the phenotype.[60,77] The susceptibility to aspergillosis is associated with a low protective T helper 1 (Th1) antifungal response. Treatment with recombinant PTX3 restores the protective Th1 response, demonstrating that PTX3 can participate in the tuning of immune responses.[60,78] Moreover, in an experimental model of chronic granulomatous disease (*p47*[phox−/−] mice), PTX3 limited the pathogenic inflammation induced by *A. fumigatus* infection. In both *p47*[phox−/−] and *p47*[phox+/+] mice, PTX3 reduced neutrophil counts and mononuclear cell recruitment to the lung parenchyma and bronchoalveolar lavage fluid.[79]

In an effort to define the molecular mechanisms underlying the opsonic activity of PTX3, it has been demonstrated that the molecule enhances the recognition and phagocytosis of conidia by neutrophils through an Fcγ receptor II (FcγRII)-, CD11b-, complement-dependent mechanism.[80] Indeed, PTX3 modulates different effector pathways involved in innate resistance to *A. fumigatus*, including complement activation[25,65,68,81] or promotion of phagocytosis by interacting with Fcγ Rs, which have been identified as pentraxin receptors.[29,82]

Recent results have indicated that PTX3 has therapeutic activity in chronic lung infection by

Pseudomonas aeruginosa, which is a major cause of morbidity and mortality in cystic fibrosis (CF) patients. C57BL/6 mice infected chronically with *P. aeruginosa* and treated with recombinant human PTX3 showed enhanced clearance of bacteria from the lungs, which was associated with reduced production of local proinflammatory cytokines and chemokines, neutrophil recruitment in the airways, and histopathological lesions.[83] In models of acute *P. aeruginosa* infection and in *in vitro* assays, the prophagocytic effect of PTX3 was shown to be maintained in C1q-deficient mice but was lost in C3- and Fcγ R-deficient mice, suggesting that PTX3-dependent facilitated recognition and phagocytosis of *P. aeruginosa* is mediated through the interplay between complement and Fcγ Rs.[83]

Ptx3-overexpressing macrophages exhibit increased phagocytosis of zymosan and *P. brasiliensis* compared with macrophages from wild-type mice.[61] In response to zymosan, *Ptx3*-transgenic macrophages had enhanced expression of dectin-1, the cellular receptor primarily involved in the interaction between macrophages and zymosan. Moreover, since zymosan induces PTX3 expression, dectin-1 upregulation by PTX3 promotes a positive feedback of phagocytosis.[61]

In *K. pneumoniae* infection, overexpression of PTX3 by transgenic mice is associated with an enhanced ability to produce proinflammatory mediators, including NO and TNF-α, and, as a consequence, leads to protection or to faster lethality, depending on the dose of the inoculum.[84]

PTX3 binds both human and murine cytomegalovirus (MCMV), reducing viral entry and infectivity of DCs *in vitro*.[62] Consistently, PTX3-deficient mice are more susceptible to MCMV infection than PTX3 wild-type mice, and PTX3 protects susceptible BALB/c mice from MCMV primary infection and reactivation *in vivo*, as well as from *A. fumigatus* superinfection.[62]

Finally, human and murine PTX3 binds influenza virus (H3N2) through the interaction of the viral hemagglutinin glycoprotein and the sialic acid residue present on the glycosidic moiety of PTX3. PTX3 inhibits virus-induced hemagglutination and viral neuraminidase activity, and neutralizes virus infectivity.[63] However, it has been recently reported that both seasonal and pandemic H1N1 influenza A viruses are resistant to the antiviral activity of PTX3.[85]

The relevance in humans of data obtained in animals on the role of PTX3 in infection has been demonstrated by Olesen *et al.*, who recently analyzed the effects of polymorphisms within the PTX3 gene on pulmonary tuberculosis (TB) and showed that the frequency of specific PTX3 haplotypes is significantly different in TB patients compared to healthy individuals.[86] The same polymorphisms studied in TB also correlated with the risk of *P. aeruginosa* infection in CF patients. PTX3 haplotype frequencies differed between CF patients colonized or not by *P. aeruginosa*, and a specific haplotype was associated with a protective effect.[87]

PTX3 in sterile inflammation and cardiovascular diseases. Data obtained in different models *in vivo* have demonstrated that PTX3 is involved in modulating inflammation in sterile conditions, for instance in acute myocardial infarction and atherosclerosis.[88] The role of PTX3 in experimental myocardial infarction was assessed in *Ptx3*-deficient mice.[45] Similar to humans, in wild-type mice PTX3 levels peaked after ischemia followed by reperfusion; and infarcts were significantly larger in *Ptx3*-deficient mice than in wild-type mice. A possible protective cardiovascular role for PTX3 has been hypothesized to occur via modulation of complement activation by PTX3, as a higher deposition of C3 was observed in *Ptx3*-deficient mice in the infarcted area. The interaction between PTX3 and FH, resulting in promotion of FH deposition on PTX3-coated surfaces, could be a mechanism for preventing tissue damage associated with exaggerated complement activation.[68] *Ptx3*-deficiency is also associated with increased atherosclerosis in apolipoprotein E (ApoE)–deficient mice, including increased macrophage accumulation in atherosclerotic lesions.[44] Furthermore, mice lacking *Ptx3* had increased expression of adhesion molecules, cytokines, and chemokines in vascular walls, thus suggesting that PTX3 may modulate the vascular-associated inflammatory response.[44]

Binding to P-selectin underlies the regulatory role of PTX3 in inflammation. Indeed, both exogenously administered PTX3 and endogenous PTX3 released from hematopoietic cells induce a negative feedback loop that prevents excessive P-selectin–dependent recruitment of neutrophils in experimental models of acute lung injury (ALI), pleurisy, mesenteric inflammation, and acute kidney injury.[71,140] Thus,

PTX3 produced by activated leukocytes might locally dampen neutrophil recruitment and regulate inflammation. In keeping with this, Liu *et al.* have suggested that PTX3 plays a protective role in the pathogenesis of ALI, and the lack of PTX3 may enhance neutrophil recruitment, cell death, and inflammatory responses in LPS instillation–induced ALI.[89] Finally, PTX3 inhibits FGF2-dependent EC proliferation *in vitro* and angiogenesis *in vivo*. In addition, *in situ*, PTX3 overexpression was associated with abrogated neointimal thickening following balloon injury of rat carotid arteries.[73] These effects were associated with the ability of PTX3 to prevent FGF2 binding to its receptor,[76] thus limiting FGF2-dependent activation, proliferation, and migration of SMCs.

These data suggest that PTX3 plays a regulatory role in inflammation and tissue damage through multiple mechanisms, including complement, P-selectin–dependent leukocyte recruitment, FGF2-dependent angiogenesis, and SMC activation.

PTX3 in autoimmunity. PRMs and complement components contribute to opsonization of apoptotic cells and their recognition by phagocytes, and thus are protective molecules in the development of autoimmune diseases. Both PTX3 and the short pentraxins SAP and CRP bind to apoptotic cells to assist their clearance.[90] When bound to self-surfaces such as apoptotic cells or damaged tissue, CRP activates the classical complement pathway through interaction with C1q, but this activation is restricted to the initial stages, with only little consumption of the terminal components C5–C9.[25,91]

PTX3 and C1q bind apoptotic cells with similar kinetics, interacting with different binding sites and remaining stably associated with the apoptotic cell membrane.[92] However, the interaction between PTX3 and C1q in the fluid phase prevents the binding of C1q and C3 deposition on apoptotic cells, as well as C1q-mediated phagocytosis of apoptotic cells by DCs and phagocytes.[91–94] In contrast, when PTX3 is incubated with apoptotic cells, it enhances the deposition of both C1q and C3 on the cell surface.[25] In addition, it has been shown that endogenous PTX3 translocates to the plasma membrane of late apoptotic neutrophils through a process that involves fusion of granules and apoptotic cell membrane. The translocated PTX3 accumulates in blebs of the plasma membrane, where it acts as

an "eat-me" molecule in promoting, rather than inhibiting, the clearance of apoptotic neutrophils by phagocytes.[95] Therefore, membrane-associated PTX3 promotes phagocytosis of late apoptotic neutrophils, in contrast to the soluble form of PTX3, which inhibits this process. Data obtained *in vivo* in a murine model of systemic lupus erythematosus are in agreement with these latter results and show that PTX3 fosters the rapid clearance of apoptotic T cells by peritoneal macrophages. This process may keep lupus autoantigens away from dendritic cells, avoiding the activation of autoreactive T cells. In agreement as well, *Ptx3*-deficiency on a lupus-prone genetic background (C57BL/6 pr) has been shown to aggravate autoimmune lung disease (peribronchial and perivascular CD3[+] T cell and macrophage infiltrates), which has been associated with selective expansion of CD4/CD8 double negative autoreactive T cells.[96]

Together, these results indicate the relevance of context of PTX3 production. On one hand, cell-bound PTX3 might serve to enhance the elimination of apoptotic cells before loss of cell-membrane permeability, release of self-antigens, and tissue damage signals.[95,97] On the other hand, rapid production and secretion of PTX3 during inflammation might avoid capture of apoptotic cells in a proinflammatory setting that is likely to trigger an immune response against self-antigens.[90] Finally, it has been reported that opsonization of apoptotic cells by factor H can limit complement-mediated lysis of these cells.[98] Through its binding to factor H, PTX3 promotes recruitment of this complement component to the surface of dying cells, therefore functioning as a negative modulator of the alternative pathway in injured tissues;[68] this effect would also prevent complement membrane attack complex-mediated bystander injury of normal cells.

Translation to the clinic

Based on the similarities with CRP—a widely used diagnostic tool in the clinic—efforts are underway to evaluate the role of PTX3 as a marker and therapeutic agent in human pathologies. PTX3 functions as an acute-phase response protein, as its level in blood, below 2 ng/mL in normal conditions, increases rapidly (peaks at 6–8 h) and dramatically (200–800 ng/mL) during endotoxic shock, sepsis, and other inflammatory and infectious conditions, including *A. fumigatus* infections, meningococcal diseases, dengue infection, tuberculosis, and leptospirosis.[60,99–104] In these cases a significant correlation has been found between PTX3 plasma levels and severity of disease and mortality. In addition, based on preclinical evidence, on-going studies are evaluating the possible use of PTX3 as an antifungal agent in immunocompromised patients.

The high levels of PTX3 expression in the heart during inflammatory reactions and its similarities with CRP prompted studies on PTX3 levels during cardiovascular diseases. A first pilot study on patients with acute myocardial infarction (AMI) showed that PTX3 increases rapidly in the plasma, with a peak at 6–8 h from symptom onset.[105] In a cohort of 748 patients with AMI and ST elevation, PTX3, measured within the first day from the onset of symptoms along with established markers including CRP, N-terminal probrain natriuretic peptide (NT-proBNP), and troponin-T, emerged as the only independent predictor of three months mortality.[106] In agreement with these results, the Cardiovascular Health Study confirmed the association of PTX3 with cardiovascular disease and all-cause mortality.[107]

The role of PTX3 as a marker of cardiovascular diseases has been extended in subjects with chronic heart failure. Two small studies suggested that best risk prediction was obtained when PTX3 levels were combined with brain natriuretic peptide and human fatty acid-binding protein.[108,109] These studies have been extended recently, when plasma levels of PTX3 were measured at randomization and after three months in 1457 patients enrolled in the Controlled Rosuvastatin Multinational Trial in Heart Failure (CORONA) and in 1233 patients from the GISSI-Heart Failure trial (GISSI-HF). In the two independent clinical trials, PTX3 was consistently associated with higher risk of all-cause mortality and cardiovascular mortality.[110] Circulating PTX3 was also significantly elevated in patients with coronary artery disease,[111] aortic valve stenosis,[112] and unstable angina,[113,114] and reflected severity of cardiovascular disease in patients with inflammatory rheumatic disease.[115] PTX3 levels correlated with the severity of carotid and femoral atherosclerosis and were highest in individuals with multiple vascular territories affected, even if they did not correlate with intima media thickness.[116,117]

Increased expression of plasma PTX3 has been observed in several inflammatory diseases, especially disorders of the immune system, such as rheumatoid arthritis,[118] progressive systemic sclerosis,[119] Churg–Straus syndrome, Wegener's granulomatosis, microscopic polyangiitis,[120] Horton's disease,[121] and systemic inflammatory response syndrome (SIRS).[104,122,123] Also, controversial results obtained by one group of authors[124,125] from patients with metabolic syndrome or obesity indicating a significant correlation between PTX3 plasma levels and body mass index were not confirmed by another study.[126] Plasma PTX3 levels were a increased in patients with ulcerative colitis but not in patients with active Crohn's disease, suggesting that the protein may be a good diagnostic marker for deterioration in patients with inflammatory bowel disease.[127,128] In addition, PTX3 levels were a predictor of mortality in patients with ischemic stroke[129] and were elevated in cerebrospinal fluid after subarachnoid hemorrhage, correlating with vasospasm.[130] In chronic kidney disease, increased PTX3 levels correlated with proteinuria, all-cause mortality, and cardiovascular mortality, indicating that the protein could have a prognostic value.[131–133]

In other contexts, PTX3 expression has been recently reported in different tumors; results obtained indicate a potential role of PTX3 as a biomarker of cancer. This is the case, for instance, in lung cancer, where proteomic analysis aimed at identifying new markers of neoplastic transformation found that PTX3 plasma levels were increased in patients with lung cancer,[134] and that these levels had diagnostic sensitivity and specificity similar to those of other clinically used lung cancer biomarkers.[135] Similarly, in myeloproliferative neoplasms (e.g., essential thrombocythemia and polycythemia vera)[136] PTX3 plasma levels were significantly increased and correlated with JAK2 V617F allele burden. In contrast to CRP, higher levels of PTX3 were inversely associated with the number of major thrombotic events, suggesting that the protein may have a protective role in preventing vascular events. PTX3 was one of the upregulated genes belonging to the stromal signature identified in ovarian cancer and associated with poor prognosis,[137] and was one of the most expressed genes in myxoid liposarcoma.[52,53] PTX3 expression is upregulated in tumor tissue from prostate carcinoma[138] but reduced in esophageal squamous cell carcinoma (ESCC).[139] In particular, recent data identified PTX3 as a new epigenetically silenced hypermethylated gene in ESCC, suggesting that the molecule may play a tumor suppressive role.

Concluding remarks

Pentraxins are multifunctional fluid phase pattern recognition molecules. CRP and PTX3 are prototypic molecules representative of the short and the long pentraxin families, respectively. While CRP lacks a strict evolutionary conservation between mouse and human, with regard to sequence, ligands recognized, and regulation, the long pentraxin PTX3 is highly conserved in evolution. Gene targeting of PTX3 has unequivocally defined functional roles of this molecule in innate immunity and inflammation. Recent progress has further defined the structure, regulation, microbial recognition, and *in vivo* activities of PTX3. PTX3 plays a role similar to that of antibodies, including in complement activation, opsonization, and glycosylation-dependent regulation of inflammation. Available evidence suggests that PTX3 not only functions as a PRM but also as a tuner of inflammatory reactions, and it may contribute to the discrimination between self, infectious nonself, and modified self.

Translational studies suggest that PTX3 may be a useful marker of human pathologies complementary to CRP, as PTX3 is directly produced by damaged tissues, and its increase precedes CRP and rapidly reflects the inflammatory process. In particular, the combination of PTX3 and classical biomarkers provides more diagnostic and prognostic value in several conditions, including sepsis, acute coronary syndrome, and chronic heart failure. In addition, emerging data indicate that further investigation is necessary to dissect the pathophysiological role of PTX3 during neoplastic transformation and its possible use as a biomarker of cancer.

The data obtained thus far suggest that PTX3 may be a novel, promising biomarker that provides useful prognostic information for clinical outcomes in different pathologic conditions. In parallel, the nonredundant role of PTX3 in various mouse and rat disease models suggests that this long pentraxin may be a novel therapeutic agent for some infectious diseases, a possibility that deserves further investigation.

Acknowledgments

The contributions of the European Commission (FP7-HEALTH-F4-2008 "TOLERAGE" 202156, FP7-HEALTH-2011-ADITEC-280873), European Research Council (project HIIS), Fondazione CARIPLO (project Nobel and Project 2009-2582), Ministero della Salute (Ricerca finalizzata), the Italian Association for Cancer Research (AIRC), and Regione Lombardia (project Metadistretti—SEPSIS) are gratefully acknowledged.

Conflicts of interest

The authors declare no conflicts of interest.

References

1. Jeannin, P. *et al.* 2005. Complexity and complementarity of outer membrane protein A recognition by cellular and humoral innate immunity receptors. *Immunity* **22:** 551–560.
2. Ip, W.K.E., K. Takahashi, K.J. Moore, *et al.* 2008. Mannose-binding lectin enhances Toll-like receptors 2 and 6 signaling from the phagosome. *J. Exp. Med.* **205:** 169–181.
3. Holmskov, U., S. Thiel & J.C. Jensenius. 2003. Collectins and ficolins: humoral lectins of the innate immune defense. *Annu. Rev. Immunol.* **21:** 547–578.
4. Endo, Y., M. Matsushita & T. Fujita. 2007. Role of ficolin in innate immunity and its molecular basis. *Immunobiology* **212:** 371–379.
5. Garlanda, C., B. Bottazzi, A. Bastone & A. Mantovani. 2005. Pentraxins at the crossroads between innate immunity, inflammation, matrix deposition and female fertility. *Annu. Rev. Immunol.* **23:** 337–366.
6. Abernethy, T.J. & O.T. Avery. 1941. The occurence during acute infections of a protein non normally present in the blood. *J. Exp. Med.* **73:** 173–182.
7. Casas, J.P., T. Shah, A.D. Hingorani, *et al.* 2008. C-reactive protein and coronary heart disease: a critical review. *J. Intern. Med.* **264:** 295–314.
8. Bottazzi, B., A. Doni, C. Garlanda & A. Mantovani. 2010. An integrated view of humoral innate immunity: pentraxins as a paradigm. *Annu. Rev. Immunol.* **28:** 157–183.
9. Emsley, J. *et al.* 1994. Structure of pentameric human serum amyloid P component. *Nature* **367:** 338–345.
10. Shrive, A.K., A.M. Metcalfe, J.R. Cartwright & T.J. Greenhough. 1999. C-reactive protein and SAP-like pentraxin are both present in *Limulus polyphemus* haemolymph: crystal structure of *Limulus* SAP. *J. Mol. Biol.* **290:** 997–1008.
11. Armstrong, P.B. *et al.* 1996. A cytolytic function for a sialic acid-binding lectin that is a member of the pentraxin family of proteins. *J. Biol. Chem.* **271:** 14717–14721.
12. Liu, T.Y., F.A. Robey & C.M. Wang. 1982. Structural studies on C-reactive protein. *Ann. N.Y. Acad. Sci USA* **389:** 151–162.
13. Pepys, M.B. & G.M. Hirschfield. 2003. C-reactive protein: a critical update. *J. Clin. Invest.* **111:** 1805–1812.

14. Rubio, N., P.M. Sharp, M. Rits, *et al.* 1993. Structure, expression, and evolution of guinea pig serum amyloid P component and C-reactive protein. *J. Biochem.* **113:** 277–284.

15. Pepys, M.B. *et al.* 1994. Human serum amyloid P component is an invariant constituent of amyloid deposits and has a uniquely homogeneous glycostructure. *Proc. Natl. Acad. Sci. USA* **91:** 5602–5606.

16. Weiss, N.G., J.W. Jarvis, R.W. Nelson & M.A. Hayes. 2011. Examining serum amyloid P component microheterogeneity using capillary isoelectric focusing and MALDI-MS. *Proteomics* **11:** 106–113.

17. Roumenina, L.T. *et al.* 2006. Interaction of C1q with IgG1, C-reactive protein and pentraxin 3: mutational studies using recombinant globular head modules of human C1q A, B, and C chains. *Biochemistry* **45:** 4093–4104.

18. Ng, P.M. *et al.* 2007. C-reactive protein collaborates with plasma lectins to boost immune response against bacteria. *EMBO J.* **26:** 3431–3440.

19. Tanio, M., K. Wakamatsu & T. Kohno. 2009. Binding site of C-reactive protein on M-ficolin. *Mol. Immunol.* **47:** 215–221.

20. Jarva, H., T.S. Jokiranta, J. Hellwage, *et al.* 1999. Regulation of complement activation by C-reactive protein: targeting of the complement inhibitory activity of factor H by an interaction with short consensus repeat domains 7 and 8–11. *J. Immunol.* **163:** 3957–3962.

21. Mihlan, M., S. Stippa, M. Jozsi & P.F. Zipfel. 2009. Monomeric CRP contributes to complement control in fluid phase and on cellular surfaces and increases phagocytosis by recruiting factor H. *Cell Death Differ.* **16:** 1630–1640.

22. Okemefuna, A.I., R. Nan, A. Miller, *et al.* 2010. Complement factor H binds at two independent sites to C-reactive protein in acute phase concentrations. *J. Biol. Chem.* **285:** 1053–1065.

23. Sjoberg, A.P., L.A. Trouw, F.D. McGrath, *et al.* 2006. Regulation of complement activation by C-reactive protein: targeting of the inhibitory activity of C4b-binding protein. *J. Immunol.* **176:** 7612–7620.

24. Garcia de Frutos, P., Y. Hardig & B. Dahlback. 1995. Serum amyloid P component binding to C4b-binding protein. *J. Biol. Chem.* **270:** 26950–26955.

25. Nauta, A.J., M.R. Daha, C. van Kooten & A. Roos. 2003. Recognition and clearance of apoptotic cells: a role for complement and pentraxins. *Trends Immunol* **24:** 148–154.

26. Bharadwaj, D., C. Mold, E. Markham & T.W. Du Clos. 2001. Serum amyloid P component binds to Fc gamma receptors and opsonizes particles for phagocytosis. *J. Immunol.* **166:** 6735–6741.

27. Bharadwaj, D., M.P. Stein, M. Volzer, *et al.* 1999. The major receptor for C-reactive protein on leukocytes is Fc-gamma receptor II. *J. Exp. Med.* **190:** 585–590.

28. Mold, C., R. Baca & T.W. Du Clos. 2002. Serum amyloid P component and C-reactive protein opsonize apoptotic cells for phagocytosis through Fc-gamma receptors. *J. Autoimmun.* **19:** 147–154.

29. Lu, J. *et al.* 2008. Structural recognition and functional activation of FcgammaR by innate pentraxins. *Nature* **456:** 989–992.

30. Szalai, A.J. 2002. The antimicrobial activity of C-reactive protein. *Microb. Infect.* **4:** 201–205.

31. Szalai, A.J., D.E. Briles & J.E. Volanakis. 1995. Human C-reactive protein is protective against fatal *Streptococcus pneumoniae* infection in transgenic mice. *J. Immunol.* **155:** 2557–2563.

32. Hind, C.R., P.M. Collins, M.L. Baltz & M.B. Pepys. 1985. Human serum amyloid P component, a circulating lectin with specificity for the cyclic 4,6-pyruvate acetal of galactose. Interactions with various bacteria. *Biochem. J.* **225:** 107–111.

33. Noursadeghi, M. *et al.* 2000. Role of serum amyloid P component in bacterial infection: protection of the host or protection of the pathogen. *Proc. Natl. Acad. Sci. USA* **97:** 14584–14589.

34. Andersen, O. *et al.* 1997. Serum amyloid P component binds to influenza A virus haemagglutinin and inhibits the virus infection in vitro. *Scand. J. Immunol.* **46:** 331–337.

35. de Haas, C.J. *et al.* 2000. Serum amyloid P component bound to gram-negative bacteria prevents lipopolysaccharide- mediated classical pathway complement activation. *Infect. Immun.* **68:** 1753–1759.

36. Horvath, A. *et al.* 2001. Serum amyloid P component inhibits influenza A virus infections: in vitro and in vivo studies. *Antiviral Res.* **52:** 43–53.

37. Suresh, M.V., S.K. Singh, D.A. Ferguson, Jr. & A. Agrawal. 2007. Human C-reactive protein protects mice from *Streptococcus pneumoniae* infection without binding to pneumococcal C-polysaccharide. *J. Immunol.* **178:** 1158–1163.

38. Szalai, A.J., J.L. VanCott, J.R. McGhee, *et al.* 2000. Human C-reactive protein is protective against fatal Salmonella enterica serovar typhimurium infection in transgenic mice. *Infect. Immun.* **68:** 5652–5656.

39. Breviario, F. *et al.* 1992. Interleukin-1-inducible genes in endothelial cells. Cloning of a new gene related to C-reactive protein and serum amyloid P component. *J. Biol. Chem.* **267:** 22190–22197.

40. Inforzato, A. *et al.* 2011. The long pentraxin PTX3 at the crossroads between innate immunity and tissue remodelling. *Tissue Antigens* **77:** 271–282.

41. Doni, A. *et al.* 2003. Production of the soluble pattern recognition receptor PTX3 by myeloid, but not plasmacytoid, dendritic cells. *Eur. J. Immunol.* **33:** 2886–2893.

42. Perrier, P. *et al.* 2004. Distinct transcriptional programs activated by interleukin-10 with or without lipopolysaccharide in dendritic cells: induction of the B cell-activating chemokine, CXC chemokine ligand 13. *J. Immunol.* **172:** 7031–7042.

43. Mantovani, A., S.K. Biswas, M.R. Galdiero, *et al.* 2013. Macrophage plasticity and polarization in tissue repair and remodelling. *J. Pathol.* **229:** 176–185.

44. Norata, G.D. *et al.* 2009. Deficiency of the long pentraxin PTX3 promotes vascular inflammation and atherosclerosis. *Circulation* **120:** 699–708.

45. Salio, M. *et al.* 2008. Cardioprotective function of the long pentraxin PTX3 in acute myocardial infarction. *Circulation* **117:** 1055–1064.

46. Doni, A. *et al.* 2008. Cell-specific regulation of PTX3 by glucocorticoid hormones in hematopoietic and non-hematopoietic cells. *J. Biol. Chem.* **283:** 29983–29992.

47. Basile, A. *et al.* 1997. Characterization of the promoter for the human long pentraxin PTX3. Role of NF-kappaB in tumor necrosis factor-alpha and interleukin-1beta regulation. *J. Biol. Chem.* **272:** 8172–8178.

48. Altmeyer, A., L. Klampfer, A.R. Goodman & J. Vilcek. 1995. Promoter structure and transcriptional activation of the murine TSG-14 gene encoding a tumor necrosis factor/interleukin-1-inducible pentraxin protein. *J. Biol. Chem.* **270:** 25584–25590.

49. Han, B. *et al.* 2005. TNF-alpha-induced long pentraxin PTX3 expression in human lung epithelial cells via JNK. *J. Immunol.* **175:** 8303–8311.

50. Norata, G.D. *et al.* 2008. Long pentraxin 3: a key component of innate immunity, is modulated by high-density lipoproteins in endothelial cells. *Arterioscler. Thromb. Vasc. Biol.* **28:** 925–931.

51. Liangos, O. *et al.* 2010. Whole blood transcriptomics in cardiac surgery identifies a gene regulatory network connecting ischemia reperfusion with systemic inflammation. *PloS One* **5:** e13658.

52. Willeke, F. *et al.* 2006. Overexpression of a member of the pentraxin family (PTX3) in human soft tissue liposarcoma. *Eur. J. Cancer* **42:** 2639–2646.

53. Germano, G. *et al.* 2010. Antitumor and anti-inflammatory effects of trabectedin on human myxoid liposarcoma cells. *Cancer Res.* **70:** 2235–2244.

54. Inforzato, A. *et al.* 2006. Structure and function of the long pentraxin PTX3 glycosidic moiety: fine-tuning of the interaction with C1q and complement activation. *Biochemistry* **45:** 11540–11551.

55. Introna, M. *et al.* 1996. Cloning of mouse ptx3, a new member of the pentraxin gene family expressed at extrahepatic sites. *Blood* **87:** 1862–1872.

56. Goodman, A.R. *et al.* 1996. Long pentraxins: an emerging group of proteins with diverse functions. *Cytokine Growth Factor Rev.* **7:** 191–202.

57. Inforzato, A. *et al.* 2008. Structural characterization of PTX3 disulfide bond network and its multimeric status in cumulus matrix organization. *J. Biol. Chem.* **283:** 10147–10161.

58. Presta, M., M. Camozzi, G. Salvatori & M. Rusnati. 2007. Role of the soluble pattern recognition receptor PTX3 in vascular biology. *J Cell Mol. Med.* **11:** 723–738.

59. Inforzato, A. *et al.* 2010. The angiogenic inhibitor long pentraxin PTX3 forms an asymmetric octamer with two binding sites for FGF2. *J. Biol. Chem.* **285:** 17681–17692.

60. Garlanda, C. *et al.* 2002. Non-redundant role of the long pentraxin PTX3 in anti-fungal innate immune response. *Nature* **420:** 182–186.

61. Diniz, S.N. *et al.* 2004. PTX3 function as an opsonin for the dectin-1-dependent internalization of zymosan by macrophages. *J. Leukoc. Biol.* **75:** 649–656.

62. Bozza, S. *et al.* 2006. Pentraxin 3 protects from MCMV infection and reactivation through TLR sensing pathways leading to IRF3 activation. *Blood* **108:** 3387–3396.

63. Reading, P.C. *et al.* 2008. Antiviral activity of the long chain pentraxin PTX3 against influenza viruses. *J. Immunol.* **180:** 3391–3398.

64. Gout, E. *et al.* 2011. M-ficolin interacts with the long pentraxin PTX3: a novel case of cross-talk between soluble pattern-recognition molecules. *J. Immunol.* **186:** 5815–5822.

65. Ma, Y.J. *et al.* 2009. Synergy between ficolin-2 and PTX3 boost innate immune recognition and complement deposition. *J. Biol. Chem.* **284:** 28263–28275.

66. Ma, Y.J. *et al.* 2011. Heterocomplexes of mannose-binding lectin and the pentraxins PTX3 or serum amyloid P component trigger cross-activation of the complement system. *J. Biol. Chem.* **286:** 3405–3417.

67. Braunschweig, A. & M. Jozsi. 2011. Human pentraxin 3 binds to the complement regulator C4b-binding protein. *PloS One* **6:** e23991.

68. Deban, L. *et al.* 2008. Binding of the long pentraxin PTX3 to factor H: interacting domains and function in the regulation of complement activation. *J. Immunol.* **181:** 8433–8440.

69. Dias, A.A. *et al.* 2001. TSG-14 transgenic mice have improved survival to endotoxemia and to CLP-induced sepsis. *J. Leukoc. Biol.* **69:** 928–936.

70. Ravizza, T. *et al.* 2001. Dynamic induction of the long pentraxin PTX3 in the CNS after limbic seizures: evidence for a protective role in seizure-induced neurodegeneration. *Neuroscience* **105:** 43–53.

71. Deban, L. *et al.* 2010. Regulation of leukocyte recruitment by the long pentraxin PTX3. *Nat. Immunol.* **11:** 328–334.

72. Rusnati, M. *et al.* 2004. Selective recognition of fibroblast growth factor-2 by the long pentraxin PTX3 inhibits angiogenesis. *Blood* **104:** 92–99.

73. Camozzi, M. *et al.* 2005. Pentraxin 3 inhibits fibroblast growth factor 2-dependent activation of smooth muscle cells *in vitro* and neointima formation *in vivo*. *Arterioscler. Thromb. Vasc. Biol.* **25:** 1837–1842.

74. Salustri, A. *et al.* 2004. PTX3 plays a key role in the organization of the cumulus oophorus extracellular matrix and in in vivo fertilization. *Development* **131:** 1577–1586.

75. Scarchilli, L. *et al.* 2007. PTX3 interacts with inter-alpha-trypsin inhibitor: implications for hyaluronan organization and cumulus oophorus expansion. *J. Biol. Chem.* **282:** 30161–30170.

76. Camozzi, M. *et al.* 2006. Identification of an antiangiogenic FGF2-binding site in the N terminus of the soluble pattern recognition receptor PTX3. *J. Biol. Chem.* **281:** 22605–22613.

77. Jaillon, S. *et al.* 2007. The humoral pattern recognition receptor PTX3 is stored in neutrophil granules and localizes in extracellular traps. *J. Exp. Med.* **204:** 793–804.

78. Gaziano, R. *et al.* 2004. Anti-*Aspergillus fumigatus* efficacy of pentraxin 3 alone and in combination with antifungals. *Antimicrob. Agents Chemother.* **48:** 4414–4421.

79. D'Angelo, C. *et al.* 2009. Exogenous pentraxin 3 restores antifungal resistance and restrains inflammation in murine chronic granulomatous disease. *J. Immunol.* **183:** 4609–4618.

80. Moalli, F. *et al.* 2010. Role of complement and Fc{gamma} receptors in the protective activity of the long pentraxin

PTX3 against Aspergillus fumigatus. *Blood* **116:** 5170–5180.

81. Bottazzi, B. *et al.* 1997. Multimer formation and ligand recognition by the long pentraxin PTX3. Similarities and differences with the short pentraxins C-reactive protein and serum amyloid P component. *J. Biol. Chem.* **272:** 32817–32823.

82. Lu, J., K.D. Marjon, C. Mold, *et al.* 2012. Pentraxins and Fc receptors. *Immunol. Rev.* **250:** 230–238.

83. Moalli, F. *et al.* 2011. The therapeutic potential of the humoral pattern recognition molecule PTX3 in chronic lung infection caused by *Pseudomonas aeruginosa. J. Immunol.* **186:** 5425–5434.

84. Soares, A.C. *et al.* 2006. Dual function of the long pentraxin PTX3 in resistance against pulmonary infection with *Klebsiella pneumoniae* in transgenic mice. *Microb. Infect.* **8:** 1321–1329.

85. Job, E.R. *et al.* 2010. Pandemic H1N1 influenza A viruses are resistant to the antiviral activities of innate immune proteins of the collectin and pentraxin superfamilies. *J. Immunol.* **185:** 4284–4291.

86. Olesen, R. *et al.* 2007. DC-SIGN (CD209), pentraxin 3 and vitamin D receptor gene variants associate with pulmonary tubercolosis risk in West-Africans. *Genes Imm.* **8:** 456–467.

87. Chiarini, M. *et al.* 2010. PTX3 genetic variations affect the risk of *Pseudomonas aeruginosa* airway colonization in cystic fibrosis patients. *Genes Immu.* **11:** 665–670.

88. Han, B. *et al.* 2012. Protective effects of long pentraxin PTX3 on lung injury in a severe acute respiratory syndrome model in mice. *Lab Invest.* **92:** 1285–1296.

89. Abraham, R. *et al.* 1995. Modulation of immunogenicity and antigenicity of proteins by maleylation to target scavenger receptors on macrophages. *J. Immunol.* **154:** 1–8.

90. Jeannin, P., S. Jaillon & Y. Delneste. 2008. Pattern recognition receptors in the immune response against dying cells. *Curr. Opin. Immunol.* **20:** 530–537.

91. Gershov, D., S. Kim, N. Brot & K.B. Elkon. 2000. C-Reactive protein binds to apoptotic cells, protects the cells from assembly of the terminal complement components, and sustains an antiinflammatory innate immune response: implications for systemic autoimmunity. *J. Exp. Med.* **192:** 1353–1364.

92. Baruah, P. *et al.* 2006. The tissue pentraxin PTX3 limits C1q-mediated complement activation and phagocytosis of apoptotic cells by dendritic cells. *J. Leukoc. Biol.* **80:** 87–95.

93. van Rossum, A.P. *et al.* 2004. The prototypic tissue pentraxin PTX3, in contrast to the short pentraxin serum amyloid P, inhibits phagocytosis of late apoptotic neutrophils by macrophages. *Arthritis Rheum.* **50:** 2667–2674.

94. Rovere, P. *et al.* 2000. The long pentraxin PTX3 binds to apoptotic cells and regulates their clearance by antigen-presenting dendritic cells. *Blood* **96:** 4300–4306.

95. Jaillon, S. *et al.* 2009. Endogenous PTX3 translocates at the membrane of late apoptotic human neutrophils and is involved in their engulfment by macrophages. *Cell Death Differ.* **16:** 465–474.

96. Lech, M. *et al.* 2011. Lack of the long pentraxin PTX3 promotes autoimmune lung disease but not glomerulonephritis in murine systemic lupus erythematosus. *PloS One* **6:** e20118.

97. Poon, I.K., M.D. Hulett & C.R. Parish. 2010. Molecular mechanisms of late apoptotic/necrotic cell clearance. *Cell Death Differ.* **17:** 381–397.

98. Trouw, L.A. *et al.* 2007. C4b-binding protein and factor H compensate for the loss of membrane-bound complement inhibitors to protect apoptotic cells against excessive complement attack. *J. Biol. Chem.* **282:** 28540–28548.

99. Biagi, E. *et al.* 2008. PTX3 as a potential novel tool for the diagnosis and monitoring of pulmonary fungal infections in immuno-compromised pediatric patients. *J. Pediatr. Hematol. Oncol.* **30:** 881–885.

100. Sprong, T. *et al.* 2009. Ptx3 and C-reactive protein in severe meningococcal disease. *Shock* **31:** 28–32.

101. Mairuhu, A.T. *et al.* 2005. Elevated plasma levels of the long pentraxin, pentraxin 3, in severe dengue virus infections. *J. Med. Virol.* **76:** 547–552.

102. Azzurri, A. *et al.* 2005. IFN-gamma-inducible protein 10 and pentraxin 3 plasma levels are tools for monitoring inflammation and disease activity in *Mycobacterium tuberculosis* infection. *Microb. Infect.* **7:** 1–8.

103. Wagenaar, J.F. *et al.* 2009. Long pentraxin PTX3 is associated with mortality and disease severity in severe Leptospirosis. *J. Infect.* **58:** 425–432.

104. Muller, B. *et al.* 2001. Circulating levels of the long pentraxin PTX3 correlate with severity of infection in critically ill patients. *Crit. Care Med.* **29:** 1404–1407.

105. Peri, G. *et al.* 2000. PTX3, a prototypical long pentraxin, is an early indicator of acute myocardial infarction in humans. *Circulation* **102:** 636–641.

106. Latini, R. *et al.* 2004. Prognostic significance of the long pentraxin PTX3 in acute myocardial infarction. *Circulation* **110:** 2349–2354.

107. Jenny, N.S., A.M. Arnold, L.H. Kuller, *et al.* 2009. Associations of pentraxin 3 with cardiovascular disease and all-cause death: the Cardiovascular Health Study. *Arterioscler. Thromb. Vasc. Biol.* **29:** 594–599.

108. Ishino, M. *et al.* 2008. Risk stratification of chronic heart failure patients by multiple biomarkers: implications of BNP, H-FABP, and PTX3. *Circ. J.* **72:** 1800–1805.

109. Kotooka, N. *et al.* 2008. Prognostic value of pentraxin 3 in patients with chronic heart failure. *Int. J. Cardiol.* **130:** 19–22.

110. Latini, R. *et al.* 2012. Pentraxin-3 in chronic heart failure: the CORONA and GISSI-HF trials. *Eur. J. Heart Failure* **14:** 992–999.

111. Kotooka, N. *et al.* 2008. Pentraxin3 is a novel marker for stent-induced inflammation and neointimal thickening. *Atherosclerosis* **197:** 368–374.

112. Naito, Y. *et al.* 2010. Increase in tissue and circulating pentraxin 3 levels in patients with aortic valve stenosis. *Am. Heart J.* **160:** 685–691.

113. Inoue, K. *et al.* 2007. Establishment of a high sensitivity plasma assay for human pentraxin 3 as a marker for unstable angina pectoris. *Arterioscler. Thromb. Vasc. Biol.* **27:** 161–167.

114. Matsui, S. *et al.* 2010. Pentraxin 3 in unstable angina and non-ST-segment elevation myocardial infarction. *Atherosclerosis* **210:** 220–225.

115. Hollan, I. *et al.* 2010. Increased levels of serum pentraxin 3, a novel cardiovascular biomarker, in patients with inflammatory rheumatic disease. *Arthritis Care Res.* **62:** 378–385.

116. Ohbayashi, H. *et al.* 2009. Pitavastatin improves plasma pentraxin 3 and arterial stiffness in atherosclerotic patients with hypercholesterolemia. *J. Atheroscler. Thromb.* **16:** 490–500.

117. Knoflach, M. *et al.* 2012. Pentraxin-3 as a marker of advanced atherosclerosis results from the Bruneck, ARMY and ARFY studies. *PloS One* **7:** e31474.

118. Luchetti, M.M. *et al.* 2000. Expression and production of the long pentraxin PTX3 in rheumatoid arthritis (RA). *Clin. Exp. Immunol.* **119:** 196–202.

119. Iwata, Y. *et al.* 2009. Increased serum pentraxin 3 in patients with systemic sclerosis. *J. Rheumatol.* **36:** 976–983.

120. Fazzini, F. *et al.* 2001. PTX3 in small-vessel vasculitides: an independent indicator of disease activity produced at sites of inflammation. *Arthritis Rheum.* **44:** 2841–2850.

121. Baldini, M. *et al.* 2011. Selective upregulation of the soluble pattern recognition receptor PTX3 and of VEGF in giant cell arteritis: relevance for recent optic nerve ischemia. *Arthritis Rheum* **64:** 854–865.

122. Mauri, T. *et al.* 2010. Persisting high levels of plasma pentraxin 3 over the first days after severe sepsis and septic shock onset are associated with mortality. *Intens. Care Med.* **36:** 621–629.

123. Mauri, T. *et al.* 2008. Pentraxin 3 in acute respiratory distress syndrome: an early marker of severity. *Crit. Care Med.* **36:** 2302–2308.

124. Zanetti, M. *et al.* 2009. Circulating pentraxin 3 levels are higher in metabolic syndrome with subclinical atherosclerosis: evidence for association with atherogenic lipid profile. *Clin. Exp. Med.* **9:** 243–248.

125. Miyaki, A. *et al.* 2010. Is pentraxin 3 involved in obesity-induced decrease in arterial distensibility? *J. Atheroscler. Thromb.* **17:** 278–284.

126. Ogawa, T. *et al.* 2010. Reciprocal contribution of pentraxin 3 and C-reactive protein to obesity and metabolic syndrome. *Obesity* **18:** 1871–1874.

127. Kato, S. *et al.* 2008. Increased expression of long pentraxin PTX3 in inflammatory bowel diseases. *Dig. Dis. Sci.* **53:** 1910–1916.

128. Savchenko, A.S. *et al.* 2011. Long pentraxin 3 (PTX3) expression and release by neutrophils in vitro and in ulcerative colitis. *Pathol. Int.* **61:** 290–297.

129. Ryu, W.-S. *et al.* 2012. Pentraxin 3: a novel and independent prognostic marker in ischemic stroke. *Atherosclerosis* **220:** 581–586.

130. Zanier, E. *et al.* 2011. Cerebrospinal fluid pentraxin 3 early after subarachnoid hemorrhage is associated with vasospasm. *Intens. Care Med.* **37:** 302–309.

131. Suliman, M.E. *et al.* 2008. Novel links between the long pentraxin 3, endothelial dysfunction, and albuminuria in early and advanced chronic kidney disease. *Clin. J. Am. Soc. Nephrol.* **3:** 976–985.

132. Tong, M.C., J. Qureshi, A.R. Anderstam, *et al.* 2007. Plasma Pentraxin 3 in chronic kidney disease patients: association with renal function, protein-energy wasting, cardiovascular disease and mortality. *Clin. J. Am. Soc. Nephrol.* **2:** 889–897.

133. Yilmaz, M.I. *et al.* 2011. Soluble TWEAK and PTX3 in non-dialysis CKD patients: impact on endothelial dysfunction and cardiovascular outcomes. *Clin. J. Am. Soc. Nephrol.* **6:** 785–792.

134. Planque, C. *et al.* 2009. Identification of five candidate lung cancer biomarkers by proteomics analysis of conditioned media of four lung cancer cell lines. *Mol. Cell. Proteom.* **8:** 2746–2758.

135. Diamandis, E.P., L. Goodglick, C. Planque & M.D. Thornquist. 2011. Pentraxin-3 is a novel biomarker of lung carcinoma. *Clin. Cancer Res.* **17:** 2395–2399.

136. Barbui, T. *et al.* 2011. Inflammation and thrombosis in essential thrombocythemia and polycythemia vera: different role of C-reactive protein and pentraxin 3. *Haematologica* **96:** 315–318.

137. Tothill, R.W. *et al.* 2008. Novel molecular subtypes of serous and endometrioid ovarian cancer linked to clinical outcome. *Clin. Cancer Res.* **14:** 5198–5208.

138. Ravenna, L. *et al.* 2009. Up-regulation of the inflammatory-reparative phenotype in human prostate carcinoma. *Prostate* **69:** 1245–1255.

139. Wang, J.X., Y.L. He, S.T. Zhu, *et al.* 2011. Aberrant methylation of the 3q25 tumor suppressor gene PTX3 in human esophageal squamous cell carcinoma. *World J. Gastroenterol.* **17:** 4225–4230.

140. Lech, M. *et al.* 2013. Endogenous and exogenous pentraxin-3 limits postischemic acute and chronic kidney injury. *Kidney Int.* Jan 16. DOI: 10.1038/ki.2012.463. [Epub ahead of print].

Ann. N.Y. Acad. Sci. ISSN 0077-8923

ANNALS OF THE NEW YORK ACADEMY OF SCIENCES

Issue: *The Year in Immunology*

The role of autoimmunity in thromboangiitis obliterans (Buerger's disease)

Siva S. Ketha and Leslie T. Cooper

Gonda Vascular Center, Mayo Clinic and Foundation, Rochester, Minnesota

Address for correspondence: Leslie T. Cooper Jr., M.D. Division of Cardiovascular Diseases Mayo Clinic, 200 First Street SW. Rochester, MN 55905. cooper.leslie@mayo.edu

Thromboangiitis obliterans (TAO), or Buerger's disease, is a nonatherosclerotic segmental vasculitis that affects the small- and medium-sized arteries and veins of the extremities and is strongly associated with tobacco exposure. The immunopathogenesis of TAO remains largely unknown. In the acute phase of the disease, macrophages and occasional giant cells are observed in the characteristic intraluminal thrombus with a relatively mild infiltration of $CD4^+$ and $CD8^+$ T cells and macrophages in the internal lamina. VCAM-1, ICAM-1, and E-selectin expression on the surface of vascular endothelial cells is increased. A variety of circulating autoreactive antibodies targeting endothelial cells and vessel wall components are associated with active disease. One recent report suggests that removal of circulating antibodies by immunoadsorption may decrease disease severity. TAO has been associated positively and negatively with various MHC class 1 and 2 genes; however, genetic testing is not currently used for clinical diagnosis or management. The possible links between tobacco exposure and loss of tolerance for vascular tissues, current management strategy for patients with TAO, and opportunities for translational science are discussed.

Keywords: Buerger's disease, peripheral arterial disease, thromboangiitis obliterans

Introduction

Thromboangiitis obliterans (TAO), or Buerger's disease, is a nonatherosclerotic segmental vasculitis that affects the small- and medium-sized arteries and veins of the extremities. TAO was first described by Felix von Winiwarter in 1879, for which he proposed the name *endarteritis obliterans*.[1] Three decades later, Leo Buerger provided a description of the gross and microscopic pathologic features of this disorder after a careful anatomical review of eleven amputated limbs.[2] When the existence of TAO as a distinct vasculopathy was challenged by Wessler *et al.* in 1960,[3] careful studies of clinical and histological features confirmed that TAO was indeed a distinct vasculopathy.[4,5]

In its earliest phase, TAO is characterized histologically by highly cellular thrombus with relative sparing of the blood vessel wall. Buerger distinguished TAO clinicopathologically from atherosclerosis and proposed the name *thromboangiitis oblit-* *erans*. In contrast, atherosclerosis (ASO) starts as an intimal infiltrative and proliferative process limited to arteries. Buerger concluded that thrombosis occurs early in medium-sized arteries and superficial veins followed by organization and recanalization, rather than a primary vasculitis with secondary thrombosis. The chronic phase of TAO is histologically characterized by segmental obliteration of involved vessels. Interestingly, thrombosis of large arteries and deep veins is rare in TAO, presumably because of a yet undefined immunologic specificity for the small- and medium-sized vessels. Other changes described such as nerve involvement and periarteritis or fibrotic thickening of tissues immediately outside the affected vessels are late and considered secondary to the initial thrombotic process.[2]

Despite more than a hundred years of descriptive research, the immunopathogenesis of TAO remains largely unknown. In particular, the trigger and pathways that lead to thrombosis and inflammation

doi: 10.1111/nyas.12048

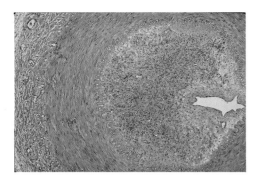

Figure 1. Buerger's disease (thromboangiitis obliterans). Involved artery, cut in cross section, shows severe luminal obstruction by active proliferative and highly cellular fibrovascular granulation tissue, without medial inflammation or destruction. (Hematoxylin and eosin, medium power.) Courtesy of Dr. William D. Edwards, Division of Anatomic Pathology, Mayo Clinic, Rochester.

for medium-sized vessels are largely unexplored. However, the clinical observation that the great majority of TAO is seen in young tobacco smokers has directed many investigations to seek clues from the pathogenesis of other tobacco-related diseases.

Histology

The highly cellular, occlusive thrombus of TAO consists mostly of polymorphonuclear leukocytes, mononuclear cells and occasional multinucleated giant cells (Fig. 1). Some macrophages expressing HLA-DR and S-100[+] dendritic cells may be located in the intima; however, the internal elastic lamina is intact and the media is structurally normal. This pattern is distinct from the much more common medium vessel vasculitis, giant cell arteritis, in which lesions start in the adventitia and evolve inwards to inflame and ultimately scar affected arteries.

The subacute phase is characterized by progressive organization of the thrombus. At this phase, fibrinoid necrosis of the vessel wall is still not observed and the architecture of the vascular wall remains relatively preserved (Fig. 2). In the chronic phase, inflammation is no longer present within the lumen of the vessel and only organized thrombus and vascular fibrosis remains. In this respect, the pathological appearance in the chronic phase resembles the chronic phases of other obliterative arterial diseases.[6]

Immunopathogenesis from studies of human tissues

A recent pathological study of TAO artery specimens demonstrated increased undulation, multiplication, and degeneration of the internal elastic lamina.[7] Several investigators confirmed that T lymphocytes infiltrate the internal layers of the vascular wall in patients with TAO. Taken together, these observations suggest that the inner layers of affected vessels may be involved in the early stages of pathogenesis. Cells observed near the internal lamina consisted of equal numbers of CD4[+] and CD8[+] T cells. At this stage, macrophages are observed in thrombi and in the intima. CD20[+] lymphocytes are scarce in acute lesions and, like T cells, are primarily seen in the intima rather than the adventitia or media. S100[+] dendritic cells also localize to the intima and to a lesser degree to the media and the adventitia.

A small study conducted on 10 patients with TAO by Gulati *et al.* revealed blood vessel specific autoantibodies (various classes of immunoglobulins IgM, IgG, IgA) and C3 component in the diseased vessels of thromboangiitis obliterans. Antiarterial antibodies were also present in the sera of these patients.[8] Other investigators have reported increased titers of antielastin antibodies in the serum of patients with TAO.[9] The functional significance of these antibodies has not been demonstrated, but yet their presence suggest that B cell-mediated, antigen-specific immunity may contribute to TAO.[8]

Adar *et al.* determined the cellular and humoral immune responses to human collagen type I and type III, common constituents of blood vessels, in 39 patients with TAO. They observed enhanced cell proliferation to collagen types I, III, and IV in affected patients using an antigen-sensitive thymidine-incorporation assay.[10,11] The variety of autoantigens observed in clinical studies suggest that the initial injury may involve more than one structure within the vessel wall and that TAO may be one phenotype resulting from injuries to a variety of vessel components.

A primary thrombotic trigger within the blood may contribute to vascular wall inflammation via inflammation at the endoluminal surface.[6,12,13] A minority of TAO cases are associated with a genetic mutation in prothrombin (prothrombin 201210A→G), suggesting that thrombophilia may promote disease susceptibility in some cases.[14]

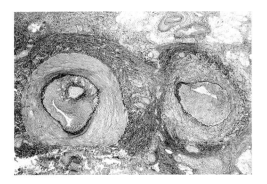

Figure 2. Buerger's disease (thromboangiitis obliterans). Involved artery (left) and vein (right), cut in cross section, show old healed severe luminal obstructions, with intact internal elastic membranes (black), normal media (tan), and secondary adventitial fibrosis (red). (Verhoeff–van Gieson stain, low power.) Courtesy of Dr. William D. Edwards, Division of Anatomic Pathology, Mayo Clinic, Rochester.

Nonetheless, the background of thrombophilia would still require a trigger from a consequence of tobacco use such as endothelial cell damage to initiate the focal vascular lesions.[12]

Because they lie at the blood–vascular interface, endothelial cells may be the site for initial damage and early expansion of the inflammatory response in TAO. Halacheva *et al.* described increased expression of adhesive molecules such as VCAM-1, ICAM-1, and E-selectin on the surface of endothelial cells and some inflammatory cells in the thickened intima of TAO patients. Ultrastructural immunohistochemistry revealed contacts between mononuclear blood cells and ICAM-1- and E-selectin–positive endothelial cells. These endothelial cells showed morphological signs of activation indicating that vascular lesions are associated with tumor necrosis factor (TNF-α) secretion by tissue-infiltrating inflammatory cells, ICAM-1, VCAM-1, and E-selectin expression on endothelial cells and leukocyte adhesion via their ligands.[15] Eichhorn *et al.* described increased levels of antiendothelial cell antibodies in the sera of TAO patients that recognized epitopes on the surface and within the cytoplasm of human endothelial cells.[16]

Nonspecific antibodies like antinuclear antibodies (ANA) may also be seen in a minority of TAO cases.[8] There are conflicting data regarding the presence of antineutrophil cytoplasmic antibodies (ANCA) in TAO. Schellong *et al.*, using indirect immunofluorescence assay (IIF), did not detect ANCA

in any of 30 analyzed cases of TAO.[17] On the other hand, Halacheva *et al.*, using a similar method, found ANCA in 15 among 27 individuals (55.5%).[18] The development of these antibodies could suggest that some TAO cases are part of a more systemic inflammatory disorder whose initial clinical feature is an unusual vasculopathy. Alternately these may be nonspecific, low affinity antibodies that are not directly related to TAO pathogenesis in the majority of cases.

Interestingly, a recent study investigating the levels of TNF-α, interleukin (IL)-1β, IL-4, IL-17, and IL-23 in the plasma of TAO patients presenting with acute clinical manifestations found increased levels of these cytokines in patients with TAO when compared to the controls, indicating an increased production of cytokines in TAO, possibly contributing to the inflammatory response.[19] In addition, the increased levels of IL-17 and IL-23 suggest that inflammation and autoimmunity play a central role in the pathogenesis of TAO.

Genetic factors

Because mechanistic investigation is not possible from cross-sectional studies of human TAO tissues and no animal model exists to dissect the initial triggers, investigators have turned to epidemiological datasets for genetic clues to early stages of pathogenesis. The prevalence of TAO is increased in Israel, India, and Japan compared to North America and Western Europe.[6,20,21] Indeed, epidemiologic data suggest that major histocompatibility complex (MHC) background may influence response to tobacco in TAO. McLoughlin *et al.* reported a greater prevalence of HLA A-9 and HLA B-5 antigens in affected persons.[22] Similarly, Otawa *et al.* reported an increased prevalence of HLA-A, HLA-BW, O, and a Japanese-specific antigen (J-1-1), together with an absence of HLA-A12 in Japanese men with TAO.[23]

Based on an association between periodontal disease and TAO, an examination by Chen *et al.* looked at whether gene polymorphisms involved in the infectious immunity were associated with TAO as the genetic factor(s). They determined polymorphisms in HLA-DPB1, DRB1, and B in 131 Japanese TAO patients and 227 healthy controls. Additionally a functional promoter polymorphism (-260 C$\rightarrow$T) of the CD14 gene, a main receptor of bacterial lipopolysaccharide, was investigated. The authors found significantly higher frequencies of the CD14

T/T genotype, DRB1*1501, and DPB1*0501 in the patients compared with the controls. Stratification analyses of three associated markers suggested synergistic roles in disease phenotype.[24]

Endothelial cells located at the interface of the vessel wall and blood may be the site for initial damage and early expansion of the inflammatory response in TAO. Endothelial nitric oxide synthase (eNOS) is a key enzyme that plays an essential role in vascular endothelial nitric oxide (NO) production, thereby affecting thrombosis and vascular inflammation. Adiguzel et al. found that the occurrence of the eNOS gene 894 T/T genotype was associated with a significant decline in the occurrence of the TAO. They concluded that the T allele of the eNOS gene 894 G→T polymorphism was a protective factor against the occurrence of TAO.[25]

Myeloid differentiation primary response protein 88 (MyD88) is a key signaling adaptor for Toll-like receptors, which have a central activation role in innate immunity. Recently, Chen et al. conducted a case–control study in Japanese study subjects, of whom 131 had TAO, 90 had Takayasu arteritis (TA), and 270 were healthy controls; all were genotyped for a single nucleotide polymorphism rs7744 A→G in the 3′-untranslated region of the MyD88 gene. They found that the frequency of G/G genotype was significantly lower in the BD patients than in the controls (6.9 vs. 15.9%, $P = 0.011$, odds ratio = 0.39, 95% confidence interval; 0.19, 0.81) and that there was no significant difference in the genotype frequencies between the TA patients and controls. MyD88 variants may modulate susceptibility to TAO in the Japanese.[26]

Environmental factors

Cigarette smoking

Tobacco exposure is central to the clinical initiation and progression of TAO in more than 95% of cases. All types of tobacco have been implicated. In one study, patients diagnosed with TAO smoked an average of 23 years. Once the disease becomes established, tobacco cessation is the only way to prevent clinical recurrence. Taking up smoking again, even years later, may trigger a new exacerbation.[6] Disease recurrence with reinstitution of the stimulus is perhaps the best evidence for a causal link.

Cigarette smoke is a highly complex mixture of more than 4,500 chemicals and many of its components are known carcinogens, cocarcinogens, muta-

gens, and other toxic substances. Chronic inhalation of tobacco smoke alters innate and adaptive immune responses.[27] It has been proposed that many of the adverse health effects of smoking might be due to its effects on the immune system.[28]

In contrast to tobacco smoke, nicotine given in isolation has been shown to have immunosuppressive properties. Animals chronically exposed to cigarette smoke have been shown to have a significant loss of antibody response and T cell proliferation.[27] Animals treated with nicotine remained immunosuppressed for several weeks after nicotine administration.[29] Nicotine inhibits the proliferation of red blood cells, fibroblasts, and macrophages. But at the same time, nicotine also increases platelet adhesiveness, raising the potential for thrombotic microvascular occlusion and tissue ischemia.[30]

Inflammation is a common feature in the pathogenesis of cigarette smoke-associated diseases. Exposure to cigarette smoke results in an inflammatory response, characterized by sequestration of neutrophils in pulmonary microvasculature, their attachment to endothelium, and flux of polymorphonuclear leukocytes and macrophages in the lung.[31–35] The recruitment of inflammatory cells into the lung and their persistence following cigarette smoke exposure present a risk of tissue damage through the release of chemotactic and toxic mediators, including proteolytic enzymes and reactive oxygen species.[36–38] The ensuing tissue damage could contribute significantly to the development of acute lung injury and chronic lung disease.[39]

Smoking induces a prothrombotic state via inhibition of tissue plasminogen activator release from the endothelium, elevation in the blood fibrinogen concentration, increased platelet activity, increased expression of tissue factor, and, in patients with advanced lung disease, elevated whole blood viscosity due to secondary polycythemia.[40–42] Smoking can also damage the vascular wall, possibly leading to impaired prostacyclin production and enhanced platelet–vessel wall interactions.[43] Although the exact components of cigarette smoke that produce microvascular dysfunction have not been characterized, nicotine and carbon monoxide may mediate damage on the vascular system.[44]

Periodontal infection

Chronic anaerobic periodontal infection has been associated with TAO. Nearly two-thirds of patients

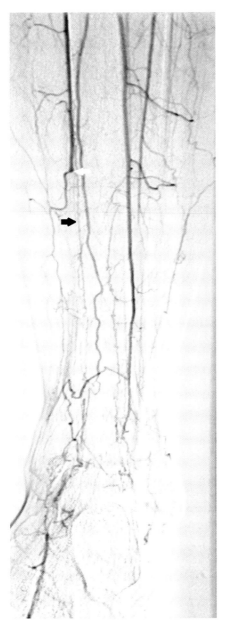

Figure 3. Left leg angiogram showing occlusion of the anterior tibial artery (yellow arrow), with collateralization "corkscrew collaterals" around the areas of occlusion (black arrow) in a patient with Buerger's disease.

with TAO have severe periodontal disease.[45] Periodontal pathogens have been detected in the occluded arteries of Buerger's disease patients. In one study, DNA fragments associated with anaerobic bacteria were found within both the arterial lesions and oral cavities of patients with thromboangiitis

obliterans.[46] These observations have been questioned as not causal because the prevalence of periodontal disease in smokers without thromboangiitis obliterans is similarly high and the presence of periodontal antigens in other thrombotic diseases is unknown.

Diagnosis

Several clinical criteria have been used to define the TAO phenotype.[47–49] Papa *et al.* recommended using a scoring system with points awarded for young age at onset, foot claudication, upper extremity involvement, superficial vein thrombosis, and vasospastic phenomena. Shionoya *et al.* proposed diagnostic criteria for TAO that included (1) smoking history; (2) onset before the age of 50 years; (3) infrapopliteal arterial occlusions; (4) either upper limb involvement or phlebitis migrans; and (5) absence of atherosclerotic risk factors other than smoking. These criteria have not been validated prospectively or in ethnically diverse populations. The erythrocyte sedimentation rate and C-reactive protein are usually normal in TAO.[50]

In practice, TAO is diagnosed using vascular laboratory data and angiography (Fig. 3) in the absence of large vessel atherosclerosis. Patients with antiphospholipid syndrome who exhibit thrombus without inflammation are excluded by definition from a diagnosis of TAO.[51] There is no specific and sensitive diagnostic test. Doppler ultrasonography and angiography are helpful in diagnosing the disease, but the findings on these studies are not pathognomonic for TAO. Histology is the gold standard to establish a definitive diagnosis but is seldom used in clinical practice due to the risk associated with biopsy and cost considerations.

Epidemiology

Because of a lack of uniform diagnostic criteria, it is difficult to determine the prevalence of TAO. The disease is worldwide in distribution but seems to have a higher prevalence in the Middle East, Asia, and the Far East than in Europe or North America.[6] It is more common in countries where tobacco is heavily used, especially among people who smoke homemade cigarettes from raw tobacco in the Indian subcontinent.[6,21] In North America, the prevalence of thromboangiitis obliterans has declined in the past 30 years, in part, due to a decline in smoking.[20] Patients with TAO now constitute no

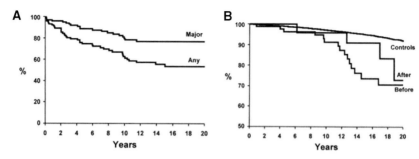

Figure 4. (A) Kaplan–Meier analysis of the rate of first amputation and major amputation in the thromboangiitis obliterans cohort from time of diagnosis. Major amputation is defined as a below the knee, above the knee, or hand amputation. (B) Observed survival in the thromboangiitis obliterans population before and after tobacco cessation compared with the expected survival in an age- and gender-matched U.S. population (controls). $P < 0.001$ by a log-rank test. Reproduced with permission from Ref. 56. Copyright © Elsevier Limited.

more than 4–5% of those with ischemic peripheral vascular disease (PAD);[52] and TAO accounts for a small minority (0.5–5.6%) of patients with PAD in Western Europe. In other parts of the world where atherosclerosis is less common, TAO may represent a higher proportion of peripheral ischemic disease, 45–63% in India, and 16–66% in Korea and Japan.[53]

TAO was initially thought to affect almost exclusively men, since less than 2% of those affected were women.[20] More recently, the proportion of female TAO patients has been noted to vary from 11% to 30%.[54,55] This may either be a true increase in the disease or it may reflect an increase in smoking among women, increased access to medical care, or a greater physician awareness of TAO.

Outcomes

Long-term outcomes, including rates of death, major and minor amputations, and mortality in patients with TAO, derive from three contemporary case series.[56–58] Olin *et al.* reported a study of 112 patients with TAO in which 27% of the study subjects underwent amputation during a mean follow-up period of 7.6 years. Interestingly, they also found that the spectrum of patients with TAO was changing, in that the male-to-female ratio was decreasing (3:1), a greater number of older patients were being diagnosed, and upper extremity involvement was commonly present. In the 48% of patients who stopped smoking, amputations and continued disease activity were uncommon.[58]

Ohta *et al.* retrospectively analyzed the outcomes of 110 patients with TAO followed for a mean of 10.6 years. The cumulative survival rate was 84%,

up to 25 years after the initial diagnosis. Forty-three percent of the study subjects underwent 108 amputation procedures, either major amputation (13 patients) or minor amputation (34 patients), of an upper or lower limb. No ischemic ulcers occurred or recurred in patients older than 60 years. Forty-one patients who stopped smoking did not undergo major amputation. Furthermore, of 69 patients who continued smoking, 13 patients (19%) underwent major amputation.

At the Mayo clinic 111 patients with proven TAO were followed for a mean of 15 years. The risk of major amputation was 11% at 5 years, 21% at 10 years and 23% at 20 years (Fig. 4A). The risk of amputation in former smokers was eliminated by eight years after smoking cessation while the risk persisted in patients that continued to smoke (Fig. 4B). In contrast to previous studies with shorter follow-up, life expectancy in patients with TAO was decreased compared to the age- and gender-matched U.S. population starting approximately 10 years after initial diagnosis. Older age at time of diagnosis was also associated with an increased risk of death.[56]

Medical management

Although altered immunity is a feature of TAO, no immune pathway-specific therapies have been tested in patients. Because the disease primarily involves small- and medium-sized arteries of the distal extremities, surgical revascularization is usually not an option. Consequently, management of TAO is still quite challenging for patients and providers. A recent review by Dargon *et al.* summarizes the various therapeutic options available.[59] The mainstay of treatment in TAO is smoking cessation.[60] Complete abstinence from tobacco products is necessary to halt disease progression and to avoid future amputations.[6] The disease may be activated by smoking as little as one or two cigarettes a day. Bupropion or varenicline should be used for smoking cessation as opposed to transdermal nicotine patches and nicotine chewing gum because they may also keep the disease active. Measurement of urinary nicotine and cotinine should be considered if the disease is active despite patient claims of tobacco cessation.[61] While it was widely believed that TAO patients have a greater degree of tobacco dependence than those with coronary atherosclerosis, a study at the Mayo clinic showed no significant difference in time to tobacco cessation after diagnosis has been demonstrated.[62]

Intermittent pneumatic compression of the foot and calves has been used to improve perfusion to the lower extremities in patients with severe claudication or critical limb ischemia (CLI) when surgical revascularization is not an option. Intermittent pneumatic compression enhances calf inflow in patients with intermittent claudication or CLI. In a study of patients with small-vessel occlusive diseases, such as scleroderma and TAO, complete healing of ischemic ulcers was achieved by 40% of patients with severely reduced transcutaneous oxygen tension, 48% with osteomyelitis or active wound infection, 46% with diabetes treated with insulin, and 28% with a previous amputation.[63]

Intravenous administration of prostanoids may reduce pain in TAO patients with CLI.[64] In a randomized controlled trial of 152 patients with TAO, patients treated with the prostanoid vasodilator iloprost had significant relief of rest pain, greater healing of ischemic ulcers, and reduced need for amputation.[65] Endothelin-1 is a vasocontrictor peptide that binds to endothelin-A (ET-A) or ET-B receptors, resulting in pulmonary vasoconstriction.[66] Bosentan, used in the treatment of pulmonary artery hypertension (PAH), is a competitive antagonist of endothelin-1 at the ET-A and ET-B receptors that decreases pulmonary vascular resistance by blocking this interaction. Treatment with Bosentan has been attempted in small studies in Buerger's disease.[67,68] Other vasodilators such as α-blockers, calcium channel blockers, and sildenafil are occasionally used, but these agents have not been studied in clinical trials.

Surgical management

Bypass surgery may be considered in selected patients with critical limb ischemia and suitable distal target vessels. TAO patients undergoing bypass surgery often have relatively low primary patency rates of only 41%, 32%, and 30% and secondary patency rates of 54%, 47%, and 39% at 1, 5, and 10 years.[57] Graft patency rates are nearly 50% lower in patients who continue smoking than in those who quit smoking after surgical intervention.[69]

Novel therapeutic strategies

The limited options for patients with severe distal peripheral artery disease and critical limb ischemia have driven a growing interest in therapeutic angiogenesis and stem cell therapy. Short-term results of therapeutic angiogenesis using growth factors or autologous bone marrow have been promising, but larger studies with longer term follow-up are needed. In one trial of six patients with nonhealing wounds (> 1 month), intramuscular vascular endothelial growth factor (VEGF)-165 was injected into seven affected limbs. Ulcers completely healed in three of five limbs. In the other two patients, nocturnal rest pain was relieved, although both continued to have claudication. In all seven limbs, perfusion was improved on magnetic resonance imaging and newly visible collateral vessels were seen on contrast angiography.[70] A third trial tested the safety of intramuscular gene transfer by using naked plasmid DNA encoding the gene for VEGF in seven patients with TAO. Ischemic pain in the affected limb was relieved or improved markedly in six of seven patients, and ischemic ulcers healed or improved in four of six patients.[71]

The therapeutic angiogenesis by cell transplantation (TACT) trial, which included patients with TAO, randomly assigned patients to autologous bone marrow mononuclear cell injection versus placebo.[72] Significant improvements were seen in leg pain scale, ulcer size, and pain-free walking distance that were maintained at two years after therapy. Other available small nonrandomized studies have shown similar short-term improvements.[73–75] In a recent pilot study, the role of immunoadsorption (IA) as a treatment option was evaluated in patients with advanced TAO.[76] Immunoadsorption therapy, which involves the selective removal of the circulating immunoglobulins and antibodies, has been used successfully for the treatment of

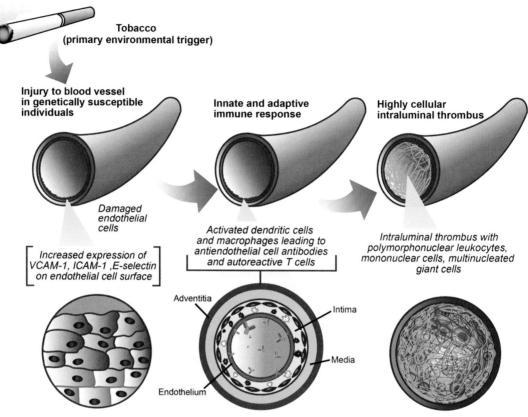

Figure 5. Pathogenesis of Buerger's Disease (thromboangiitis obliterans).

several autoimmune diseases including removal of antiglomerular basement membrane antibodies in Goodpasture's syndrome,[77] antiacetylcholine antibodies in myasthenia gravis,[78] dsDNA antibodies in systematic lupus erythematosus[79] and autoantibodies in idiopathic dilated cardiomyopathy.[80,81] Baumann *et al.* studied 10 TAO patients with chronic ischemic rest pain and evidence of ischemic lesions despite medical therapy. All the study subjects underwent IA over five consecutive days. All patients experienced a significant improvement in pain immediately after the treatment and remained pain free at one- and six-month intervals. There was also a significant increase in the maximum walking distance, transcutaneous oxygen tension, transcutaneous carbon dioxide tension, and photoplethysmography measurements after IA at one- and six-month intervals. These data support the theory that autoreactive antibodies are central to the pathogenesis of TAO.

Future directions

More than 100 years after TAO was initially described, the pathogenesis is still poorly understood. Available data suggest interplay between hereditary susceptibility identified by genetic polymorphisms, tobacco exposure, and immune-mediated responses (Fig. 5). The spectrum of antibodies associated with the disease may reflect a variable immune response toward tobacco and may provide clues to pathway-specific therapy. Further translational science may follow the encouraging response to immunoadsorption, a therapy that allows for elution and *in vitro* study of the adsorbed material.[76] The gaps in our understanding could be addressed if a murine model resembling human disease could be constructed. Without a new model, multicenter longitudinal registries linked to serum and tissue biobanks, consistent phenotyping, and adjudicated outcomes probably hold the best hope for new insights in the next few years.

Conflicts of interest

The authors declare no conflicts of interest.

References

1. Von Winiwarter, F. 1879. Ueber eine eigenthumliche from von endarteritis und endophlephitis mit gangran des fusses. *Arch. Klin. Chir.* **23:** 202–226.

2. Buerger. 1908. Thrombo-angiits obliterans: a study of the vascular lesions leading to presenile spontaneous gangrene. *Am. J. Med. Sci.* **136:** 567–580.

3. Wessler, S., S.C. Ming, V. Gurewich & D.G. Freiman. 1960. A critical evaluation of thromboangitis obliterans. The case against Buerger's disease. *N. Engl. J. Med.* **262:** 1149–1160 (in English).

4. McKusick, V.A. 1962. Buerger's disease: a distinct clinical and pathologic entity. *JAMA* **181:** 5–12.

5. McPherson, J.R., J.L. Juergens & R.W. Gifford Jr. 1963. Thromboangiitis obliterans and arteriosclerosis obliterans. Clinical and prognostic differences. *Ann. Intern. Med.* **59:** 288–296 (in English).

6. Olin, J.W. 2000. Thromboangiitis obliterans (Buerger's disease). *N. Engl. J. Med.* **343:** 864–869 (in English).

7. Kim, E.J., B.S. Cho, *et al.* 2000. Morphologic change of the internal elastic lamina in Buerger's disease. *J. Korean Med. Sci.* **15:** 44–48 (in English).

8. Gulati, S.M., K. Madhra, T.K. Thusoo, *et al.* 1982. Autoantibodies in thromboangiitis obliterans (Buerger's disease). *Angiology* **33:** 642–651 (in English).

9. Berlit, P., C. Kessler, R. Reuther & K.H. Krause. 1984. New aspects of thromboangiitis obliterans (von Winiwarter–Buerger's disease). *Eur. Neurol.* **23:** 394–399 (in English).

10. Adar, R. *et al.* 1983. Cellular sensitivity to collagen in thromboangiitis obliterans. *N. Engl. J. Med.* **308:** 1113–1116 (in English).

11. Hada, M., T. Sakihama, K. Kamiya, *et al.* 1993. Cellular and humoral immune responses to vascular components in thromboangiitis obliterans. *Angiology* **44:** 533–540 (in English).

12. Kobayashi, M., M. Ito, A. Nakagawa, N. Nishikimi & Y. Nimura. 1999. Immunohistochemical analysis of arterial wall cellular infiltration in Buerger's disease (endarteritis obliterans). *J. Vasc. Surg.* **29:** 451–458 (in English).

13. Mills, J.L., Sr. 2003. Buerger's disease in the 21st century: diagnosis, clinical features, and therapy. *Semin. Vasc. Surg.* **16:** 179–189 (in English).

14. Avcu, F. *et al.* 2000. The role of prothrombotic mutations in patients with Buerger's disease. *Thromb. Res.* **100:** 143–147 (in English).

15. Halacheva, K., M.V. Gulubova, I. Manolova & D. Petkov. 2002. Expression of ICAM-1, VCAM-1, E-selectin and TNF-alpha on the endothelium of femoral and iliac arteries in thromboangiitis obliterans. *Acta. Histochem.* **104:** 177–184 (in English).

16. Eichhorn, J. *et al.* 1998. Antiendothelial cell antibodies in thromboangiitis obliterans. *Am. J. Med. Sci.* **315:** 17–23 (in English).

17. Schellong, S.M., A. Rautmann, W.L. Gross & K. Alexander. 1993. No ANCA in thromboangiitis obliterans (Burger's disease). *Adv. Exp. Med. Biol.* **336:** 327–330 (in English).

18. Halacheva, K.S., I.M. Manolova, D.P. Petkov & A.P. Andreev. 1998. Study of anti-neutrophil cytoplasmic antibodies in patients with thromboangiitis obliterans (Buerger's disease). *Scand. J. Immunol.* **48:** 544–550 (in English).

19. Dellalibera-Joviliano, R., E.E. Joviliano, J.S. Silva & P.R.B. Evora. 2012. Activation of cytokines corroborate with development of inflammation and autoimmunity in thromboangiitis obliterans patients. *Clin. Exp. Immunol.* **170:** 28–35 (in English).

20. Lie, J.T. 1989. The rise and fall and resurgence of thromboangiitis obliterans (Buerger's disease). *Acta. Pathol. Jpn.* 39: 153–158 (in English).

21. Grove, W.J. & G.P. Stansby. 1992. Buerger's disease and cigarette smoking in Bangladesh. *Ann. R. Coll. Surg. Engl.* 74: 115–117; discussion 118 (in English).

22. McLoughlin, G.A., C.R. Helsby, *et al.* 1976. Association of HLA-A9 and HLA-B5 with Buerger's disease. *Br. Med. J.* **2:** 1165–1166 (in English).

23. Otawa, T., T. Jugi, N. Kawano, *et al.* 1974. Letter: HL-A antigens in thromboangiitis obliterans. *JAMA* **230:** 1128 (in English).

24. Chen, Z. *et al.* 2007. Synergistic contribution of CD14 and HLA loci in the susceptibility to Buerger disease. *Hum. Genet.* **122:** 367–372 (in English).

25. Adiguzel, Y., E. Yilmaz & N. Akar. 2010. Effect of eNOS and ET-1 polymorphisms in thromboangiitis obliterans. *Clin. Appl. Thromb. Hemost.* **16:** 103–106 (in English).

26. Chen, Z. *et al.* 2011. A single nucleotide polymorphism in the 3'-untranslated region of MyD88 gene is associated with Buerger disease but not with Takayasu arteritis in Japanese. *J. Hum. Genet.* **56:** 545–547 (in English).

27. Sopori, M. 2002. Effects of cigarette smoke on the immune system. *Nat. Rev. Immunol.* **2:** 372–377 (in English).

28. Holt, P.G. & D. Keast. 1977. Environmentally induced changes in immunological function: acute and chronic effects of inhalation of tobacco smoke and other atmospheric contaminants in man and experimental animals. *Bacteriol. Rev.* **41:** 205–216 (in English).

29. Geng, Y., S.M. Savage, S. Razani-Boroujerdi & M.L. Sopori. 1996. Effects of nicotine on the immune response. II. Chronic nicotine treatment induces T cell anergy. *J. Immunol.* **156:** 2384–2390 (in English).

30. Silverstein, P. 1992. Smoking and wound healing. *Am. J. Med.* **93:** 22S–24S (in English).

31. Gairola, C.G. 1986. Free lung cell response of mice and rats to mainstream cigarette smoke exposure. *Toxicol. Appl. Pharmacol.* **84:** 567–575 (in English).

32. Ludwig, P.W., B.A. Schwartz, J.R. Hoidal & D.E. Niewoehner. 1985. Cigarette smoking causes accumulation of polymorphonuclear leukocytes in alveolar septum. *Am. Rev. Respir. Dis.* **131:** 828–830 (in English).

33. MacNee, W., B. Wiggs, A.S. Belzberg & J.C. Hogg. 1989. The effect of cigarette smoking on neutrophil kinetics in human lungs. *N. Engl. J. Med.* **321:** 924–928 (in English).

34. Lehr, H.A. 1993. Adhesion-promoting effects of cigarette smoke on leukocytes and endothelial cells. *Ann. N.Y. Acad. Sci.* **686:** 112–118; discussion 118–119 (in English).

35. van der Vaart, H., D.S. Postma, W. Timens & N.H. ten Hacken. 2004. Acute effects of cigarette smoke on

inflammation and oxidative stress: a review. *Thorax* **59:** 713–721 (in English).

36. Morrison, D., I. Rahman, S. Lannan & MacNee W. 1999. Epithelial permeability, inflammation, and oxidant stress in the air spaces of smokers. *Am. J. Respir. Crit. Care Med.* **159:** 473–479 (in English).

37. Dhami, R. *et al.* 2000. Acute cigarette smoke-induced connective tissue breakdown is mediated by neutrophils and prevented by alpha1-antitrypsin. *Am. J. Respir. Cell. Mol. Biol.* **22:** 244–252 (in English).

38. Churg, A. *et al.* 2002. Acute cigarette smoke-induced connective tissue breakdown requires both neutrophils and macrophage metalloelastase in mice. *Am. J. Respir. Cell. Mol. Biol.* **27:** 368–374 (in English).

39. Bhalla, D.K., F. Hirata, A.K. Rishi & C.G. Gairola. 2009. Cigarette smoke, inflammation, and lung injury: a mechanistic perspective. *J. Toxicol. Environ. Health B Crit. Rev.* **12:** 45–64 (in English).

40. Newby, D.E. *et al.* 1999. Endothelial dysfunction, impaired endogenous fibrinolysis, and cigarette smoking: a mechanism for arterial thrombosis and myocardial infarction. *Circulation* **99:** 1411–1415 (in English).

41. Fusegawa, Y., S. Goto, S. Handa, *et al.* 1999. Platelet spontaneous aggregation in platelet-rich plasma is increased in habitual smokers. *Thromb. Res.* **93:** 271–278 (in English).

42. Matetzky, S. *et al.* 2000. Smoking increases tissue factor expression in atherosclerotic plaques: implications for plaque thrombogenicity. *Circulation* **102:** 602–604 (in English).

43. Nowak, J., J.J. Murray, J.A. Oates & G.A. FitzGerald. 1987. Biochemical evidence of a chronic abnormality in platelet and vascular function in healthy individuals who smoke cigarettes. *Circulation* **76:** 6–14 (in English).

44. Leone, A. 2005. Biochemical markers of cardiovascular damage from tobacco smoke. *Curr. Pharm. Des.* **11:** 2199–2208.

45. Iwai, T. *et al.* 2005. Oral bacteria in the occluded arteries of patients with Buerger disease. *J. Vasc. Surg.* **42:** 107–115 (in English).

46. Chen, Y.W. *et al.* 2009. Association between periodontitis and anti-cardiolipin antibodies in Buerger disease. *J. Clin. Periodontol.* **36:** 830–835 (in English).

47. Mills, J.L. & J.M. Porter. 1993. Buerger's disease: a review and update. *Semin. Vasc. Surg.* **6:** 14–23 (in English).

48. Papa, M.Z., I. Rabi & R. Adar. 1996. A point scoring system for the clinical diagnosis of Buerger's disease. *Eur. J. Vasc. Endovasc. Surg.* **11:** 335–339 (in English).

49. Shionoya, S. 1998. Diagnostic criteria of Buerger's disease. *Int. J. Cardiol.* **66** Suppl 1: S243–S245; discussion S247 (in English).

50. Olin, J.W. & A. Shih. 2006. Thromboangiitis obliterans (Buerger's disease). *Curr. Opin. Rheumatol.* **18:** 18–24 (in English).

51. Maslowski, L., R. McBane, P. Alexewicz & W.E. Wysokinski. 2002. Antiphospholipid antibodies in thromboangiitis obliterans. *Vasc. Med.* **7:** 259–264 (in English).

52. Ansari, A. 1990. Thromboangiitis obliterans: current perspectives and future directions. *Tex. Heart Inst. J.* **17:** 112–117 (in English).

53. Arkkila, P.E. 2006. Thromboangiitis obliterans (Buerger's disease). *Orphanet. J. Rare. Dis.* **1:** 14 (in English).

54. Mills, J.L., L.M. Taylor, Jr. & J.M. Porter. 1987. Buerger's disease in the modern era. *Am. J. Surg.* **154:** 123–129 (in English).

55. Sasaki, S., M. Sakuma, T. Kunihara & K. Yasuda. 1999. Current trends in thromboangiitis obliterans (Buerger's disease) in women. *Am. J. Surg.* **177:** 316–320 (in English).

56. Cooper, L.T. *et al.* 2004. Long-term survival and amputation risk in thromboangiitis obliterans (Buerger's disease). *J. Am. Coll. Cardiol.* **44:** 2410–2411 (in English).

57. Ohta, T., H. Ishioashi, M. Hosaka & I. Sugimoto. 2004. Clinical and social consequences of Buerger disease. *J. Vasc. Surg.* **39:** 176–180 (in English).

58. Olin, J.W., J.R. Young, R.A. Graor, W.F. Ruschhaupt & J.R. Bartholomew. 1990. The changing clinical spectrum of thromboangiitis obliterans (Buerger's disease). *Circulation* **82**(5 Suppl): IV3–8 (in English).

59. Dargon, P.T. & G.J. Landry. 2012. Buerger's disease. *Ann. Vasc. Surg.* **26:** 871–880 (in English).

60. Corelli, F. 1973. Buerger's disease: cigarette smoker disease may always be cured by medical therapy alone. Uselessness of operative treatment. *J. Cardiovasc. Surg.* **14:** 28–36 (in English).

61. Hurt, R.D. & J.T. Hays. 2008. Urinary tobacco alkaloid measurement in patients having thromboangiitis obliterans. *Mayo. Clin. Proc.* **83:** 1187–1188; author reply. 1188 (in English).

62. Cooper, L.T. *et al.* 2006. A prospective, case-control study of tobacco dependence in thromboangiitis obliterans (Buerger's Disease). *Angiology* **57:** 73–78 (in English).

63. Montori, V.M., S.J. Kavros, E.E. Walsh & T.W. Rooke. 2002. Intermittent compression pump for nonhealing wounds in patients with limb ischemia. The Mayo Clinic experience (1998–2000). *Int. Angiol.* **21:** 360–366 (in English).

64. Anonymous. 1998. Oral iloprost in the treatment of thromboangiitis obliterans (Buerger's disease): a double-blind, randomised, placebo-controlled trial. The European TAO Study Group. *Eur. J. Vasc. Endovasc. Surg.* **15:** 300–307 (in English).

65. Fiessinger, J.N. & M. Schafer. 1990. Trial of iloprost versus aspirin treatment for critical limb ischaemia of thromboangiitis obliterans. The TAO study. *Lancet* **335:** 555–557 (in English).

66. Watts, S.W. 2010. Endothelin receptors: what's new and what do we need to know? *Am. J. Physiol. Regul. Integr. Comp. Physiol.* **298:** R254–260 (in English).

67. Todoli Parra, J.A., M.M. Hernandez & M.A. Arrebola Lopez. 2010. Efficacy of bosentan in digital ischemic ulcers. *Ann. Vasc. Surg.* **24:** 690 e691–694 (in English).

68. De Haro, J., F. Acin, S. Bleda, *et al.* 2012. Treatment of thromboangiitis obliterans (Buerger's disease) with bosentan. *BMC Cardiovasc. Disord.* **12:** 5 (in English).

69. Sasajima, T., Y. Kubo, M. Inaba, K. Goh & N. Azuma. 1997. Role of infrainguinal bypass in Buerger's disease: an eighteen-year experience. *Eur. J. Vasc. Endovasc. Surg.* **13:** 186–192 (in English).

70. Isner, J.M. *et al.* 1998. Treatment of thromboangiitis obliterans (Buerger's disease) by intramuscular gene transfer of vascular endothelial growth factor: preliminary clinical results. *J. Vasc. Surg.* **28:** 964–973; discussion 973–965 (in English).

71. Kim, H.J. *et al.* 2004. Vascular endothelial growth factor-induced angiogenic gene therapy in patients with peripheral artery disease. *Exp. Mol. Med.* **36:** 336–344 (in English).

72. Matoba, S. *et al.* 2008. Long-term clinical outcome after intramuscular implantation of bone marrow mononuclear cells (Therapeutic Angiogenesis by Cell Transplantation [TACT] trial) in patients with chronic limb ischemia. *Am. Heart J.* **156:** 1010–1018 (in English).

73. Saito, Y. *et al.* 2007. Effect of autologous bone-marrow cell transplantation on ischemic ulcer in patients with Buerger's disease. *Circ. J.* **71:** 1187–1192 (in English).

74. Durdu, S. *et al.* 2006. Autologous bone-marrow mononuclear cell implantation for patients with Rutherford grade II-III thromboangiitis obliterans. *J. Vasc. Surg.* **44:** 732–739 (in English).

75. Motukuru, V., K.R. Suresh, V. Vivekanand, S. Raj & K.R. Girija. 2008. Therapeutic angiogenesis in Buerger's disease (thromboangiitis obliterans) patients with critical limb ischemia by autologous transplantation of bone marrow mononuclear cells. *J. Vasc. Surg.* **48**(6 Suppl)**:** 53S–60S; discussion 60S (in English).

76. Baumann, G. *et al.* 2011. Successful treatment of thromboangiitis obliterans (Buerger's disease) with immunoadsorption: results of a pilot study. *Clin. Res. Cardiol.* **100:** 683–690 (in English).

77. Laczika, K. *et al.* 2000. Immunoadsorption in Goodpasture's syndrome. *Am. J. Kidney. Dis.* **36:** 392–395 (in English).

78. Gajdos, P., S. Chevret & K. Toyka. 2002. Plasma exchange for myasthenia gravis. *Cochrane Database Syst. Rev.* (4)**:** CD002275 (in English)

79. Stummvoll, G.H. 2011. Immunoadsorption (IAS) for systemic lupus erythematosus. *Lupus* **20:** 115–119 (in English).

80. Burgstaler, E.A., L.T. Cooper & J.L. Winters. 2007. Treatment of chronic dilated cardiomyopathy with immunoadsorption using the staphylococcal A-agarose column: a comparison of immunoglobulin reduction using two different techniques. *J. Clin. Apher.* **22:** 224–232 (in English).

81. Cooper, L.T. *et al.* 2007. A pilot study to assess the use of protein a immunoadsorption for chronic dilated cardiomyopathy. *J. Clin. Apher.* **22:** 210–214 (in English).

Ann. N.Y. Acad. Sci. ISSN 0077-8923

ANNALS OF THE NEW YORK ACADEMY OF SCIENCES

Issue: *The Year in Immunology*

Wiskott-Aldrich syndrome: a comprehensive review

Michel J. Massaad, Narayanaswamy Ramesh, and Raif S. Geha

Division of Immunology, Boston Children's Hospital, and Department of Pediatrics, Harvard Medical School, Boston, Massachusetts

Address for correspondence: Michel J. Massaad, Ph.D., M.Sc., Division of Immunology, Boston Children's Hospital, Karp Building 10th floor, One Blackfan Circle, Boston, MA, 02115. michel.massaad@childrens.harvard.edu

Wiskott-Aldrich syndrome (WAS) is a rare X-linked primary immunodeficiency characterized by microthrombocytopenia, eczema, recurrent infections, and an increased incidence of autoimmunity and malignancies. The disease is caused by mutations in the *WAS* gene expressed exclusively in hematopoietic cells. WAS protein (WASp) is a multidomain protein that exists in complex with several partners that play important roles in its function. WASp belongs to a family of proteins that relay signals from the surface of the cell to the actin cytoskeleton. Mutations in the *WAS* gene have various effects on the level of WASp, which, in turn, correlates with the severity of the disease. In addition to WAS, mutations in the *WAS* gene can result in the mild variant X-linked thrombocytopenia, or in X-linked neutropenia, characterized by neutropenia with myelodysplasia. The absence of functional WASp leads to a severe clinical phenotype that can result in death if not diagnosed and treated early in life. The treatment of choice with the best outcome is hematopoietic stem cell transplantation, preferably from a matched related donor.

Keywords: Wiskott-Aldrich syndrome; primary immunodeficiency; hematopoietic cells; F-actin; immune cell function; hematopoietic stem cell transplantation; gene therapy

Introduction

In 1937, Alfred Wiskott described three brothers with a condition characterized by microthrombocytopenia, bloody diarrhea, eczema, episodes of fever, and recurrent ear infections. Because their sisters were not affected, he concluded that these boys had a novel hereditary thrombopathy and not idiopathic thrombocytopenic purpura.[1] Robert Aldrich reported a similar clinical phenotype in sixteen out of forty males, but not females, over six generations of a single family he studied in 1954, clearly showing an X-linked mode of inheritance.[2] This condition was named Wiskott-Aldrich syndrome (WAS) after the two physicians who described it. The gene for WAS (*WAS*) was identified on the X chromosome (position Xp11.22–p11.23) by positional cloning,[3] and the family that was initially described by Wiskott was confirmed to have a deletion of two nucleotides at positions 73–74 (AC73–74del) of *WAS*, resulting in frameshift and premature termination of the protein.[4]

WAS protein (WASp) is a multifaceted protein associated with several clinical disorders. Mutations that result in absent WASp cause classic WAS characterized by thrombocytopenia with small platelets, eczema, recurrent infections because of immunodeficiency, and an increased incidence of autoimmunity and malignancies.[5,6] Mutations that result in decreased, but not absent, protein expression cause the milder disease X-linked thrombocytopenia (XLT) that is characterized mainly by thrombocytopenia and sometimes is associated with milder eczema and immunodeficiency.[7,8] In addition, a third disorder termed X-linked neutropenia (XLN), characterized by neutropenia and variable myelodysplasia, has been attributed to activating mutations in the GTPase-binding domain (GBD) of WASp.[9–11]

In this review, we will focus on WASp structure and interactions, the defects in the different immune compartments, the genotype/phenotype association, and on the therapy of WAS and XLT.

doi: 10.1111/nyas.12049

Ann. N.Y. Acad. Sci. 1285 (2013) 26–43 © 2013 New York Academy of Sciences.

WASp family and domain structure

WASp was the first identified member of a family of actin nucleation-promoting factors (NPFs) that relay surface signals to actin polymerization through the actin-related protein (Arp)2/3 complex.[12] The other members of this family include neural-WASp (N-WASp),[13,14] suppressor of cAR/WASp family verprolin-homologous proteins (SCAR/WAVE1–3),[15,16] WAS protein and SCAR homologue (WASH),[17] WASp homologue associated with actin, membranes, and microtubules (WHAMM),[18] junction-mediated and regulator protein (JMY),[19] as well as the two hypothetical proteins WASp without WH1 domain (WAWH) and WASp- and MIM-like (WAML).[20] WASp is exclusively expressed in hematopoietic cells,[21,22] whereas the distribution of N-WASp and SCAR/WAVE1–3, the closest members of the family to WASp, is broader.[13,16]

WASp is a 502 amino acid (aa) multidomain protein encoded by twelve exons on the X-chromosome (Fig. 1). Members of this family of proteins share a high degree of homology at the C-terminal end, whereas the N-terminal end varies. Because WASp and N-WASp are the most similar proteins in the family, with $\sim$ 50% overall identity and $\sim$ 80% identity in the conserved domains, they can substitute for each other in many *in vitro* assays. We will restrict our description to WASp and N-WASp because most of our knowledge of the structure and function comes from work on these two proteins.

At the N-terminus, WASp and N-WASp possess an Ena-VASP homology domain (EVH1)/WASp homology domain 1 (WH1), followed by a basic region (BR), a Cdc42/Rac GBD, a proline-rich region (PPP), a globular actin (G-actin)–binding verprolin homology (V) domain, a cofilin homology or central (C) domain, and a C-terminal acidic (A) domain (Fig. 1).[3,12]

WASp/N-WASp interactions

The EVH1/WH1 domain

The EVH1/WH1 domain is the binding site of WASp-interacting protein (WIP). WIP is a 503 aa ubiquitously expressed protein that was cloned in a yeast two-hybrid screen using WASp as bait.[23] WASp exists in a constitutive complex with WIP, and WIP is crucial for the stability of WASp, but not N-WASp.[24,25] Most of the missense mutations identified in WAS patients are found in the EVH1/WH1 domain,[26] and some have been shown to decrease the affinity of WASp to WIP, leading to dissociation of the complex and degradation of WASp.[27,28] NMR studies have precisely mapped the N-WASp binding sites on human WIP to aa 451–485.[29,30] We have shown that a 40 aa peptide that covers this region of WIP is sufficient to interact with WASp and to stabilize the otherwise degradation-prone EVH1/WH1 mutant WASp.[31]

WIP maintains the autoinhibitory conformation of WASp *in vivo*[32] and decreases N-WASp–mediated actin polymerization *in vitro*.[33] The inhibition of N-WASp by WIP can be released by the transducer of Cdc42-dependent actin assembly (Toca)-1, although a direct interaction between WIP and Toca-1 has yet to be shown.[32,34] WIP is important for the localization of WASp to podosomes in dendritic cells (DCs),[24] and for podosome and phagocytic cup formation in macrophages.[35,36] In addition, WIP interacts with the adaptor molecules Nck and CrkL, and is important for the recruitment of WASp to the T cell receptor (TCR).[37,38] In sum, WIP stabilizes WASp and keeps it in an inactive state and correctly localized, thus maintaining a proper spatial and temporal regulation of its activity.

The BR and GBD

In resting cells, WASp/N-WASp exist in the cytoplasm in an auto-inhibited inactive state, maintained by intramolecular interaction among the BR, GBD, and VCA domain,[39,40] and stabilized by WIP.[32,33] Stimulation of the cell leads to the cooperative binding of phophatidylinositol(4,5)-biphosphate (PIP_2) with the BR, and of the activated form of Cdc42 (Cdc42-GTP) with the GBD. This releases the autoinhibition and liberates the VCA domain for activation of the Arp2/3 complex.[41–45] The activation of WASp/N-WASp by Cdc42-GTP and PIP_2 is maintained by the phosphorylation of a tyrosine residue at position 291 (Y291) in the GBD of WASp (Y253 or Y256 in N-WASp) by the protein tyrosine kinases Lyn, Btk, Hck, or Fyn.[46–52]

The PPP

The PPP of WASp/N-WASp is the binding site of many Src homology 3 (SH3) domain–containing proteins (reviewed in Ref. 53). Protein tyrosine kinases such as Btk, Tec, Itk, Hck, and Fyn associate with WASp/N-WASp through interaction of one or more of their SH3 domains with the PPP of WASp/

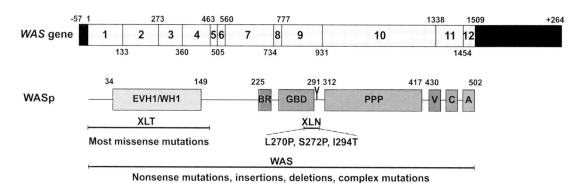

Figure 1. Schematic representation of the *WAS* gene exon structure and protein domains. The 12 exons of the *WAS* gene are indicated. The numbers above and below the *WAS* gene indicate the starting nucleotide number of each exon. The untranslated regions of the first and last exon are shows in black. The domain structure of WASp is shown below the respective exons. The amino acid numbers are shown above the domains. Most missense mutations are located in exons 1 through 4 resulting in X-linked thrombocytopenia (XLT). Mutations L270P and S272P are in the GBD, whereas I294T is C-terminal to the GBD and results in X-linked neutropenia (XLN). Nonsense mutations, insertions, deletions, and complex mutations are distributed throughout the *WAS* gene and result in Wiskott-Aldrich syndrome (WAS). Most splice-site mutations are found in introns 6 to 10 (not shown). EVH1/WH1, Ena-Vasp homology domain/WASp homology domain 1; BR, basic region; GBD, Cdc42/Rac GTPase binding domain; Y, tyrosine at position 291; PPP, proline-rich region; V, verprolin homology domain; C, cofilin homology or central domain; A, acidic domain; WIP, WASp-interacting protein; PIP_2, phosphatidylinositol(4,5)-biphosphate; Cdc42, cell division control protein 42 homolog; SH3, Src homology 3 domain; Arp2/3, actin-related proteins 2 and 3.

N-WASp.[47,50,54–56] One set of studies showed that Btk, Hck, and Fyn interact with the proline-rich domain of WASp/N-WASp and phosphorylate the protein, resulting in its activation.[46,47,50] In contrast, a recent study by Sato *et al.* showed that Fyn binds to the EVH1/WH1 domain rather than the PPP of WASp.[57] The reason for the difference obtained in these studies is not clear, but the loss of Fyn binding to the proline-rich domain–deleted WASp mutant used by Badour *et al.*[50] could be, in part, because of misfolding of the protein.

In addition to tyrosine kinases, the PPP of WASp/N-WASp serves as a docking region for the SH3 domain of several adaptor molecules with no intrinsic kinase activity. The best studied of these include Nck1, Grb2, and PSTPIP1.[50,58,59] The association of Nck and PIP_2 with N-WASp increases its actin polymerization activity independent of Cdc42-GTP, providing a mechanism for N-WASp activation independent of the GTPase.[60] In support of this, phosphorylation of Y291 in the absence of the GBD is sufficient to activate WASp.[50] These two studies suggest that Y291 phosphorylation, or Nck/PIP_2 binding to the PPP, is sufficient to activate WASp/N-WASp. On the other hand, Grb2 synergizes with Cdc42 to activate WASp/N-WASp and recruit it to epidermal growth factor receptor upon stimulation with EGF.[59,61] Furthermore, Nck, Grb2, PIP_2, and WIP are important for N-WASp–mediated intracellular vesicle movement.[62] This process occurs in the absence of Cdc42, suggesting that the presence of Nck in this complex is enough to activate N-WASp.

Although the binding and phosphorylation of WASp/N-WASp by the molecules described above results in its activation, binding of PSTPIP1 to the PPP of WASp results in its deactivation.[63] This occurs through the recruitment of PTP-PEST, which dephosphorylates WASp, resulting in its deactivation.[50]

The VCA domain

The Arp2/3 complex is composed of seven proteins critical for *de novo* actin polymerization in mammalian cells. In this complex, Arp2 and Arp3 share structural features with G-actin and can bind monomeric actin molecules to create the minimal basic nucleus required for the initiation of actin polymerization. However, the Arp2/3 complex cannot by itself initiate actin polymerization; it requires the activity of NPFs to enhance its function.[64] The VCA domain of WASp/N-WASP is the functional unit that interacts with and activates the Arp2/3 complex to initiate filamentous actin (F-actin) polymerization. Deletion of the VCA domain results in complete loss of WASp/N-WASp-mediated actin polymerization.[40,65,66]

The VCA domain is kept in an inactive state by intramolecular interactions with the BR/GBD.[39,40] Upon release from inhibition, the V domain binds a monomer of G-actin, and the A domain interacts with the Arp2/3 complex. The C domain assists both the V and A domains in their respective interactions. WASp/N-WASp then feeds G-actin to the Arp2/3 complex, facilitating the nucleation of actin filaments and branches.[13,67] Thus, the combination of cytosolic G-actin, G-actin bound to the V domain, Arp2, and Arp3 form the minimal nuclear unit onto which more G-actin molecules are added to form longer F-actin filaments. In accordance with this, short F-actin units make better nuclei than G-actin and greatly accelerate the elongation and branching of actin filaments.[65]

Mechanism of WASp activation

The understanding of its structure and function and the identification of interacting proteins provided solid evidence with which to propose a mechanism of WASp/N-WASp function (Fig. 2). WASp/N-WASp exists in a closed auto-inhibited conformation in the cytoplasm, maintained by the interaction with WIP. Upon cellular activation, WASp/N-WASp is recruited to the site of membrane signaling through the binding of adaptor molecules to their PPP, and/or through the interaction of Nck or CrkL with WIP.[37,38] Depending on the microenvironment where the complex has been recruited, one or more signals that include binding of Cdc42-GTP to the GBD, binding of PIP_2 to the BR, phosphorylation of Y291 (Y253 or Y256 in N-WASp), binding of Toca-1 to the PPP and Cdc42-GTP, and binding of adaptor molecules, such as Nck and Grb2 to the PPP, result in the release of the auto-inhibition of WASp/N-WASp, exposing the VCA domain. The V domain then binds G-actin whereas the A domain binds the Arp2/3 complex, and G-actin is transferred to the Arp2/3 complex to initiate localized elongation and/or branching of actin filaments. Phosphorylated WASp is then ubiquitinated and degraded in a proteasome- and calpain-dependent manner, thus providing a plausible mechanism for its inactivation.[68–72]

Immune cell function in WAS

WASp is expressed exclusively in hematopoietic cells.[3,21,22] There is a strong correlation between the level of WASp and the severity of WAS. Complete WASp absence leads to a pronounced defect in the function of multiple hematopoietic cell lineages, resulting in thrombocytopenia with small platelets and progressive lymphopenia with abnormal lymphoid and myeloid cell function.[73] On the other hand, decreases in WASp levels have variable effects on the function of the different cell types, with platelets being the most affected in humans.[74]

WAS T cells

Studies using WAS patients and mouse models have shown that the T cell defect is a major cause of the immunodeficiency observed in WAS. WAS patients suffer from T cell lymphopenia, which manifests during childhood and adolescence, because of abnormal T cell development and thymic output, as well as increased rate of apoptosis.[73,75–78] The surface architecture of T cells from WAS patients displays abnormal projections, with a paucity in the number and structure of surface microvilli, pointing to a defect in the architecture of the actin cytoskeleton.[79,80] Consistent with this observation, T cells from WAS patients fail to polymerize actin and rearrange their actin cytoskeleton when stimulated with immobilized anti-CD3 monoclonal antibodies (mAb).[31,81]

Peripheral blood mononuclear cell (PBMC) proliferation to mitogen varies among different WAS patients;[73,82] these differences could be due to either variability of the T cell counts in the PBMC population or to a residual level of WASp per cell. Primary T cells and T cell lines generated from WAS patients invariably fail to upregulate the activation markers CD69 and CD25, proliferate, and secrete interleukin (IL)-2 when stimulated with immobilized anti-CD3 mAb (our unpublished data and Refs. 81, 83, and 84). Also defective are interferon (IFN)-γ and tumor necrosis factor-α secretion. These defects are likely due to a reduction in *T-bet* mRNA expression and failure of translocation of NFAT1/2 to the nucleus.[85,86] It has also been shown that cytotoxic T cells from WAS patients fail to effectively kill B cell lymphoma target cells because of inefficient polarization of cytotoxic granules toward the tumor, providing a possible explanation for the development

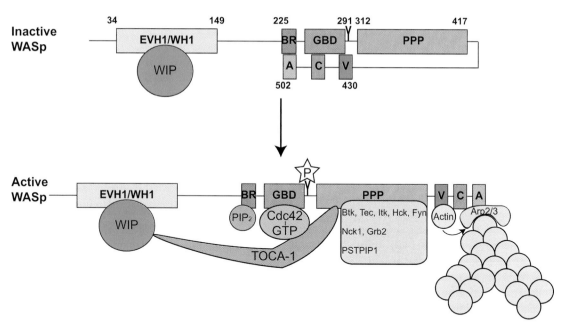

Figure 2. Schematic representation of WASp in the inactive and active conformations. WASp exists in a closed autoinhibited conformation. Binding of Cdc42-GTP to the GBD, PIP_2 to the BR, phosphorylation of Y291, binding of Toca-1 to the proline-rich region and Cdc42-GTP, or binding of adaptor molecules, such as Nck and Grb2 to the proline-rich region, release the autoinhibition of WASp, thus exposing the VCA domain, and leading to the localized elongation and/or branching of actin filaments. WASp also interacts with several SH3-containing proteins through the proline-rich region (most, but not all, are represented in the schematic). EVH1/WH1, Ena-Vasp homology domain/WASp homology domain 1; BR, basic region; GBD, Cdc42/Rac GTPase binding domain; Y, tyrosine at position 291; PPP, proline-rich region; V, verprolin homology domain; C, cofilin homology or central domain; A, acidic domain; WIP, WASp-interacting protein; PIP_2, phophatidylinositol(4,5)-biphosphate; Cdc42, cell division control protein 42 homolog; SH3, Src homology 3 domain; Arp2/3, actin-related proteins 2 and 3.

of hematological malignancies in WAS patients.[87] Deletion of the *WAS* gene in a murine model ($WASp^{-/-}$) confirmed the results observed in T cells from WAS patients[88,89] and showed that T cells expressing a TCRα chain specific for an ovalbumin peptide proliferate normally when stimulated with antigen-presenting cells (APCs) presenting the ovalbumin peptide, whereas their proliferation to plate-bound anti-CD3 mAb is severely affected.[90] In addition, the N-terminal domain of WASp is important for IL-2 signaling mediated by NFAT, whereas the C-terminal domain is responsible for actin polymerization.[86,91,92]

Activation of T cells requires the formation of a stable interaction between T cell and APC. The interface between the T cell and APC is known as the immune synapse (IS), a structure rich in F-actin and signaling molecules.[93,94] IS formation is a dynamic process that involves the clustering of lipid rafts containing signaling molecules.[95] Following T cell activation, WASp is required for the transport of lipid raft marker GM1 to the cell surface

and for the movement of lipid rafts in the membrane that leads to their aggregation.[84] WASp itself is recruited to the IS with the adaptor protein Nck, where it colocalizes with the tyrosine kinase Zap70 in a mechanism that requires phosphorylation of the TCR and the involvement of the adaptors LAT and SLP-76.[38,84,96] CD4+ T cells from WAS patients have a slightly increased IS length, fail to fully polarize their microtubule organizing center (MTOC) toward the center of the IS, and fail to enrich phosphorylated CD3ε molecules at the IS, resulting in reduced T cell activation.[97] A deeper understanding of the structure of the IS in murine T cells showed that the IS is a very dynamic structure that depends on PKC-θ to break, and on WASp to reform, and that cycles of symmetry-breaking and relocation are important for cell migration and IL-2 production.[98]

T cells isolated from a WAS patient fail to migrate toward SDF-1α *in vitro* via a mechanism that requires the phosphorylation of WASp and its interaction with Cdc42-GTP and Nck.[99,100] Studies conducted in mice showed that $WASp^{-/-}$ T cells tether less efficiently to the substratum and migrate less than their wild-type (WT) counterparts toward lymphoid organs *in vivo*, or in a transwell system *in vitro*, despite normal expression of the chemokine receptors on their surface.[101,102]

WAS regulatory T cells

A large proportion of WAS patients are affected by at least one autoimmune episode,[103,104] raising the possibility of a defect in regulatory T (T_{reg}) cells, a population of T cells that attenuates the immune system's reaction to nonself antigens and promotes tolerance toward self antigens.[105,106] Although T_{reg} cell development is not impaired in WAS patients, T_{reg} cells isolated from WAS patients show decreased suppression of effector T cell proliferation and IFN-γ production *in vitro*.[107,108] Similarly, WASp$^{-/-}$ mouse T_{reg} cells develop normally, despite decreased homeostasis and tissue distribution owing to aberrant expression of tissue-homing receptors. However, they fail to suppress the proliferation of WT T cells *in vitro*, a function that can be corrected by preincubating WASp$^{-/-}$ T_{reg} cells with IL-2. WASp$^{-/-}$ mouse T_{reg} cells also fail to prevent the development of colitis in an *in vivo* model, as well as fail to protect *scurfy* mice (Foxp3-deficient) from the development of autoimmunity.[107–110] In addition, WASp$^{-/-}$ mouse T_{reg} cells fail to suppress B cells proliferation and apoptosis owing to a decrease in granzyme B secretion.[111]

The inability of WASp-deficient T_{reg} cells to control T effector cell and B cell function could contribute to the autoimmunity observed in WAS patients and in WASp$^{-/-}$ mice.[103,112] However, the intrinsic role of T_{reg} cells can only be determined using a mouse model in which WASp expression is exclusively abolished in the T_{reg} compartment.

WAS B cells

Although B cell development is not greatly affected in patients with WAS or in WASp$^{-/-}$ mice, WASp$^{-/-}$ B cells have a selective disadvantage compared to WT B cells; consequently, peripheral B cell counts, especially marginal zone (MZ) B cells, are severely reduced in WASp$^{-/-}$ mice.[113–117] B cells from WAS patients and WASp$^{-/-}$ mice have fewer and shorter surface microvilli. In addition, they have defective actin cytoskeletons, fail to make filopodia, are less motile, spread less, and aggregate less than normal B cells on Ab-coated surfaces.[115,118–120] This cytoskeletal defect could be the cause of the decreased migra-

tion of WAS-deficient B cells *in vitro* and *in vivo* and the poor homeostasis of peripheral B cells, mostly MZ B cells.[115–117]

Primary B cells from WAS patients and WASp$^{-/-}$ mice proliferate normally and have normal signaling downstream of the B cell receptor.[88,89,121] However, B cell lines immortalized by infection of WAS PBMCs with Epstein Bar virus (EBV-B) proliferated poorly and showed less Ca$^+$2 mobilization when stimulated with antibodies directed against surface immunoglobulins.[122] The basis of the difference in this study and the study of Henriquez *et al.*[121] is not clear but could be due to the type of cells used and/or the intensity of the stimulation. On the other hand, both selective deletion of WASp in B cells[114] and bone marrow (BM) chimeric mice with selective defect of WASp expression in the B cell compartment[123] showed that WASp-deleted B cells are hyperproliferative.

Patients with WAS show multiple autoimmune manifestations.[6,103,104,124] Selective deletion of WASp in B cells leads to production of autoantibodies and the development of autoimmunity.[112,114] Furthermore, BM chimeric mice with selective defect of WASp expression in B cells develop autoimmunity that is CD4$^+$ T cell– and MyD88-dependent.[123]

These results indicate that the absence of WASp leads to hyperresponsive B cells and intrinsic breaks of tolerance, which contribute to the autoimmunity observed in WAS patients and WASp$^{-/-}$ mice, especially in the context of normal T cell and TLR signaling.

WAS platelets

Microthrombocytopenia is a consistent feature of WAS and XLT and is associated with the bleeding diathesis observed in patients.[6] It is most likely due to the absence of WASp in platelets, even in cases where an adequate WASp level is detected in other cell types.[74] WASp is phosphorylated upon platelet activation by a mechanism that involves Btk, Grb2, PLC-γ2, PKC-θ, and SGK1.[69,125–128] Platelet activation and aggregation alter the binding of WASp to the actin cytoskeleton and results in its degradation in a calpain-dependent manner, thus providing a plausible mechanism for WASp inactivation.[68,69,71]

Initial studies have shown that platelets from WAS patients are irregular in shape and structure, lack pseudopodia, and spread poorly; their F-actin content is also decreased. They also have fewer α-granules in their cytoplasm, are less metabolically active, and aggregate poorly.[129–132] Contrary to these observations, several later studies reported normal platelet activation and aggregation, procoagulant activity, α-granule secretion, filopodia extension, lamellae spreading, F-actin increase, and Arp2/3 complex activation.[74,78,126,133–135] One difference between the earlier and later studies is in the method of isolation of the platelets, as well as their stimulation. Another difference could be that the groups that reported normal platelet structure and function obtained their samples from patients who had undergone splenectomy, as removal of the spleen has been shown to improve the count and quality of the platelets in patients with WAS.[136–139]

Low platelet levels exist in WAS patients and WASp$^{-/-}$ mice because of decreased platelet production and increased platelet clearance from the circulation. First, while the number of megakaryocytes in the BM of WAS patients and WASp$^{-/-}$ mice is normal to increased,[73,130,140,141] their ability to produce proplatelets and platelets *in vitro* is not grossly affected.[133] Megakaryocytes from WASp$^{-/-}$ mice migrate poorly in response to SDF-1α and tend to prematurely produce platelets in the BM.[141,142] Second, platelets in WAS patients and WASp$^{-/-}$ mice are cleared at a faster rate from the blood circulation. This could be because the abnormal shape and structure of the platelets results in their phagocytosis by BM or spleen macrophages, or to platelet-associated immunoglobulins that coat their surface and lead to their trapping in the spleen or other organs and increased opsonization by macrophages.[129,130,135,143–145]

WAS natural killer (NK) cells

Patients with WAS and XLT have normal to elevated levels of NK cells in their peripheral blood; however, the cytotoxic activity of WAS NK cells is severely decreased, whereas that of XLT NK cells is heterogeneous depending on the level of residual WASp present.[146,147] NK cells from WAS patients have a disorganized NK immune synapse because of impaired localization of F-actin, CD2, LFA-1, and Mac1 at the IS,[147–149] which affects their ability to form stable conjugates with target cells.[146] This also results in delayed activation of the signaling molecules NFAT2, NF-κB, PLC-γ, and calcineurin.[149] Furthermore, MTOC and lytic granule polarization to the IS is severely decreased in NK cells from WAS patients, which decreases target cell lysis;[147,148] this might also contribute to the development of tumors observed in some WAS patients.[6,124,150] The interaction between the microtubules and F-actin network at the NK IS is mediated by Cdc42-interacting protein 4 (CIP4), which could bridge the two networks for proper transfer of lytic granules to the NK cell membrane.[151] In addition to the role played by WASp, WIP forms a complex with actin and myosin IIA, associates with lytic granules, and mediates NK cell interaction with, and killing of, target cells.[152,153]

NK cells isolated from a WAS patient treated subcutaneously with IL-2, or *ex vivo* addition of recombinant IL-2 to NK cells isolated from WAS patients, results in complete correction of F-actin distribution to the NK IS, binding to target cells, and cytotoxic activity in a mechanism that involves WAVE2; this provides a parallel mechanism of NK cell activation.[146,149,154]

In addition, NK cells isolated from WAS patients have decreased migration through ICAM-1- and VCAM-1-coated filters owing to their failure to upregulate the β2-integrin LFA-1 high affinity state.[155] NK cell activation results in Cdc42 activation, as well as phosphorylation of WASp and its association with Fyn and Pyk-2, which is important for NK cell migration.[146,152,155]

WAS NKT cells

Invariant NKT (iNKT) cells are absent in patients with WAS and severely decreased in patients with XLT.[156] WASP$^{-/-}$ mice have decreased iNKT cell numbers in the peripheral organs (mainly spleen and liver) because of an intrinsic defect in iNKT cell maturation and migration to, or retention within, peripheral organs. Furthermore, WASP$^{-/-}$ iNKT cell proliferation and production of IL-4 and IFN-γ are severely decreased.[156,157] Therefore, WASp plays a key role in iNKT cell homeostasis and function, and decreased iNKT function may contribute to the global defect observed in WAS.

WAS DCs

DCs from patients with WAS express normal surface protein markers. However, F-actin is abnormally distributed in WAS DCs and they fail to make sustained ruffles, lamellopodia, and filopodia; they also have reduced translocational mobility *in vitro*, possibly because of a decrease in the recruitment of

Cdc42 into these structure.[158,159] In addition, the ability of WAS DCs to induce IFN-γ production by normal PBMCs is greatly reduced.[160]

DCs isolated from WASp$^{-/-}$ mice fail to form a leading edge and are unable to detach the trailing edge, which results in a relatively static hyperextended morphology where the DC body oscillates between two poles. They migrate less efficiently in response to chemotactic signals *in vitro*, are retained longer in the skin following *in vivo* challenge, and migrate less efficiently into the lymph nodes T cell zone.[161,162] In addition, WASp$^{-/-}$ DCs form transient unstable ISs with WT T cells, resulting in poor signal transduction and T cell activation *in vitro* and T cell proliferation, especially at low antigen strength, *in vivo*.[160,163,164] Furthermore, WASp is important for the adhesion and formation of stable ISs with NK cells and for polarization of IL-12–containing granules at the DC side of the IS, leading to decreased NK cell activation, IFN-γ production, and cytotoxic activity.[165] Therefore, WASp is important for the reorganization of the actin cytoskeleton required for efficient DC migration, IS formation, and activation of effector cells. Dysfunction of WASp-deficient DCs could contribute to the high incidence of infections observed in WAS patients through poor activation of effector cells.

WAS monocytes/marcophages

Monocytes and macrophages from WAS patients display fewer filopodia, have a severe defect in podosome formation and cell polarization, and fail to migrate to a chemokine gradient despite having normal expression of chemokine receptors.[166–168] Upon cell stimulation, WASp localizes to the podosomes along with actin, WIP, Cdc42, Arp2/3, and vinculin in a molecular complex where the function of WASp depends on its phosphorylation and interaction with WIP.[35,168,169] The failure of directional migration of WASp$^{-/-}$ macrophages is not because of the inability to form filopodia but to the instability of the filopodia, which tend to retract faster.[170]

In addition, WASp forms a complex with signaling molecules at the site of active phagocytosis, and its absence or dissociation from WIP results in reduced phagocytic cup formation, as well as reduced engulfment of apoptotic cells and IgG-coated antigens.[36,171,172] Therefore, cytoskeletal rearrangement mediated by WASp is required for the migration of monocytes and macrophages to the infected or inflamed tissue, and for the binding and phagocytosis of antigen.

WAS neutrophils

Neutrophils from a WAS patient and WASp$^{-/-}$ mice attach less to adhesive surfaces and cellular monolayers under shear flow, and fail to rearrange their surface integrins and spread. They fail to polymerize actin and migrate normally *in vitro* and *in vivo*, degranulate upon stimulation, and have reduced activation of respiratory burst. In addition, signaling downstream from leukocyte integrins after ligand engagement and clustering are severely diminished in WASp$^{-/-}$ neutrophils owing to aberrant localization of β2-integrins with phospho-Syk and phospho-Pyk2.[173]

Clinical manifestations

Mutations in the *WAS* gene result in a broad range of disease severity. A scoring system on a scale of one to five was introduced to differentiate XLT from WAS patients based solely on the severity of the clinical phenotype.[174] Patients considered to have XLT are assigned a score of one to two, whereas patients considered to have WAS are assigned a score of three to four. XLT and WAS patients who develop autoimmunity and/or malignancies at a later stage in life progress to a score of five.

Around 300 unique mutations spanning the *WAS* gene have been described (from the Resource of Asian Primary Immunodeficiency Diseases). The most frequent are missense mutations, followed by splice-site mutations, deletions, nonsense mutations, insertions, and complex mutations.[175,176] Most missense mutations are located in exons one to four, splice-site mutations are predominantly in introns six to ten, whereas nonsense mutations, insertions/deletions, and complex mutations are distributed throughout the *WAS* gene (Fig. 1).[26,124,174,177]

The effect of a given mutation on WASp expression correlates with severity of disease, albeit with some exceptions. In general, mutations that cause decreased WASp levels result in XLT, whereas mutations that abolish WASp expression or result in the expression of a truncated protein are associated with WAS.[174,178–180]

Patients with XLT who present with microthrombocytopenia but no other immunologic defects are assigned a score of one, whereas those who present with platelet defects, mild transient eczema, and minor infections are assigned a score of two. The survival rate of these two groups is similar to healthy individuals, yet XLT is associated with severe disease-related events such as serious hemorrhage episodes, life-threatening infections, autoimmunity, and cancer.[177] Because diagnosis could be before the full manifestation of the disease, patients with XLT should be reevaluated at a later stage in life and their clinical scores updated accordingly.

Patients with WAS who present with thrombocytopenia and small platelets, persistent but manageable eczema, and/or recurrent infections are assigned a score of three, whereas those who present with difficult-to-treat eczema and multiple severe infections are assigned a score of four. Microthrombocytopenia is associated with increased risk of bleeding diathesis, the most severe being intracranial, gastrointestinal, and oral bleeding.[6] Eczema does not usually manifest exclusively, but is frequently associated with one or more of symptoms, and its incidence is higher in patients with complete absence of WASp.[6,124] Decreased lymphocyte counts and defects in T cell and B cell function result in serious bacterial, viral, and fungal infections. Furthermore, the defects in cytotoxic T cell and NK cell function contribute both to the increased risk of infections and to the development of tumor cells.

Patients with WAS exhibit variable levels of serum IgM, normal to high levels of serum IgA, and high levels of serum IgD, IgG, and IgE.[103,181–185] The elevated levels of serum IgE, usually associated with allergic diseases[186] such as the eczema observed in WAS, could be due to the imbalance of Th1/Th2 cytokine production reported in these patients.[85,187] Upon immunization, WAS patients produce a normal Ab response to protein antigens but exibit a selective defect of their Ab response to polysaccharide antigens.[181,182,188] Patients with WAS are at a higher risk of developing autoimmunity, the most frequent being autoimmune hemolytic anemia, autoimmune neutropenia, vasculitis, IgA nephropathy, arthritis, and inflammatory bowel disease.[6,103,104,124] Furthermore, WAS patients often develop malignancies, mostly lymphomas, and their risk of development is increased in patients with autoimmunity.[6,124,150] The development of malignancies could be due to decreased cytotoxic T cell killing of cancer cells.[87] And despite lack of direct evidence, decreased NK cell function and genomic instability might contribute to the development of malignancies.

Although XLT and WAS are caused by mutations that negatively affect the level and/or function of WASp, XLN results from activating mutations of WASp. Thus patients with XLN are not included in the scoring system assigned for XLT and WAS. The mutations identified in XLN patients (L270P, S272P, and I294T) are located in the GBD, or C-terminal to it, decreasing its affinity to the VCA domain and affecting the autoinhibited state of the protein.[9–11] Patients with XLN suffer from recurrent major bacterial infections, severe neutropenia and monocytopenia, decreased NK and B cell levels, and low-to-normal platelets and serum IgA levels. In addition, they suffer from myelodysplasia because of abnormal F-actin formation during mitosis, which results in genomic instability, aborted cytokinesis, and accumulation of multinucleated cells that undergo apoptosis.[9,189,190]

Treatment of WAS

Despite advances in diagnosis and clinical care, the prognosis of WAS remains poor. Diagnosis should take into account protein expression level and clinical phenotype at the time of presentation. Conventional management can be used for mild cases such as XLT; however, hematopoietic stem cell transplantation (HSCT) remains the treatment of choice for WAS, and should be considered for XLT cases as well, as will be discussed later. In addition, recent advances in gene therapy make it an attractive alternative to HSCT for WAS, especially in cases where no matched donor is available.

Conventional treatment

Microthrombocytopenia is a common feature of XLT and WAS. Splenectomy has been shown to increase the level of platelets to normal, and, in some cases, corrects the mean platelet volume in patients with XLT. Because patients with WAS are deficient in Ab production to polysaccharide antigens, regimented use of prophylactic antibiotics and intravenous immunoglobulin (IVIG) decrease the risk of infections in splenectomized patients.[137–139,177] However, splenectomy does not decrease the risks of autoimmunity and lymphoproliferative disorders, and T and B cell function are reduced in patients who undergo HSCT following splenectomy, making it a less desirable intervention if HSCT is considered.[191] Nevertheless, because of the introduction of efficient vaccines and antibiotics, splenectomy remains a reasonable treatment for XLT patients with mild disease.

Hematopoietic stem cell transplantation

HSCT is the treatment of choice for WAS and can correct all aspects of the disease provided hematologic and immune reconstitution is achieved.[192] The use of HSCT for XLT is still controversial, considering the excellent long-term survival with conventional treatment. However, in light of possible severe infections, autoimmunity, and lymphoproliferative disorders in some XLT patients, HSCT can be considered, especially if a human leukocyte antigen (HLA)–identical related sibling donor is available.[177]

Several criteria affect the level of success of HSCT, most important of which are the conditioning regimen, the donor source, and the age and clinical status of the recipient at the time of HSCT.[193] The standard approach to curative therapy requires both myeloablation with busulfan and immunosuppression with cyclophosphamide to ensure high level donor chimerism.[194] Traditionally, the best transplantation outcome has been achieved with HLA-identical sibling donors and matched-unrelated donors when the age of the recipient is less than five years at the time of the transplant,[191,195–197] whereas lower survival rates are achieved with mismatched unrelated donors.[191,196,198] With the improvement of supportive care and high resolution HLA-typing methods, better success rates have been achieved in the last decade especially with matched-unrelated donors when the patient is more than five years of age, or by using matched cord blood as a source of stem cells.[199,200]

Patients who undergo transplantation in better clinical conditions have a lower rate of pos-HSCT complications. Acute or chronic graft-versus-host disease (GVHD) is observed especially in the first year after HSCT but can persist longer, and is treated with immunosuppression. Recently, autoimmunity independent of GVHD has been observed in patients with WAS following HSCT, and is associated with reduced donor chimerism.[199,200] The highest degree of donor chimerism is observed in T lymphocytes, followed by B lymphocytes, then myeloid cells. Co-existence of recipient and donor B cells could account for the autoimmunity, whereas low myeloid donor chimerism could account for persistent thrombocytopenia observed in some patients.[199,200] Mixed chimerism could occur when reduced intensity conditioning regimens are used. Therefore, because complete and stable multilineage donor engraftment is required to fully correct the disease, novel conditioning strategies and infusion of a larger number of donor stem cells might be needed in the future treatment of WAS.

Gene therapy

Gene therapy is an alternative to HSCT in the treatment of WAS. The protocol consists of isolating autologous HSCs (CD34[+]) from the patient, transducing them *ex vivo* with a retrovirus that expresses WASp as a transgene, then reinfusing them back into the patient following myelosuppressive treatment. Patients likely to benefit most from the development of gene therapy are those with a high clinical score and/or absent protein, and with no HLA-matched donor.

The first gene therapy for ten WAS patients was conducted in Hanover, Germany using a gammaretroviral vector (GV) derived from a Moloney murine leukaemia virus expressing WASp as a transgene.[201] A report on two of the patients demonstrated stable engraftment and production of WASp[+] T cells, B cells, monocytes, and platelets. In addition, their T and NK cell functions were corrected, and the ability of monocytes to make podosomes was increased. The patients responded normally to immunization and had decreased infections and autoimmunity significantly; eczema was ameliorated in one patient. Insertional analysis demonstrated that vector integration occurred preferentially in the vicinity of transcription start sites and was clustered in regions proximal to protooncogenes. Unfortunately, at least one patient from the Hanover study was reported to have developed acute T cell leukemia because of insertion near the T cell oncogene LMO2.[202,203]

One of the downfalls of gene therapy is that the viruses used for therapy integrate in the host genome, which raises the fear of serious consequences. In general, GV shows preferential insertion at transcription start sites, promoters, and enhancer regions of active genes and at conserved noncoding DNA, resulting in a high rate of transformations.[204,205] The genotoxic risk of GV can be reduced by replacing the strong promoter/enhancer long terminal repeat (LTR) of the virus with promoters derived from endogenous genes to produce a self inactivating (SIN) vector.[206] Recently, a recombinant lentiviral vector (LV) derived from the human immunodeficiency virus and carrying the *WAS* cDNA under the control of 1.6 kb derived from the endogenous *WAS* promoter (WAS-LV) was developed for treatment of WAS.[207,208] The use of WAS-LV presents a major advantage compared to the GV used previously. First, LVs are among the most versatile of all integrating vectors, in that they are stable, easy to produce and concentrate, and they have broad tropism, including quiescent cells, thus eliminating the need for extended activation periods that might affect the characteristics of the HSCs and are associated with loss of long-term engraftment.[202,208,209] Second, LVs randomly integrate into DNA with no bias to a specific area in the genome, and they have lower rates of insertional mutagenesis.[205,210] Third, elimination of the LTR and the expression of the *WAS* transgene under the control of its own promoter decreases the risk of insertional-mediated oncogene activation, and ensures physiologic levels of expression of the transgene restricted to the hematopoietic lineages.[210,211]

Several clinical studies are currently open in Europe and the United States for the use of WAS-LV in the gene therapy of WAS. Pre-clinical studies demonstrated high transduction efficiency and survival advantage of human PBMCs and HSCs transduced with WAS-LV, with no cytotoxicity. This resulted in normal T cell proliferation and IL-2 production, as well as normal podosome formation by DCs. In addition, WAS-LV–transduced HSCs from a patient with WAS, transplanted into immunodeficient mice, showed normal engraftment and differentiation ability toward lymphoid and myeloid cells.[208,212,213] In addition, murine BM cells isolated from WASp$^{-/-}$ mice, transduced *ex vivo* with WAS-LV and then transplanted into irradiated WASp$^{-/-}$ mice, demonstrated high transduction efficiency, long-term engraftment, and expression of the transgene in the lymphoid and myeloid compartments.[214–216] This resulted in correction of F-actin polarization, T cell proliferation and cytokine production, enhanced migration of B cells and DCs, and increased podosome formation and turnover in DCs. Gene therapy also resulted in the improvement of the splenic architecture, increased *in vivo*

B cell immunoglobulin production against polysaccharide Ags, and decreased autoantibody production.[217] Furthermore, DC phagocytosis, *in vivo* migration, and Ag presentation to effector cells was increased.[218] Importantly, gene therapy was tolerated and did not result in abnormalities in hematopoietic cell counts. These data are encouraging for the use of WAS-LV in the gene therapy of WAS.

On the other hand, a recent study showed that the WAS promoter is not very efficient in sustaining adequate levels of WASp expression in human and murine HSCs, and that this might lead to less effective rescuing of WASp-dependent defects and to the development of autoimmune manifestations *in vivo*, suggesting the need to explore more robust promoters for the clinical trial.[219]

We have used a different approach to stabilize mutant WASp in XLT patients by expressing a small peptide derived from the WASp-binding domain of WIP (nWIP).[31] We have shown that nWIP can interact with the mutant WASp and stabilize it, resulting in correction of the cytoskeletal rearrangement in primary T cells isolated from patients with XLT. This approach would stabilize endogenous WASp, thus eliminating the risk of too little or too much expression. However, it would not be applicable in cases of complete WASp absence and in patients expressing truncated WASp.

Concluding remarks

WASp is a promiscuous protein with multiple interacting partners that cooperate and compete for its stabilization, activation, localization, and degradation. WASp expression is restricted to the hematopoietic compartment, where it plays a role in almost all actin-mediated cellular processes. WASp dysfunction manifests in a range of phenotypes, from mild XLP to more severe WAS or XLN. Treatment is mostly restricted to antibiotics, IVIG therapy, in some cases splenectomy, and, when possible, BM transplantation. Current advances in HSCT and gene therapy provide treatments with highly favorable results.

Acknowledgments

This work was supported in part by USPHS Grant 5PO1HL059561.

Conflicts of interest

The authors declare no conflicts of interest.

References

1. Wiskott, A. 1937. Familiarer, angeborener Morbus Werlhofii? *Monatsschr. Kinderheilkd.* **68:** 212–216.
2. Aldrich, R., A. Steinberg & D. Campbell. 1954. Pedigree demonstrating a sex-linked recessive condition characterized by draining ears, eczematoid dermatits and bloody diarrhea. *Pediatrics* **13:** 133–139.
3. Derry, J.M., H.D. Ochs & U. Francke. 1994. Isolation of a novel gene mutated in Wiskott-Aldrich syndrome. *Cell* **78:** 635–644.
4. Binder, V. *et al.* 2006. The genotype of the original Wiskott phenotype. *N. Engl. J. Med.* **355:** 1790–1793.
5. Kirchhausen, T. & F.S. Rosen. 1996. Disease mechanism: unravelling Wiskott-Aldrich syndrome. *Curr. Biol.* **6:** 676–678.
6. Sullivan, K.E. *et al.* 1994. A multiinstitutional survey of the Wiskott-Aldrich syndrome. *J. Pediatr.* **125:** 876–885.
7. Villa, A. *et al.* 1995. X-linked thrombocytopenia and Wiskott-Aldrich syndrome are allelic diseases with mutations in the WASP gene. *Nat. Genet.* **9:** 414–417.
8. Zhu, Q. *et al.* 1995. The Wiskott-Aldrich syndrome and X-linked congenital thrombocytopenia are caused by mutations of the same gene. *Blood.* **86:** 3797–3804.
9. Ancliff, P.J. *et al.* 2006. Two novel activating mutations in the Wiskott-Aldrich syndrome protein result in congenital neutropenia. *Blood.* **108:** 2182–2189.
10. Beel, K. *et al.* 2009. A large kindred with X-linked neutropenia with an I294T mutation of the Wiskott-Aldrich syndrome gene. *Br. J. Haematol.* **144:** 120–126.
11. Devriendt, K. *et al.* 2001. Constitutively activating mutation in WASP causes X-linked severe congenital neutropenia. *Nat. Genet.* **27:** 313–317.
12. Snapper, S.B. & F.S. Rosen. 1999. The Wiskott-Aldrich syndrome protein (WASP): roles in signaling and cytoskeletal organization. *Annu. Rev. Immunol.* **17:** 905–929.
13. Miki, H., K. Miura & T. Takenawa. 1996. N-WASP, a novel actin-depolymerizing protein, regulates the cortical cytoskeletal rearrangement in a PIP2-dependent manner downstream of tyrosine kinases. *EMBO J.* **15:** 5326–5335.
14. Miki, H. *et al.* 1998. Induction of filopodium formation by a WASP-related actin-depolymerizing protein N-WASP. *Nature.* **391:** 93–96.
15. Bear, J.E., J.F. Rawls & C.L. Saxe, 3rd. 1998. SCAR, a WASP-related protein, isolated as a suppressor of receptor defects in late Dictyostelium development. *J. Cell Biol.* **142:** 1325–1335.
16. Suetsugu, S., H. Miki & T. Takenawa. 1999. Identification of two human WAVE/SCAR homologues as general actin regulatory molecules which associate with the Arp2/3 complex. *Biochem. Biophys. Res. Commun.* **260:** 296–302.
17. Linardopoulou, E.V. *et al.* 2007. Human subtelomeric WASH genes encode a new subclass of the WASP family. *PLoS Genet.* **3:** 2477–2485.
18. Campellone, K.G. *et al.* 2008. WHAMM is an Arp2/3 complex activator that binds microtubules and functions in ER to Golgi transport. *Cell.* **134:** 148–161.
19. Zuchero, J.B. *et al.* 2009. p53-cofactor JMY is a multifunctional actin nucleation factor. *Nat. Cell Biol.* **11:** 451–459.
20. Kollmar, M., D. Lbik & S. Enge. 2012. Evolution of the eukaryotic ARP2/3 activators of the WASP family: WASP,
WAVE, WASH, and WHAMM, and the proposed new family members WAWH and WAML. *BMC Res. Notes.* **5:** 1–23.
21. Parolini, O. *et al.* 1997. Expression of Wiskott-Aldrich syndrome protein (WASP) gene during hematopoietic differentiation. *Blood.* **90:** 70–75.
22. Stewart, D.M. *et al.* 1996. Studies of the expression of the Wiskott-Aldrich syndrome protein. *J. Clin. Invest.* **97:** 2627–2634.
23. Ramesh, N. *et al.* 1997. WIP, a protein associated with wiskott-aldrich syndrome protein, induces actin polymerization and redistribution in lymphoid cells. *Proc. Natl. Acad. Sci. U.S.A.* **94:** 14671–14676.
24. Chou, H.C. *et al.* 2006. WIP regulates the stability and localization of WASP to podosomes in migrating dendritic cells. *Curr. Biol.* **16:** 2337–2344.
25. de la Fuente, M.A. *et al.* 2007. WIP is a chaperone for Wiskott-Aldrich syndrome protein (WASP). *Proc. Natl. Acad. Sci. U.S.A.* **104:** 926–931.
26. Jin, Y. *et al.* 2004. Mutations of the Wiskott-Aldrich Syndrome Protein (WASP): hotspots, effect on transcription, and translation and phenotype/genotype correlation. *Blood.* **104:** 4010–4019.
27. Luthi, J.N., M.J. Gandhi & J.G. Drachman. 2003. X-linked thrombocytopenia caused by a mutation in the Wiskott-Aldrich syndrome (WAS) gene that disrupts interaction with the WAS protein (WASP)-interacting protein (WIP). *Exp. Hematol.* **31:** 150–158.
28. Stewart, D.M., L. Tian & D.L. Nelson. 1999. Mutations that cause the Wiskott-Aldrich syndrome impair the interaction of Wiskott-Aldrich syndrome protein (WASP) with WASP interacting protein. *J. Immunol.* **162:** 5019–5024.
29. Volkman, B.F. *et al.* 2002. Structure of the N-WASP EVH1 domain-WIP complex: insight into the molecular basis of Wiskott-Aldrich Syndrome. *Cell.* **111:** 565–576.
30. Peterson, F.C. *et al.* 2007. Multiple WASP-interacting protein recognition motifs are required for a functional interaction with N-WASP. *J. Biol. Chem.* **282:** 8446–8453.
31. Massaad, M.J. *et al.* 2010. A peptide derived from the Wiskott-Aldrich syndrome (WAS) protein-interacting protein (WIP) restores WAS protein level and actin cytoskeleton reorganization in lymphocytes from patients with WAS mutations that disrupt WIP binding. *J. Allergy Clin. Immunol.* **127:** 998–1005 e1001–1002.
32. Lim, R.P. *et al.* 2007. Analysis of conformational changes in WASP using a split YFP. *Biochem. Biophys. Res. Commun.* **362:** 1085–1089.
33. Martinez-Quiles, N. *et al.* 2001. WIP regulates N-WASP-mediated actin polymerization and filopodium formation. *Nat. Cell Biol.* **3:** 484–491.
34. Ho, H.Y. *et al.* 2004. Toca-1 mediates Cdc42-dependent actin nucleation by activating the N-WASP-WIP complex. *Cell.* **118:** 203–216.
35. Tsuboi, S. 2007. Requirement for a complex of Wiskott-Aldrich syndrome protein (WASP) with WASP interacting protein in podosome formation in macrophages. *J. Immunol.* **178:** 2987–2995.
36. Tsuboi, S. & J. Meerloo. 2007. Wiskott-Aldrich syndrome protein is a key regulator of the phagocytic cup formation in macrophages. *J. Biol. Chem.* **282:** 34194–34203.

37. Anton, I.M. *et al.* 1998. The Wiskott-Aldrich syndrome protein-interacting protein (WIP) binds to the adaptor protein Nck. *J. Biol. Chem.* **273:** 20992–20995.

38. Sasahara, Y. *et al.* 2002. Mechanism of recruitment of WASP to the immunological synapse and of its activation following TCR ligation. *Mol. Cell.* **10:** 1269–1281.

39. Kim, A.S. *et al.* 2000. Autoinhibition and activation mechanisms of the Wiskott-Aldrich syndrome protein. *Nature* **404:** 151–158.

40. Rohatgi, R. *et al.* 1999. The interaction between N-WASP and the Arp2/3 complex links Cdc42-dependent signals to actin assembly. *Cell.* **97:** 221–231.

41. Symons, M. *et al.* 1996. Wiskott-Aldrich syndrome protein, a novel effector for the GTPase CDC42Hs, is implicated in actin polymerization. *Cell.* **84:** 723–734.

42. Hemsath, L. *et al.* 2005. An electrostatic steering mechanism of Cdc42 recognition by Wiskott-Aldrich syndrome proteins. *Mol. Cell.* **20:** 313–324.

43. Higgs, H.N. & T.D. Pollard. 2000. Activation by Cdc42 and PIP(2) of Wiskott-Aldrich syndrome protein (WASp) stimulates actin nucleation by Arp2/3 complex. *J. Cell Biol.* **150:** 1311–1320.

44. Prehoda, K.E. *et al.* 2000. Integration of multiple signals through cooperative regulation of the N-WASP-Arp2/3 complex. *Science.* **290:** 801–806.

45. Rohatgi, R., H.Y. Ho & M.W. Kirschner. 2000. Mechanism of N-WASP activation by CDC42 and phosphatidylinositol 4, 5-bisphosphate. *J. Cell Biol.* **150:** 1299–1310.

46. Guinamard, R. *et al.* 1998. Tyrosine phosphorylation of the Wiskott-Aldrich syndrome protein by Lyn and Btk is regulated by CDC42. *FEBS Lett.* **434:** 431–436.

47. Baba, Y. *et al.* 1999. Involvement of wiskott-aldrich syndrome protein in B-cell cytoplasmic tyrosine kinase pathway. *Blood.* **93:** 2003–2012.

48. Cory, G.O. *et al.* 2002. Phosphorylation of tyrosine 291 enhances the ability of WASp to stimulate actin polymerization and filopodium formation. Wiskott-Aldrich Syndrome protein. *J. Biol. Chem.* **277:** 45115–45121.

49. Torres, E. & M.K. Rosen. 2003. Contingent phosphorylation/dephosphorylation provides a mechanism of molecular memory in WASP. *Mol. Cell.* **11:** 1215–1227.

50. Badour, K. *et al.* 2004. Fyn and PTP-PEST-mediated regulation of Wiskott-Aldrich syndrome protein (WASp) tyrosine phosphorylation is required for coupling T cell antigen receptor engagement to WASp effector function and T cell activation. *J. Exp. Med.* **199:** 99–112.

51. Suetsugu, S. *et al.* 2002. Sustained activation of N-WASP through phosphorylation is essential for neurite extension. *Dev. Cell* **3:** 645–658.

52. Cai, G.Q. *et al.* 2012. Neuronal Wiskott-Aldrich syndrome protein (N-WASP) is critical for formation of alpha-smooth muscle actin filaments during myofibroblast differentiation. *Am. J. Physiol. Lung Cell Mol. Physiol.* **303:** L692–702.

53. Blundell, M.P. *et al.* 2010. The Wiskott-Aldrich syndrome: the actin cytoskeleton and immune cell function. *Dis. Markers.* **29:** 157–175.

54. Cory, G.O. *et al.* 1996. Evidence that the Wiskott-Aldrich syndrome protein may be involved in lymphoid cell signaling pathways. *J. Immunol.* **157:** 3791–3795.

55. Bunnell, S.C. *et al.* 1996. Identification of Itk/Tsk Src homology 3 domain ligands. *J. Biol. Chem.* **271:** 25646–25656.

56. Banin, S., I. Gout & P. Brickell. 1999. Interaction between Wiskott-Aldrich Syndrome protein (WASP) and the Fyn protein-tyrosine kinase. *Mol. Biol. Rep.* **26:** 173–177.

57. Sato, M. *et al.* 2011. Identification of Fyn as the binding partner for the WASP N-terminal domain in T cells. *Int. Immunol.* **23:** 493–502.

58. Rivero-Lezcano, O.M. *et al.* 1995. Wiskott-Aldrich syndrome protein physically associates with Nck through Src homology 3 domains. *Mol. Cell. Biol.* **15:** 5725–5731.

59. She, H.Y. *et al.* 1997. Wiskott-Aldrich syndrome protein is associated with the adapter protein Grb2 and the epidermal growth factor receptor in living cells. *Mol. Biol. Cell.* **8:** 1709–1721.

60. Rohatgi, R. *et al.* 2001. Nck and phosphatidylinositol 4,5-bisphosphate synergistically activate actin polymerization through the N-WASP-Arp2/3 pathway. *J. Biol. Chem.* **276:** 26448–26452.

61. Carlier, M.F. *et al.* 2000. GRB2 links signaling to actin assembly by enhancing interaction of neural Wiskott-Aldrich syndrome protein (N-WASp) with actin-related protein (ARP2/3) complex. *J. Biol. Chem.* **275:** 21946–21952.

62. Benesch, S. *et al.* 2002. Phosphatidylinositol 4,5-biphosphate (PIP2)-induced vesicle movement depends on N-WASP and involves Nck, WIP, and Grb2. *J. Biol. Chem.* **277:** 37771–37776.

63. Badour, K. *et al.* 2003. The Wiskott-Aldrich syndrome protein acts downstream of CD2 and the CD2AP and PST-PIP1 adaptors to promote formation of the immunological synapse. *Immunity.* **18:** 141–154.

64. Higgs, H.N. & T.D. Pollard. 2001. Regulation of actin filament network formation through ARP2/3 complex: activation by a diverse array of proteins. *Annu. Rev. Biochem.* **70:** 649–676.

65. Higgs, H.N., L. Blanchoin & T.D. Pollard. 1999. Influence of the C terminus of Wiskott-Aldrich syndrome protein (WASp) and the Arp2/3 complex on actin polymerization. *Biochemistry.* **38:** 15212–15222.

66. Machesky, L.M. & R.H. Insall. 1998. Scar1 and the related Wiskott-Aldrich syndrome protein, WASP, regulate the actin cytoskeleton through the Arp2/3 complex. *Curr. Biol.* **8:** 1347–1356.

67. Marchand, J.B. *et al.* 2001. Interaction of WASP/Scar proteins with actin and vertebrate Arp2/3 complex. *Nat. Cell Biol.* **3:** 76–82.

68. Lutskiy, M.I. *et al.* 2007. WASP localizes to the membrane skeleton of platelets. *Br. J. Haematol.* **139:** 98–105.

69. Oda, A. *et al.* 1998. Collagen induces tyrosine phosphorylation of Wiskott-Aldrich syndrome protein in human platelets. *Blood* **92:** 1852–1858.

70. Blundell, M.P. *et al.* 2009. Phosphorylation of WASp is a key regulator of activity and stability in vivo. *Proc. Natl. Acad. Sci. U.S.A.* **106:** 15738–15743.

71. Shcherbina, A. *et al.* 2001. WASP and N-WASP in human platelets differ in sensitivity to protease calpain. *Blood.* **98:** 2988–2991.

72. Reicher, B. *et al.* 2012. Ubiquitylation-Dependent Negative Regulation of WASp Is Essential for Actin Cytoskeleton Dynamics. *Mol. Cell. Biol.* **32:** 3153–3163.

73. Ochs, H.D. *et al.* 1980. The Wiskott-Aldrich syndrome: studies of lymphocytes, granulocytes, and platelets. *Blood* **55:** 243–252.

74. Shcherbina, A., F.S. Rosen & E. Remold-O'Donnell. 1999. WASP levels in platelets and lymphocytes of wiskott-aldrich syndrome patients correlate with cell dysfunction. *J. Immunol.* **163:** 6314–6320.

75. Kawabata, K. *et al.* 1996. Decreased alpha/beta heterodimer among CD8 molecules of peripheral blood T cells in Wiskott-Aldrich syndrome. *Clin. Immunol. Immunopathol.* **81:** 129–135.

76. Park, J.Y. *et al.* 2004. Early deficit of lymphocytes in Wiskott-Aldrich syndrome: possible role of WASP in human lymphocyte maturation. *Clin. Exp. Immunol.* **136:** 104–110.

77. Rawlings, S.L. *et al.* 1999. Spontaneous apoptosis in lymphocytes from patients with Wiskott-Aldrich syndrome: correlation of accelerated cell death and attenuated bcl-2 expression. *Blood* **94:** 3872–3882.

78. Rengan, R. *et al.* 2000. Actin cytoskeletal function is spared, but apoptosis is increased, in WAS patient hematopoietic cells. *Blood.* **95:** 1283–1292.

79. Kenney, D. *et al.* 1986. Morphological abnormalities in the lymphocytes of patients with the Wiskott-Aldrich syndrome. *Blood.* **68:** 1329–1332.

80. Molina, I.J. *et al.* 1992. T cell lines characterize events in the pathogenesis of the Wiskott-Aldrich syndrome. *J. Exp. Med.* **176:** 867–874.

81. Gallego, M.D. *et al.* 1997. Defective actin reorganization and polymerization of Wiskott-Aldrich T cells in response to CD3-mediated stimulation. *Blood.* **90:** 3089–3097.

82. Zabay, J.M. *et al.* 1984. Disorders of regulatory T cell function in patients with the Wiskott-Aldrich syndrome. *Clin. Exp. Immunol.* **56:** 23–28.

83. Molina, I.J. *et al.* 1993. T cells of patients with the Wiskott-Aldrich syndrome have a restricted defect in proliferative responses. *J. Immunol.* **151:** 4383–4390.

84. Dupre, L. *et al.* 2002. Wiskott-Aldrich syndrome protein regulates lipid raft dynamics during immunological synapse formation. *Immunity.* **17:** 157–166.

85. Trifari, S. *et al.* 2006. Defective Th1 cytokine gene transcription in CD4+ and CD8+ T cells from Wiskott-Aldrich syndrome patients. *J. Immunol.* **177:** 7451–7461.

86. Cianferoni, A. *et al.* 2005. Defective nuclear translocation of nuclear factor of activated T cells and extracellular signal-regulated kinase underlies deficient IL-2 gene expression in Wiskott-Aldrich syndrome. *J. Allergy Clin. Immunol.* **116:** 1364–1371.

87. De Meester, J. *et al.* 2010. The Wiskott-Aldrich syndrome protein regulates CTL cytotoxicity and is required for efficient killing of B cell lymphoma targets. *J. Leukoc. Biol.* **88:** 1031–1040.

88. Snapper, S.B. *et al.* 1998. Wiskott-Aldrich syndrome protein-deficient mice reveal a role for WASP in T but not B cell activation. *Immunity* **9:** 81–91.

89. Zhang, J. *et al.* 1999. Antigen receptor-induced activation and cytoskeletal rearrangement are impaired in Wiskott-Aldrich syndrome protein-deficient lymphocytes. *J. Exp. Med.* **190:** 1329–1342.

90. Le Bras, S. *et al.* 2009. WIP is critical for T cell responsiveness to IL-2. *Proc. Natl. Acad. Sci. U.S.A.* **106:** 7519–7524.

91. Silvin, C., B. Belisle & A. Abo. 2001. A role for Wiskott-Aldrich syndrome protein in T-cell receptor-mediated transcriptional activation independent of actin polymerization. *J. Biol. Chem.* **276:** 21450–21457.

92. Cannon, J.L. & J.K. Burkhardt. 2004. Differential roles for Wiskott-Aldrich syndrome protein in immune synapse formation and IL-2 production. *J. Immunol.* **173:** 1658–1662.

93. Grakoui, A. *et al.* 1999. The immunological synapse: a molecular machine controlling T cell activation. *Science.* **285:** 221–227.

94. Monks, C.R. *et al.* 1998. Three-dimensional segregation of supramolecular activation clusters in T cells. *Nature* **395:** 82–86.

95. Simons, K. & E. Ikonen. 1997. Functional rafts in cell membranes. *Nature* **387:** 569–572.

96. Barda-Saad, M. *et al.* 2005. Dynamic molecular interactions linking the T cell antigen receptor to the actin cytoskeleton. *Nat. Immunol.* **6:** 80–89.

97. Calvez, R. *et al.* 2011. The Wiskott-Aldrich syndrome protein permits assembly of a focused immunological synapse enabling sustained T-cell receptor signaling. *Haematologica.* **96:** 1415–1423.

98. Sims, T.N. *et al.* 2007. Opposing effects of PKCtheta and WASp on symmetry breaking and relocation of the immunological synapse. *Cell* **129:** 773–785.

99. Haddad, E. *et al.* 2001. The interaction between Cdc42 and WASP is required for SDF-1-induced T-lymphocyte chemotaxis. *Blood* **97:** 33–38.

100. Okabe, S., S. Fukuda & H.E. Broxmeyer. 2002. Activation of Wiskott-Aldrich syndrome protein and its association with other proteins by stromal cell-derived factor-1alpha is associated with cell migration in a T-lymphocyte line. *Exp. Hematol.* **30:** 761–766.

101. Gallego, M.D. *et al.* 2006. WIP and WASP play complementary roles in T cell homing and chemotaxis to SDF-1alpha. *Int. Immunol.* **18:** 221–232.

102. Snapper, S.B. *et al.* 2005. WASP deficiency leads to global defects of directed leukocyte migration in vitro and in vivo. *J. Leukoc. Biol.* **77:** 993–998.

103. Dupuis-Girod, S. *et al.* 2003. Autoimmunity in Wiskott-Aldrich syndrome: risk factors, clinical features, and outcome in a single-center cohort of 55 patients. *Pediatrics.* **111:** e622–627.

104. Schurman, S.H. & F. Candotti. 2003. Autoimmunity in Wiskott-Aldrich syndrome. *Curr. Opin. Rheumatol.* **15:** 446–453.

105. Sakaguchi, S. 2005. Naturally arising Foxp3-expressing CD25+CD4+ regulatory T cells in immunological tolerance to self and non-self. *Nat. Immunol.* **6:** 345–352.

106. Shevach, E.M. 2002. CD4+ CD25+ suppressor T cells: more questions than answers. *Nat. Rev. Immunol.* **2:** 389–400.

107. Adriani, M. *et al.* 2007. Impaired in vitro regulatory T cell function associated with Wiskott-Aldrich syndrome. *Clin. Immunol.* **124:** 41–48.

108. Marangoni, F. *et al.* 2007. WASP regulates suppressor activity of human and murine CD4(+)CD25(+)FOXP3(+) natural regulatory T cells. *J. Exp. Med.* **204:** 369–380.

109. Humblet-Baron, S. *et al.* 2007. Wiskott-Aldrich syndrome protein is required for regulatory T cell homeostasis. *J. Clin. Invest.* **117:** 407–418.

110. Maillard, M.H. *et al.* 2007. The Wiskott-Aldrich syndrome protein is required for the function of CD4(+)CD25(+)Foxp3(+) regulatory T cells. *J. Exp. Med.* **204:** 381–391.

111. Adriani, M. *et al.* 2011. Defective inhibition of B-cell proliferation by Wiskott-Aldrich syndrome protein-deficient regulatory T cells. *Blood* **117:** 6608–6611.

112. Shimizu, M. *et al.* 2011. Development of IgA nephropathy-like glomerulonephritis associated with Wiskott-Aldrich syndrome protein deficiency. *Clin. Immunol.* **142:** 160–166.

113. Park, J.Y. *et al.* 2005. Phenotypic perturbation of B cells in the Wiskott-Aldrich syndrome. *Clin. Exp. Immunol.* **139:** 297–305.

114. Recher, M. *et al.* 2012. B cell-intrinsic deficiency of the Wiskott-Aldrich syndrome protein (WASp) causes severe abnormalities of the peripheral B-cell compartment in mice. *Blood* **119:** 2819–2828.

115. Westerberg, L. *et al.* 2005. Wiskott-Aldrich syndrome protein deficiency leads to reduced B-cell adhesion, migration, and homing, and a delayed humoral immune response. *Blood* **105:** 1144–1152.

116. Westerberg, L.S. *et al.* 2008. WASP confers selective advantage for specific hematopoietic cell populations and serves a unique role in marginal zone B-cell homeostasis and function. *Blood* **112:** 4139–4147.

117. Westerberg, L.S. *et al.* 2012. Wiskott-Aldrich syndrome protein (WASP) and N-WASP are critical for peripheral B-cell development and function. *Blood* **119:** 3966–3974.

118. Andreu, N., J.M. Aran & C. Fillat. 2007. Novel membrane cell projection defects in Wiskott-Aldrich syndrome B cells. *Int. J. Mol. Med.* **20:** 445–450.

119. Westerberg, L. *et al.* 2001. Cdc42, Rac1, and the Wiskott-Aldrich syndrome protein are involved in the cytoskeletal regulation of B lymphocytes. *Blood* **98:** 1086–1094.

120. Sato, R. *et al.* 2012. Impaired cell adhesion, apoptosis, and signaling in WASP gene-disrupted Nalm-6 pre-B cells and recovery of cell adhesion using a transducible form of WASp. *Int. J. Hematol.* **95:** 299–310.

121. Henriquez, N.V., G.T. Rijkers & B.J. Zegers. 1994. Antigen receptor-mediated transmembrane signaling in Wiskott-Aldrich syndrome. *J. Immunol.* **153:** 395–399.

122. Simon, H.U. *et al.* 1992. Evidence for defective transmembrane signaling in B cells from patients with Wiskott-Aldrich syndrome. *J. Clin. Invest.* **90:** 1396–1405.

123. Becker-Herman, S. *et al.* 2011. WASp-deficient B cells play a critical, cell-intrinsic role in triggering autoimmunity. *J. Exp. Med.* **208:** 2033–2042.

124. Imai, K. *et al.* 2004. Clinical course of patients with WASP gene mutations. *Blood* **103:** 456–464.

125. Miki, H. *et al.* 1997. Tyrosine kinase signaling regulates Wiskott-Aldrich syndrome protein function, which is essential for megakaryocyte differentiation. *Cell Growth Differ.* **8:** 195–202.

126. Gross, B.S. *et al.* 1999. Regulation and function of WASp in platelets by the collagen receptor, glycoprotein VI. *Blood.* **94:** 4166–4176.

127. Schmidt, E.M. *et al.* 2012. SGK1 Sensitivity of Platelet Migration. *Cell. Physiol. Biochem.* **30:** 259–268.

128. Soriani, A. *et al.* 2006. A role for PKCtheta in outside-in alpha(IIb)beta3 signaling. *J. Thromb. Haemost.* **4:** 648–655.

129. Grottum, K.A. *et al.* 1969. Wiskott-Aldrich syndrome: qualitative platelet defects and short platelet survival. *Br. J. Haematol.* **17:** 373–388.

130. Baldini, M.G. 1972. Nature of the platelet defect in the Wiskott-Aldrich syndrome. *Ann. N.Y. Acad. Sci.* **201:** 437–444.

131. Semple, J.W. *et al.* 1997. Flow cytometric analysis of platelets from children with the Wiskott-Aldrich syndrome reveals defects in platelet development, activation and structure. *Br. J. Haematol.* **97:** 747–754.

132. Tsuboi, S., S. Nonoyama & H.D. Ochs. 2006. Wiskott-Aldrich syndrome protein is involved in alphaIIb beta3-mediated cell adhesion. *EMBO reports.* **7:** 506–511.

133. Haddad, E. *et al.* 1999. The thrombocytopenia of Wiskott Aldrich syndrome is not related to a defect in proplatelet formation. *Blood* **94:** 509–518.

134. Falet, H. *et al.* 2002. Normal Arp2/3 complex activation in platelets lacking WASp. *Blood* **100:** 2113–2122.

135. Falet, H. *et al.* 2009. Platelet-associated IgAs and impaired GPVI responses in platelets lacking WIP. *Blood* **114:** 4729–4737.

136. Corash, L., B. Shafer & R.M. Blaese. 1985. Platelet-associated immunoglobulin, platelet size, and the effect of splenectomy in the Wiskott-Aldrich syndrome. *Blood* **65:** 1439–1443.

137. Litzman, J. *et al.* 1996. Intravenous immunoglobulin, splenectomy, and antibiotic prophylaxis in Wiskott-Aldrich syndrome. *Arch. Dis. Child.* **75:** 436–439.

138. Lum, L.G. *et al.* 1980. Splenectomy in the management of the thrombocytopenia of the Wiskott-Aldrich syndrome. *N. Engl. J. Med.* **302:** 892–896.

139. Mullen, C.A., K.D. Anderson & R.M. Blaese. 1993. Splenectomy and/or bone marrow transplantation in the management of the Wiskott-Aldrich syndrome: long-term follow-up of 62 cases. *Blood* **82:** 2961–2966.

140. Notarangelo, L.D. *et al.* 1991. Presentation of Wiskott Aldrich syndrome as isolated thrombocytopenia. *Blood* **77:** 1125–1126.

141. Sabri, S. *et al.* 2006. Deficiency in the Wiskott-Aldrich protein induces premature proplatelet formation and platelet production in the bone marrow compartment. *Blood* **108:** 134–140.

142. Pearson, H.A. *et al.* 1966. Platelet survival in Wiskott-Aldrich syndrome. *J. Pediatr.* **68:** 754–760.

143. Prislovsky, A. *et al.* 2008. Rapid platelet turnover in WASP(-) mice correlates with increased ex vivo phagocytosis of opsonized WASP(-) platelets. *Exp. Hematol.* **36:** 609–623.

144. Marathe, B.M. *et al.* 2009. Antiplatelet antibodies in WASP(-) mice correlate with evidence of increased in vivo platelet consumption. *Exp. Hematol.* **37:** 1353–1363.

145. Prislovsky, A. *et al.* 2012. Platelets from WAS patients show an increased susceptibility to ex vivo phagocytosis. *Platelets.* Epub ahead of print. DOI:10.3109/09537104.2012.693991.

146. Gismondi, A. *et al.* 2004. Impaired natural and CD16-mediated NK cell cytotoxicity in patients with WAS and XLT: ability of IL-2 to correct NK cell functional defect. *Blood* **104:** 436–443.

147. Orange, J.S. *et al.* 2002. Wiskott-Aldrich syndrome protein is required for NK cell cytotoxicity and colocalizes with actin to NK cell-activating immunologic synapses. *Proc. Natl. Acad. Sci. U.S.A.* **99:** 11351–11356.

148. Orange, J.S. *et al.* 2003. The mature activating natural killer cell immunologic synapse is formed in distinct stages. *Proc. Natl. Acad. Sci. U.S.A.* **100:** 14151–14156.

149. Huang, W. *et al.* 2005. The Wiskott-Aldrich syndrome protein regulates nuclear translocation of NFAT2 and NF-kappa B (RelA) independently of its role in filamentous actin polymerization and actin cytoskeletal rearrangement. *J. Immunol.* **174:** 2602–2611.

150. Shcherbina, A. *et al.* 2003. High incidence of lymphomas in a subgroup of Wiskott-Aldrich syndrome patients. *Br. J. Haematol.* **121:** 529–530.

151. Banerjee, P.P. *et al.* 2007. Cdc42-interacting protein-4 functionally links actin and microtubule networks at the cytolytic NK cell immunological synapse. *J. Exp. Med.* **204:** 2305–2320.

152. Krzewski, K. *et al.* 2006. Formation of a WIP-, WASp-, actin-, and myosin IIA-containing multiprotein complex in activated NK cells and its alteration by KIR inhibitory signaling. *J. Cell Biol.* **173:** 121–132.

153. Krzewski, K., X. Chen & J.L. Strominger. 2008. WIP is essential for lytic granule polarization and NK cell cytotoxicity. *Proc. Natl. Acad. Sci. U.S.A.* **105:** 2568–2573.

154. Orange, J.S. *et al.* 2011. IL-2 induces a WAVE2-dependent pathway for actin reorganization that enables WASp-independent human NK cell function. *J. Clin. Invest.* **121:** 1535–1548.

155. Stabile, H. *et al.* 2010. Impaired NK-cell migration in WAS/XLT patients: role of Cdc42/WASp pathway in the control of chemokine-induced beta2 integrin high-affinity state. *Blood* **115:** 2818–2826.

156. Locci, M. *et al.* 2009. The Wiskott-Aldrich syndrome protein is required for iNKT cell maturation and function. *J. Exp. Med.* **206:** 735–742.

157. Astrakhan, A., H.D. Ochs & D.J. Rawlings. 2009. Wiskott-Aldrich syndrome protein is required for homeostasis and function of invariant NKT cells. *J. Immunol.* **182:** 7370–7380.

158. Binks, M. *et al.* 1998. Intrinsic dendritic cell abnormalities in Wiskott-Aldrich syndrome. *Eur. J. Immunol.* **28:** 3259–3267.

159. Burns, S. *et al.* 2001. Configuration of human dendritic cell cytoskeleton by Rho GTPases, the WAS protein, and differentiation. *Blood* **98:** 1142–1149.

160. Bouma, G. *et al.* 2011. Cytoskeletal remodeling mediated by WASp in dendritic cells is necessary for normal immune synapse formation and T-cell priming. *Blood* **118:** 2492–2501.

161. de Noronha, S. *et al.* 2005. Impaired dendritic-cell homing in vivo in the absence of Wiskott-Aldrich syndrome protein. *Blood* **105:** 1590–1597.

162. Bouma, G., S. Burns & A.J. Thrasher. 2007. Impaired T-cell priming in vivo resulting from dysfunc-tion of WASp-deficient dendritic cells. *Blood* **110:** 4278–4284.

163. Pulecio, J. *et al.* 2008. Expression of Wiskott-Aldrich syndrome protein in dendritic cells regulates synapse formation and activation of naive CD8+ T cells. *J. Immunol.* **181:** 1135–1142.

164. Westerberg, L. *et al.* 2003. Efficient antigen presentation of soluble, but not particulate, antigen in the absence of Wiskott-Aldrich syndrome protein. *Immunology* **109:** 384–391.

165. Borg, C. *et al.* 2004. NK cell activation by dendritic cells (DCs) requires the formation of a synapse leading to IL-12 polarization in DCs. *Blood* **104:** 3267–3275.

166. Badolato, R. *et al.* 1998. Monocytes from Wiskott-Aldrich patients display reduced chemotaxis and lack of cell polarization in response to monocyte chemoattractant protein-1 and formyl-methionyl-leucyl-phenylalanine. *J. Immunol.* **161:** 1026–1033.

167. Zicha, D. *et al.* 1998. Chemotaxis of macrophages is abolished in the Wiskott-Aldrich syndrome. *Br. J. Haematol.* **101:** 659–665.

168. Linder, S. *et al.* 1999. Wiskott-Aldrich syndrome protein regulates podosomes in primary human macrophages. *Proc. Natl. Acad. Sci. U.S.A.* **96:** 9648–9653.

169. Linder, S. *et al.* 2000. The polarization defect of Wiskott-Aldrich syndrome macrophages is linked to dislocalization of the Arp2/3 complex. *J. Immunol.* **165:** 221–225.

170. Ishihara, D. *et al.* 2012. The chemotactic defect in Wiskott-Aldrich syndrome macrophages is due to the reduced persistence of directional protrusions. *PloS One.* **7:** e30033.

171. Lorenzi, R. *et al.* 2000. Wiskott-Aldrich syndrome protein is necessary for efficient IgG-mediated phagocytosis. *Blood* **95:** 2943–2946.

172. Leverrier, Y. *et al.* 2001. Cutting edge: the Wiskott-Aldrich syndrome protein is required for efficient phagocytosis of apoptotic cells. *J. Immunol.* **166:** 4831–4834.

173. Zhang, H. *et al.* 2006. Impaired integrin-dependent function in Wiskott-Aldrich syndrome protein-deficient murine and human neutrophils. *Immunity* **25:** 285–295.

174. Zhu, Q. *et al.* 1997. Wiskott-Aldrich syndrome/X-linked thrombocytopenia: WASP gene mutations, protein expression, and phenotype. *Blood* **90:** 2680–2689.

175. Ochs, H.D. & A.J. Thrasher. 2006. The Wiskott-Aldrich syndrome. *J. Allergy Clin. Immunol.* **117:** 725–738; quiz 739.

176. Albert, M.H., L.D. Notarangelo & H.D. Ochs. 2011. Clinical spectrum, pathophysiology and treatment of the Wiskott-Aldrich syndrome. *Curr. Opin. Hematol.* **18:** 42–48.

177. Albert, M.H. *et al.* 2010. X-linked thrombocytopenia (XLT) due to WAS mutations: clinical characteristics, long-term outcome, and treatment options. *Blood* **115:** 3231–3238.

178. Wengler, G.S. *et al.* 1995. High prevalence of nonsense, frame shift, and splice-site mutations in 16 patients with full-blown Wiskott-Aldrich syndrome. *Blood* **86:** 3648–3654.

179. Lemahieu, V., J.M. Gastier & U. Francke. 1999. Novel mutations in the Wiskott-Aldrich syndrome protein gene and

their effects on transcriptional, translational, and clinical phenotypes. *Hum. Mutat.* **14:** 54–66.

180. Lutskiy, M.I., F.S. Rosen & E. Remold-O'Donnell. 2005. Genotype-proteotype linkage in the Wiskott-Aldrich syndrome. *J. Immunol.* **175:** 1329–1336.

181. Blaese, R.M. *et al.* 1968. The Wiskott-Aldrich syndrome. A disorder with a possible defect in antigen processing or recognition. *Lancet* **1:** 1056–1061.

182. Cooper, M.D. *et al.* 1968. Wiskott-Aldrich syndrome. An immunologic deficiency disease involving the afferent limb of immunity. *Am. J. Med.* **44:** 499–513.

183. Belohradsky, B.H. *et al.* 1978. [The Wiskott-Aldrich syndrome]. *Ergeb. Inn. Med. Kinderheilkd.* **41:** 85–184.

184. Berglund, G. *et al.* 1968. Wiskott-Aldrich syndrome. A study of 6 cases with determination of the immunoglobulins A, D, G, M and ND. *Acta Paediatr. Scand.* **57:** 89–97.

185. Waldmann, T.A. *et al.* 1972. Immunoglobulin E in immunologic deficiency diseases. II. Serum IgE concentration of patients with acquired hypogammaglobulinemia, thymoma and hypogammaglobulinemia, myotonic dystrophy, intestinal lymphangiectasia and Wiskott-Aldrich syndrome. *J. Immunol.* **109:** 304–310.

186. Leung, D.Y. *et al.* 2004. New insights into atopic dermatitis. *J. Clin. Invest.* **113:** 651–657.

187. Ozcan, E., L.D. Notarangelo & R.S. Geha. 2008. Primary immune deficiencies with aberrant IgE production. *J. Allergy Clin. Immunol.* **122:** 1054–1062; quiz 1063–1054.

188. Oppenheim, J.J., R.M. Blaese & T.A. Waldmann. 1970. Defective lymphocyte transformation and delayed hypersensitivity in Wiskott-Aldrich syndrome. *J. Immunol.* **104:** 835–844.

189. Moulding, D.A. *et al.* 2007. Unregulated actin polymerization by WASp causes defects of mitosis and cytokinesis in X-linked neutropenia. *J. Exp. Med.* **204:** 2213–2224.

190. Westerberg, L.S. *et al.* 2010. Activating WASP mutations associated with X-linked neutropenia result in enhanced actin polymerization, altered cytoskeletal responses, and genomic instability in lymphocytes. *J. Exp. Med.* **207:** 1145–1152.

191. Ozsahin, H. *et al.* 1996. Bone marrow transplantation in 26 patients with Wiskott-Aldrich syndrome from a single center. *J. Pediatr.* **129:** 238–244.

192. Parkman, R. *et al.* 1978. Complete correction of the Wiskott-Aldrich syndrome by allogeneic bone-marrow transplantation. *N. Engl. J. Med.* **298:** 921–927.

193. Pai, S.Y. & L.D. Notarangelo. 2010. Hematopoietic cell transplantation for Wiskott-Aldrich syndrome: advances in biology and future directions for treatment. *Immunol. Allergy Clin. North Am.* **30:** 179–194.

194. Kapoor, N. *et al.* 1981. Reconstitution of normal megakaryocytopoiesis and immunologic functions in Wiskott-Aldrich syndrome by marrow transplantation following myeloablation and immunosuppression with busulfan and cyclophosphamide. *Blood* **57:** 692–696.

195. Antoine, C. *et al.* 2003. Long-term survival and transplantation of haemopoietic stem cells for immunodeficiencies: report of the European experience 1968–99. *Lancet* **361:** 553–560.

196. Filipovich, A.H. *et al.* 2001. Impact of donor type on outcome of bone marrow transplantation for Wiskott-Aldrich syndrome: collaborative study of the International Bone Marrow Transplant Registry and the National Marrow Donor Program. *Blood* **97:** 1598–1603.

197. Pai, S.Y. *et al.* 2006. Stem cell transplantation for the Wiskott-Aldrich syndrome: a single-center experience confirms efficacy of matched unrelated donor transplantation. *Bone Marrow Transplant.* **38:** 671–679.

198. Fischer, A. *et al.* 1994. Bone marrow transplantation (BMT) in Europe for primary immunodeficiencies other than severe combined immunodeficiency: a report from the European Group for BMT and the European Group for Immunodeficiency. *Blood* **83:** 1149–1154.

199. Ozsahin, H. *et al.* 2008. Long-term outcome following hematopoietic stem-cell transplantation in Wiskott-Aldrich syndrome: collaborative study of the European Society for Immunodeficiencies and European Group for Blood and Marrow Transplantation. *Blood* **111:** 439–445.

200. Moratto, D. *et al.* 2011. Long-term outcome and lineage-specific chimerism in 194 patients with Wiskott-Aldrich syndrome treated by hematopoietic cell transplantation in the period 1980–2009: an international collaborative study. *Blood* **118:** 1675–1684.

201. Boztug, K. *et al.* 2010. Stem-cell gene therapy for the Wiskott-Aldrich syndrome. *N. Engl. J. Med.* **363:** 1918–1927.

202. Galy, A. & A.J. Thrasher. 2011. Gene therapy for the Wiskott-Aldrich syndrome. *Curr. Opin. Allergy Clin. Immunol.* **11:** 545–550.

203. Avedillo Diez, I. *et al.* 2011. Development of novel efficient SIN vectors with improved safety features for Wiskott-Aldrich syndrome stem cell based gene therapy. *Mol. Pharm.* **8:** 1525–1537.

204. Cattoglio, C. *et al.* 2010. High-definition mapping of retroviral integration sites identifies active regulatory elements in human multipotent hematopoietic progenitors. *Blood* **116:** 5507–5517.

205. Modlich, U. *et al.* 2009. Insertional transformation of hematopoietic cells by self-inactivating lentiviral and gammaretroviral vectors. *Mol. Ther.* **17:** 1919–1928.

206. Zychlinski, D. *et al.* 2008. Physiological promoters reduce the genotoxic risk of integrating gene vectors. *Mol. Ther.* **16:** 718–725.

207. Dupre, L. *et al.* 2004. Lentiviral vector-mediated gene transfer in T cells from Wiskott-Aldrich syndrome patients leads to functional correction. *Mol. Ther.* **10:** 903–915.

208. Merten, O.W. *et al.* 2011. Large-scale manufacture and characterization of a lentiviral vector produced for clinical ex vivo gene therapy application. *Hum. Gene Ther.* **22:** 343–356.

209. Zufferey, R., *et al.* 1998. Self-inactivating lentivirus vector for safe and efficient in vivo gene delivery. *J. Virol.* **72:** 9873–9880.

210. Mantovani, J. *et al.* 2009. Diverse genomic integration of a lentiviral vector developed for the treatment of Wiskott-Aldrich syndrome. *J. Gene Med.* **11:** 645–654.

211. Martin, F. *et al.* 2005. Lentiviral vectors transcriptionally targeted to hematopoietic cells by WASP gene proximal promoter sequences. *Gene Ther.* **12:** 715–723.

212. Charrier, S. *et al.* 2007. Lentiviral vectors targeting WASp expression to hematopoietic cells, efficiently transduce and correct cells from WAS patients. *Gene Ther.* **14:** 415–428.

213. Scaramuzza, S. *et al.* 2013. Preclinical safety and efficacy of human CD34(+) cells transduced with lentiviral vector for the treatment of Wiskott-Aldrich syndrome. *Mol. Ther.* **21:** 175–184.

214. Blundell, M.P. *et al.* 2008. Improvement of migratory defects in a murine model of Wiskott-Aldrich syndrome gene therapy. *Mol Ther*. **16:** 836–844.

215. Dupre, L. *et al.* 2006. Efficacy of gene therapy for Wiskott-Aldrich syndrome using a WAS promoter/cDNA-containing lentiviral vector and nonlethal irradiation. *Hum. Gene Ther.* **17:** 303–313.

216. Marangoni, F. *et al.* 2009. Evidence for long-term efficacy and safety of gene therapy for Wiskott-Aldrich syndrome in preclinical models. *Mol. Ther.* **17:** 1073–1082.

217. Bosticardo, M. *et al.* 2011. Lentiviral-mediated gene therapy leads to improvement of B-cell functionality in a murine model of Wiskott-Aldrich syndrome. *J. Allergy Clin. Immunol.* **127:** 1376–1384 e1375.

218. Catucci, M. *et al.* 2012. Dendritic cell functional improvement in a preclinical model of lentiviral-mediated gene therapy for Wiskott-Aldrich syndrome. *Gene Ther.* **19:** 1150–1158.

219. Astrakhan, A. *et al.* 2012. Ubiquitous high-level gene expression in hematopoietic lineages provides effective lentiviral gene therapy of murine Wiskott-Aldrich syndrome. *Blood* **119:** 4395–4407.

Ann. N.Y. Acad. Sci. ISSN 0077-8923

ANNALS OF THE NEW YORK ACADEMY OF SCIENCES

Issue: *The Year in Immunology*

Anti-β₂-glycoprotein I antibodies

Rohan Willis[1,2] and Silvia S. Pierangeli[1]

[1]Antiphospholipid Standardization Laboratory, Division of Rheumatology, Department of Internal Medicine, University of Texas Medical Branch, Galveston, Texas. [2]Department of Microbiology, University of the West Indies, Kingston, Jamaica

Address for correspondence: Silvia S. Pierangeli, APLS Laboratory, Brackenridge Hall 2.108, 301 University Boulevard, Galveston, TX 77555-003. sspieran@utmb.edu.

Anti-β_2-glycoprotein I (anti-β_2GPI) antibodies are the main antiphospholipid antibodies, along with anticardiolipin and lupus anticoagulant, that characterize the autoimmune disease antiphospholipid syndrome (APS). While the exact physiological functions of β_2GPI are unknown, there is overwhelming evidence that anti-β_2GPI antibodies are pathogenic, contributing to thrombosis, pregnancy morbidity, and accelerated atherosclerosis in APS and systemic lupus erythematosus patients. The revelation that these antibodies play a central role in the pathogenesis and pathophysiology of APS has driven research to characterize the physiology and structure of β_2GPI as well as the pathogenic effects of anti-β_2GPI antibodies. It has also resulted in the development of improved testing methodologies for detecting these antibodies. In this review we discuss the characteristics of β_2GPI; the generation, pathogenic effects, and standardized testing of anti-β_2GPI antibodies; and the potential use of therapies that target the β_2GPI/anti-β_2GPI interaction in the treatment of APS.

Keywords: β_2-glycoprotein I; anti-β_2-glycoprotein I antibodies; antiphospholipid antibodies; antiphospholipid syndrome

Introduction

Antiphospholipid syndrome (APS) is an autoimmune multisystem disorder characterized clinically by recurrent thrombosis and pregnancy morbidity, and serologically by the presence of antiphospholipid antibodies (aPLs), including anticardiolipin (aCL) and anti-β_2-glycoprotein I (anti-β_2GPI) antibodies as well as a positive lupus anticoagulant test.[1–3] It is now widely accepted that aPLs are a large group of heterogeneous antibodies that interact with an array of phospholipids (PLs), PL–protein complexes, and PL binding proteins, and that the action of aPLs on these numerous antigenic targets forms the basis of the pathophysiology of APS.[4,5] In spite of this diversity of antibodies, it is now generally accepted that only one class of aPL, those directed against β_2-glycoprotein I (β_2GPI), are largely responsible for the clinical manifestations that characterize the syndrome.[4,5]

The presence of aPLs has been closely related to the development of thrombosis and pregnancy complications in APS. Increased propensity for thrombosis occurs as a result of the activation of platelets, monocytes, and endothelial cells, and also as a consequence of disruptions in natural anticoagulant and fibrinolytic systems mediated by aPLs.[6–8] In addition to thrombosis, abnormal cellular proliferation and differentiation processes underlie the noninflammatory pathogenic role of aPLs in the development of obstetric APS.[9] Inflammation is a central pathogenic factor in APS; it serves as an inciting factor for thrombosis in the presence of the procoagulant phenotype that characterizes the disease. Additionally, inflammation is an alternative mediator of the placental injury typical of aPL-induced obstetric complications.[10]

The discovery, in the 1990s, that β_2GPI was an antigen of central importance in APS was accompanied by the development of assays in an ELISA format to detect antibodies targeting this antigen.[5,11] The standardization of these assays has generated much debate and has been the subject of many international workshops and multinational collaborations, but is still an ongoing process.[12] Refinements in testing methodologies have allowed for the

doi: 10.1111/nyas.12080

Ann. N.Y. Acad. Sci. 1285 (2013) 44–58 © 2013 New York Academy of Sciences.

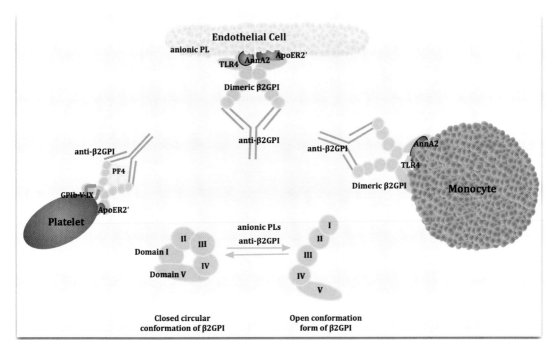

Figure 1. Cell surface interactions of β-2 glycoprotein I. Abbreviations: AnnA2, annexin A2; ApoER2, apolipoprotein endothelial receptor 2; β₂GPI, β-2 glycoprotein I; GPIb-V-IX, glycoprotein Ib-V-IX; PF4, platelet factor 4; TLR4, Toll-like receptor 4.

detection of oxidized or reduced anti-β₂GPI antibodies, antibodies with low and high avidity, as well as those specific for domains I, IV, and V, each apparently having distinct clinical associations.[11–14]

The specific interaction of anti-β₂GPI with domain I of β₂GPI, and that of β₂GPI with exposed PLs and protein receptors on the cell membrane, are important in the pathophysiology of APS.[14,15] The targeted inhibition of these specific β₂GPI interactions has shown promise in preliminary studies for limiting autoantibody-mediated activation of cells and humoral factors.[16] It could potentially provide an effective approach to the management of APS patients with limited side effects. In this review, we discuss the characteristics of β₂GPI; the generation, pathogenic effects, and standardized testing of anti-β₂GPI antibodies; and the potential use of therapies that target the specific interactions of β₂GPI in the treatment of APS.

β₂-Glycoprotein I

β₂-GPI is a 50 kDa PLs–plasma glycoprotein that consists of five homologous complement control protein domains. Domains I–IV each consist of 62 amino acids in the regular, conserved sequence, but domain V is unique in that it also possesses a 6-residue insertion, a 19-residue C-terminal extension, and an additional disulfide bond that includes a C-terminal cysteine.[17–19] The aberrant domain V structure, with a high content of lysine residues, results in the formation of a positively charged region at the bottom side of this domain that determines its affinity for anionic PLs. There is also a flexible hydrophobic loop that gives domain V the ability to insert into lipid membranes.[18,19] Studies have shown that dimerization of β₂GPI increases its affinity for anionic PLs 1000-fold, and the importance of the bivalent interactions of β₂GPI with anionic PLs in inducing thrombosis in hamsters.[20,21] β₂GPI interacts with the cell surface receptors of diverse cell types, including endothelial cells, monocytes, platelets, trophoblasts, and decidual cells, as well as coagulation factors with important consequences related to the pathophysiology of APS (Fig. 1).[22]

Plasma levels of β₂GPI range from 50 to 500 μg/mL and are reduced in patients with acute cerebrovascular accidents, myocardial infarctions, and pregnant women, while levels increase with age and in patients with APS.[23,24] The crystal structure of β_2GPI was solved at the end of the 1990s and revealed a hockey stick–like arrangement, with domains I–IV stretched and domain V at a right angle to the other domains.[19,25] This structure predicts that β_2GPI could bind to lipid membranes via domain V, with domains I to IV pointing away from the membrane with exposed epitopes for binding to anti-β_2GPI antibodies.[26] Interestingly, a potential binding site for autoantibodies reacting to β_2GPI has been located on domain I of the β_2GPI molecule.[14] Results of X-ray scattering studies and electron microscopy have suggested that β_2GPI exists in closed and open conformations *in vivo*, and that interaction of the molecule with its environment determines its conformational structure at any given time.[27] This is intriguing since, in the closed-loop conformation, the epitope recognized by anti-β_2GPI antibodies is hidden, while this binding site becomes exposed in the open hockey stick–like conformation.[27,28] It has been postulated that β_2GPI exists in the closed-loop conformation in plasma but adopts the hockey stick–like open conformation once it binds to anionic PLs, exposing cryptic epitopes in domain I and allowing for anti-β_2GPI binding.[28]

The function of β_2GPI is still unknown, and neither humans nor mice deficient in this protein exhibit any clear abnormalities in hemostasis or pregnancy.[29] Ten years after the first description of β_2GPI null mice, no additional information on the phenotypic manifestations that occur as a consequence of the genetic abnormality seen in these mice have been published, and we can therefore only guess at the unique physiological role for β_2GPI. However, *in vitro* studies have demonstrated a putative role for β_2GPI in the regulation of hemostasis, since it can inhibit adenosine diphosphate (ADP)-induced platelet aggregation and regulate contact activation, which is important in the intrinsic coagulation pathway.[30] Recent evidence has suggested that β_2GPI may function as a particularly efficient lipopolysaccharide (LPS) scavenger protein, working in concert with phagocytes, such as monocytes, to clear LPS from the circulation.[31]

How are anti-β₂-glycoprotein antibodies generated in APS?

The processes underlying the production of aPLs in APS patients remain undetermined. When these antibodies were first described, aPLs were defined as antibodies reacting to cardiolipin; however, it is now well accepted that the majority of pathogenic antibodies in APS patients recognize various proteins that interact with PLs, the most important being β_2GPI.[4,5] Indeed, efforts to induce high-titer production of pathogenic aPLs in animal models succeeded only after immunization with heterologous β_2GPI rather than pure PLs.[32] This led researchers to believe that perhaps *in vivo* binding of foreign PL-binding proteins resembling β_2GPI to self PLs in APS patients may lead to the formation of immunogenic complexes against which aPLs are produced.

Infections, molecular mimicry, and anti-β₂-glycoprotein I antibodies

Many infections may be accompanied by aPL elevations (particularly aCL antibodies) and, in some instances, these elevations may be accompanied by clinical manifestations of APS (Table 1). Several reviews on the association of aPLs with infections have been published and highlight the prevalence of aPLs in the presence of certain viral, bacterial, and even parasitic infections. These include organisms, such as cytomegalovirus, parvovirus B19, human immunodeficiency virus (HIV), hepatitis B and C (HCV) viruses, human T cell lymphoma/leukemia virus, varicella zoster virus, and *Mycobacterium leprae*, among others.[33,34] Antiphospholipid antibodies have been associated with skin infections (18%), HIV infection (17%), pneumonia (14%), HCV infections (13%), and urinary tract infections.[33–35]

Following the discovery that a synthesized 15 amino acid peptide, GDKV, which spanned an area of the fifth domain of β_2GPI known to be a major PL-binding site of the molecule, could induce pathogenic anti-β_2GPI production in mice, candidate peptides from microorganisms with functional and sequence similarity to that of the PL-binding site of β_2GPI were found (Fig. 2).[36,37] The peptides TIFI and VITT from cytomegalovirus (CMV), TADL from adenovirus (AdV), and SGDF from *Bacillus subtilis*, all had greater degrees of PL-binding compared to GDKV and induced high titer aPL and anti-β_2GPI production in mice. Subsequent *in vivo* and *in vitro* experiments confirmed the pathogenicity of antibodies induced in TIFI-immunized mice.[38–40]

Further supporting evidence for molecular mimicry as a possible mechanism for APS development was provided by a study evaluating the

Table 1. Proposed mechanisms for the involvement of infectious agents in the pathogenesis of the antiphospholipid syndrome

Proposed mechanisms	Evidence
Foreign PL-binding structures similar to β_2GPI bind to self PLs to induce autoantibody production	• Pathogenic aPLs induced in mice immunized with heterologous β_2GPI or GDKV peptide (found in PL-binding domain of β_2GPI) but NOT in mice immunized with pure PLs
Foreign triggering antigens may be found on infectious agents	• Peptides TIFI and VITT (CMV), TADL (adenovirus), and SGDF (*Bacillus subtillis*) structurally similar to GDKV and induce pathogenic aPL able to induce thrombosis in murine models
	• Immunization of mice with several preparations of infectious agents (with peptide TLRVYK) induced pathogenic anti-β_2GPI antibodies able to induce fetal loss in naive mice
Infectious agents/inflammation may induce conformational changes in antigens exposing hidden epitopes to enable autoantibody production	• Protein H of *Streptococcus pyogenes* induces conformational changes in β_2GPI and anti-β_2GPI production
	• Oxidation of β_2GPI (by various oxidative and nitrosative reactive species) results in its increased immunogenicity utilizing Th1 cells
TLR4—role in inducing break in tolerance to β_2GPI and epitope spread to other autoantigens	• Mice immunized with pathogen-derived TLR ligand (LPS—ligand for TLR4) and β_2GPI produce high levels of aPL and develop other SLE-associated autoantibodies
TLR7 and 9—role in autoantibody production	• Lupus-prone TLR7- and/or TLR9-deficient mice unable to produce pathogenic anti-β_2GPI compared to normal counterparts

APS-related pathogenic potential of microorganisms carrying sequences related to a hexapeptide, TLRVYK, known to be specifically recognized by a pathogenic monoclonal anti-β_2GPI.[41] Following immunization with *Haemophilus influenzae, Neisseria gonorrhoeae,* or tetanus toxoid, high affinity antipeptide (TLRVYK) and anti-β_2GPI were observed in BALB/c immunized mice. TLRVYK affinity-purified antibodies were then infused into naive mice at day 0 of pregnancy. At day 15, these mice had significant thrombocytopenia, prolonged activated partial thromboplastin times, and increased frequency of fetal loss compared to controls. An additional example was provided by peptide A (NTLK-TPRVGGC), a synthetic peptide that shares structural similarities with common bacterial antigens and regions of β_2GPI, which reversed aPL-mediated thrombosis in mice *in vivo*.[42]

In addition to molecular mimicry, infectious agents can potentially induce production of autoreactive anti-β_2GPI antibodies by acting as adjuvants, that is, selectively activating or destroying unique lymphocyte subsets, directing cytokine/chemokine release, or exposing cryptic autoantigens. Recent evidence has suggested that exposure of cryptic antigens on domain I of β_2GPI due to conformational changes could induce production of anti-β_2GPI antibodies.[43] Subsequently, *in vivo* mouse studies have highlighted the possible role of protein H from *Streptococcus pyogenes* in inducing conformational changes in β_2GPI and enabling anti-β_2GPI antibody production in this capacity.[44] Similarly, lipopolysaccharide (LPS) can induce conformational changes in β_2GPI and potentially contribute to the development of anti-β_2GPI antibodies.[31] Studies have highlighted the central part played by TLR4, the cell surface receptor that binds LPS, in inducing a break in tolerance and subsequent aPL production with epitope spread to several autoantigens.[45] Quite recently, our group demonstrated for the first time that both TLR7 and TLR9 are involved in pathogenic aPL production by utilizing lupus-prone mice treated with CMV-derived peptides in the presence of TLR7 or TLR9 agonists, and other lupus-prone mice deficient in TLR7, or both TLR7 and TLR9.[46]

In addition to exposing hidden epitopes of β_2GPI, infections could increase the immunogenicity of this glycoprotein by altering its redox potential. It has

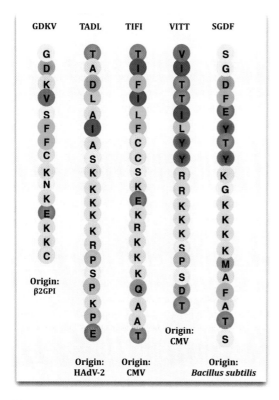

Figure 2. Candidate peptides found in various microorganisms with structural similarity to β-2 glycoprotein I. Abbreviations: β₂GPI, β-2 glycoprotein I; CMV, cytomegalovirus; HAdV-2, adenovirus.

been shown that the majority of circulating β₂GPI exists in a reduced form containing unpaired cysteines (free thiols), which interact with platelets and endothelial cells, serving as an antioxidant reservoir protecting cells or critical molecules from oxidative stress.[47] Oxidation of β₂GPI has been shown to confer an increase in its immunogenicity through a Th1 immunological mechanism.[48] It is possible that the generation of reactive oxidative and nitrosative species by certain infectious agents could allow for generation of an abundance of oxidized β₂GPI and foster autoantibody production. Indeed, serum from patients with APS assessed by a novel ELISA assay have a significant increase in oxidized β₂GPI.[48]

Are anti-β₂-glycoprotein I antibodies pathogenic?

There is strong evidence indicating that aPL antibodies and, more specifically, anti-β₂GPI antibodies enhance thrombus formation in animal models.

First, Pierangeli *et al.* have shown that human and murine monoclonal and polyclonal aPL antibodies with specificity for β₂GPI enhance thrombus formation in a mouse model of induced thrombosis.[49] This effect was abrogated when the immunoglobulin preparations were depleted of their anti-β₂GPI activity. In addition, Jankowski *et al.* and Fischetti *et al.* showed thrombogenic effects of monoclonal and polyclonal anti-β₂GPI antibodies in induced thrombosis models in hamsters and rats.[21,50] In a recent publication, Ramesh *et al.* confirmed the thrombogenicity of polyclonal aPL preparations in mice utilizing a model in which the thrombogenic injury is induced with ferric chloride.[51] Similarly, Arad *et al.* confirmed the thrombogenic effects of affinity purified anti-β₂GPI antibodies in a dose-dependent manner in mice, utilizing an *in vivo* model of induced thrombosis in which thrombus formation was induced with a micropoint laser system.[52] Hence, several groups of investigators have examined the causal relationship that likely exists between anti-β₂GPI auto-antibodies and thromboembolic complications. However, the mechanism by which anti-β₂GPI antibodies induce an increased risk of thrombosis and fetal loss is not completely understood. Further human studies are also needed to provide direct evidence for the role that aPLs play in causing thrombosis in APS patients.

How do anti-β₂-glycoprotein I antibodies exert their pathogenic effects on target cells?

Patients with APS can present with widely divergent clinical features, since, in addition to the classical thrombotic and obstetric manifestations, these patients can develop thrombocytopenia, chorea, livedo reticularis, and heart valve abnormalities.[3] These manifestations are not included in the classical definition of the syndrome, but these features are frequently observed in patients with APS. A thrombotic cause for most of these additional manifestations seems unlikely, because treatment of the thrombotic complications rarely results in the disappearance of these phenomena.[9,52] The simultaneous presence of thrombotic and nonthrombotic clinical manifestations in patients with APS suggests that anti-β₂GPI antibodies do not simply interfere with mechanisms affecting hemostasis, but also with unique biological pathways affecting several organ systems.

As is indicated by their name, aPL antibodies were originally thought to be directed against anionic PLs. From this perspective, it was logical to study the interaction of β_2GPI with cellular membranes and cells. Numerous *in vitro* and *in vivo* experiments have demonstrated that β_2GPI, in complex with specific antibodies, can bind to and activate myriad cells involved in maintaining hemostasis, including endothelial cells,[53] monocytes,[54] and platelets.[55] Intracellular signaling that originates from the interaction of extracellular moieties with membrane components is mediated by protein receptors embedded in the membrane rather than membrane PLs themselves. Several receptors have thus far been identified as mediators in β_2GPI-induced cell activation, including TLR2,[56] TLR4,[57] TLR8,[58] annexin A2,[59] glycoprotein Ib,[60] and a member of the LDL-receptor family, LRP8 (ApoER2),[61] and the idea of a multiprotein receptor complex has recently been proposed.[62]

Endothelial cell activation

It has been firmly established that aPL antibodies activate endothelial cells and induce a proinflammatory and procoagulant endothelial phenotype. However, the mechanism through which endothelial cells are activated by these antibodies is much less clear. There are reports that indicate involvement of TLR2, TLR4, annexin A2, and more recently, LRP8.[53,56–59,61] Several studies on endothelial cell activation report the activation of a signal transduction pathway, but the reported signaling events, for example, NFκB and p38MAPK activation,[63,64] are usually too far downstream to be specific to one receptor. A role of aPLs in tissue factor (TF) upregulation and expression has been confirmed by many investigators in endothelial cells, in monocytes *in vitro* and *in vivo*.[54,65] Nevertheless, there are data that show activation of the general TLR signaling pathway in endothelial cells upon activation with aPL antibodies, with downstream activation of TRAF6 and myeloid differentiation factor 88 (MyD88).[57]

More compelling evidence comes from studies that used specific receptor blockade,[59] knockdown with interfering RNA,[62] or receptor-deficient endothelial cell lines.[57] Raschi *et al.* demonstrated that the MyD88 signaling cascade (an adaptor molecule for TLR4 that transduces TLR-mediated intracellular signaling terminating in the translocation

of NF-κB, phosphorylation of p38MAPK, or upregulation of pro-inflammatory cytokines) is triggered by anti-β_2GPI on human endothelial cells *in vitro*.[57] In order to evaluate the role of TLR4 in aPL-mediated endothelial cell activation and thrombosis *in vivo*, Pierangeli *et al.* carried out experiments in LPS-nonresponsive $(^{-/-})$ and LPS-responsive $(^{+/+})$ mice. LPS$^{-/-}$ mice display a point mutation of the *Tlr4* gene leading to the expression of a TLR4 that does not recognize LPS.[66] IgG-aPL isolated from two APS patients produced significantly larger thrombi and induced higher TF activity in carotid artery homogenates and increased adherence of leukocytes (WBC) to endothelial cells in the microcirculation of the cremaster muscle of LPS$^{+/+}$ mice when compared to control IgG-normal human serum (NHS) (as an indication of endothelial cell activation). These effects were abrogated after removal of the anti-β_2GPI activity from the IgG-aPL preparations.[66] The two IgG-aPLs induced significantly smaller thrombus sizes, lower numbers of WBC adhering to endothelial cells and decreased TF activity in LPS$^{-/-}$ compared to LPS$^{+/+}$ mice.[66] Altogether, the group demonstrated involvement of TLR4 in aPL-mediated *in vivo* pathogenic effects in mice.

In additional unpublished studies, a TLR4 ligand antagonist inhibited the binding of anti-β_2GPI and the upregulation of intercellular adhesion molecule (ICAM)-1 in human decidual and endothelial cells (Pierangeli *et al.* unpublished data). In another set of experiments,[67] cultured human umbilical vein endothelial cells (HUVEC) were treated with IgG-aPL (200 μg/mL), IgG-aPL plus 1 mg/mL anti-TLR4, IgG-normal human serum (IgG-NHS), or culture medium for four hours. TF activity was determined in lysates of the cells. In HUVEC, IgG-aPL induced a significant upregulation of TF activity when compared to cells treated with IgG-NHS (180.8 pM/mg/mL vs. 69.8 pM/mg/mL, respectively). The treatment with anti-TLR4 decreased that activity by 38% (112.0 pM/mg/mL). In another set of experiments, cultured HUVEC were treated with 200 μg/mL IgG-APS or IgG-NHS in the presence or absence of 1 μg/mL TLR4 ligand antagonist or 4 μg/mL anti-TLR4 antibody, for four hours. ICAM-1 and E-selectin expression were determined by cyto-ELISA. The data showed significant inhibition of aPL-induced ICAM-1 expression by the TLR-4 antagonist (30%) and the anti-TLR4 antibody (39%). Similarly, E-selectin expression was inhibited by 23% and 42%. β_2GPI has been shown to bind to trophoblasts and induce human chorionic gonadotrophin hormone (hCG) production. These effects were abrogated by a TLR4 inhibitor.[67]

A role has been proposed for annexin A2, a receptor for tissue plasminogen activator, in endothelial cell activation induced by aPL antibodies. In addition, aPL-mediated pathogenic effects are partially but significantly ameliorated in annexin A2–deficient mice and diminished *in vitro* and *in vivo* by an anti-annexin A2 antibody, confirming the importance of annexin A2 in aPL-mediated thrombosis.[59] Since this PLs binding protein lacks a transmembrane domain, it is unlikely that it conveys activation signals across the plasma membrane by itself. It could, however, function as a docking site for β_2GPI on endothelial cells, as part of a multiprotein receptor signaling complex with TLR4.[62] Zhang *et al.* identified a protein of 83 kD that appeared to be TLR4 among those that bound to immobilized β_2GPI by affinity-purification in Affi-Gel HZ columns followed by elution, SDS-PAGE, and LC-MS analysis.[62] In addition, Sorice *et al.* confirmed the involvement of TLR4 and annexin A2 as a receptor for anti-β_2GPI in monocyte cell surface lipid rafts.[68]

Other molecules such as the apolipoprotein E receptor 2 (ApoER2) also might act as receptors for β_2GPI on various cells. ApoER2 is a member of the low-density lipoprotein (LDL) receptor family and is present on endothelial cells and many other cells in the body.[69] In addition to its function as a scavenger receptor for lipoproteins, ApoER2 induces intracellular signaling. Recently, Romay-Penabad *et al.* showed that ApoER2 plays a role in APS *in vivo*, since ApoER2-deficient mice are protected from aPL-induced thrombophilia and TF upregulation in endothelial cells and monocytes.[61]

Monocyte activation

Monocyte activation in relation to aPL antibodies has been studied extensively, with cytokine production[54] and TF expression[70–72] as the primary indicators of activation. Several members of the Toll-like receptor family, including TLR2, TLR4, and TLR8 have been implicated in monocyte activation, as well as LRP8.[56–58,61] Again, downstream signaling pathways were studied, providing evidence of the involvement of TLRs in mediating the effects

of aPL antibodies.[73] However, none of these studies provide conclusive evidence on the identity of the TLR most likely to be responsible for mediating signals initiated by pathogenic anti-β_2GPI antibodies. Annexin A2 may also serve as a receptor for aPL-mediated signaling in monocytes. Interestingly, knockdown experiments of annexin A2 were performed with a monocytic cell line, providing evidence of involvement of annexin A2 in monocyte activation by aPL antibodies.[74] It remains unclear how a protein that is incapable of transmembrane signaling contributes to cellular activation; however, molecular mechanisms involving transduction of signals through co-receptors with intracellular domains, particularly TLR4,[75] are likely.

Platelet activation

Platelets are key players in arterial thrombosis and, as such, are of interest as mediators of aPL antibody–induced thrombosis. Platelet activation by aPL antibodies is well documented,[55,71] and great progress was made in recent years in unraveling the mechanisms through which platelets are influenced by aPL antibodies. Two receptors for anti-β_2GPI/β_2GPI complexes were identified on the platelet surface: GPIbα[76] and LRP8.[77] Because platelets are anucleate cell fragments that cannot be cultured *in vitro*, they are impossible to modify with recombinant DNA techniques. In platelets, dimers of β_2GPI—which mimic anti-β_2GPI/β_2GPI complexes—bind to apoER2, leading to phosphorylation of p38MAPK, thromboxane production, and cell activation. Van Lummel *et al.* showed that domain V of β_2GPI is involved in both binding of β_2GPI to anionic PL and also in interaction with ApoER2 with subsequent activation of platelets.[78] Lutters *et al.* also demonstrated that when the ApoER2 receptor on platelets is blocked using receptor-associated protein, the anti-β_2GPI/β_2GPI–mediated increase in platelet adhesion to collagen is lost.[77] The ApoER2 was able to coprecipitate with dimerized β_2GPI, providing evidence for a direct interaction between β_2GPI and the receptor. These findings suggest that the ApoER2 is involved in the activation of platelets mediated by aPLs. The role of GPIbα in aPL-mediated platelet activation was shown with well-characterized antibodies against ligand-binding domains of this receptor. Further evidence of the involvement of both receptors was provided with the delineation of the initial signaling events upon stimulation of platelets with β_2GPI/anti-β_2GPI antibody complexes.[60,76]

Platelet factor-4 (PF4) is a member of the CXC chemokine family and is secreted by activated platelets but also has the ability to bind to the platelet surface. PF4 has also been shown to have a procoagulant and prothrombotic effect.[79] Sikara *et al.* showed that β_2GPI forms stable complexes with PF4, leading to the stabilization of the dimeric β_2GPI structure, facilitating the recognition of anti-β_2GPI antibodies. The authors demonstrated that the interaction of PF4, anti-β_2GPI/β_2GPI complexes, and platelets leads to the phosphorylation of p38MAPK and the production of thromboxane A2.[79]

The role of cell surface signaling in determining clinical outcomes

Interestingly, functional or absolute deficiencies of most of these proposed receptors in mouse models of APS lead to decreased thrombus formation, suggesting that all these receptors are involved in the development of the various clinical manifestations that characterize the syndrome. However, the extent to which any of these receptors contribute individually or collectively to the pathogenesis of APS *in vivo* is unknown. The myriad cell surface receptors that bind β_2GPI in different tissues allow for selective signaling through different receptors that could potentially result in distinct clinical sequelae.[80,81] Furthermore, there is some presumptive evidence that functional or structural differences in anti-β_2GPI antibodies could determine the intracellular signaling cascades that are activated, quite possibly by selective signaling through the different cell surface receptors for β_2GPI, and could therefore determine clinical phenotypes. For example, Giles *et al.* showed that purified IgG from APS patients with thrombosis alone but no pregnancy morbidity caused TLR4-mediated phosphorylation of NF-κB and p38MAPK, and upregulation of TF activity in monocytes, while IgG from APS patients with pregnancy morbidity alone, aPL-positive patients without APS, or healthy controls, did not.[82] Further affinity purification of the IgG from these patients confirmed that these effects were specific to the anti-β_2GPI subfraction. Similar experiments utilizing trophoblast cells showed that IgG from patients with a history of pregnancy morbidity alone significantly increased the release of sEndoglin, whereas

aPLs from patients with a thrombotic history increased trophoblast sFlt-1 production.[83]

An important clue toward the elucidation of the mechanisms of action of aPL antibodies lies in the observation that anti-β_2GPI/β_2GPI complexes have an increased affinity for cellular surfaces compared to unbound β_2GPI.[28] The interaction of β_2GPI with many different cell types is well documented and it is attractive to speculate that anti-β_2GPI/β_2GPI complexes could function as general cellular activators. The universal cell-triggering activity of anti-β_2GPI antibodies could very well be the basis of the clinical manifestations in APS. As stated before, β_2GPI can exist in two different conformations, a circular conformation in solution and an open hockey stick–like conformation after interaction with anti-β_2GPI or anionic PLs.[19,25,26] The conformational change in β_2GPI induced by anti-β_2GPI antibodies likely results in the exposure of a pattern recognition site that increases the binding potential of β_2GPI to cell surface protein receptors. In this respect, it is of interest that TLRs, GPIbα, and LRP8 are all multiligand receptors that recognize structurally and functionally dissimilar ligands. Although this might explain why β_2GPI/anti-β_2GPI antibody complexes can interact with many different receptors, it does not help to identify the importance of the different receptors in the pathophysiology of APS. This question will need to be addressed in future studies.

The role of β_2GPI and anti-β_2GPI in accelerated atherosclerosis in APS

A number of studies have indicated that aPLs trigger an inflammatory cascade[31,32] and are associated with atherosclerosis (AT), as well as cerebrovascular and peripheral arterial diseases.[84,85] Recent studies have shown that nontraditional risk factors are involved in APS-associated atherogenesis. For example, aPLs may crossreact with oxidized low-density lipoprotein (ox-LDL), and both aPL and anti-oxLDL antibodies have been implicated in the pathogenesis of atherosclerosis associated with SLE and APS (Fig. 3). It has been shown that aPLs, in particular anti-β_2GPI antibodies, can accelerate the influx of oxLDL into macrophages, a major step in the development of atheromatous plaques.[86] Other autoantibodies, such as anti-high-density lipoprotein (anti-HDL) and anti-apolipoprotein A-I, have also been detected in APS. The β_2GPI cofactor has

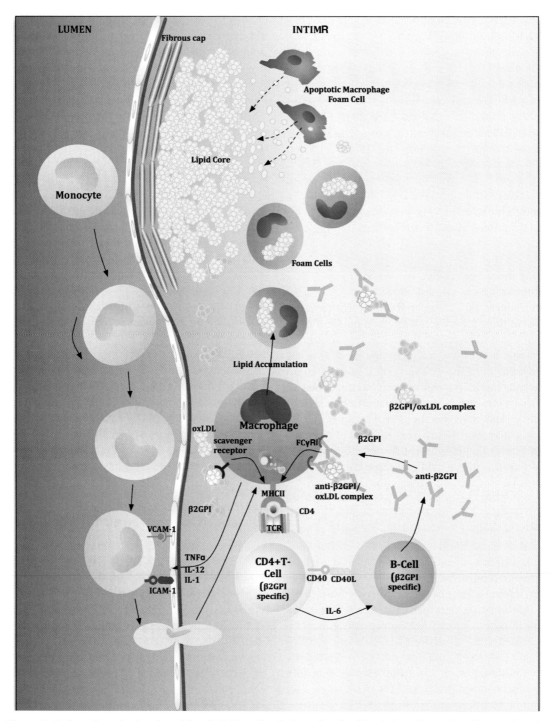

Figure 3. Pathogenic mechanisms in antiphospholipid-mediated atherosclerosis. Abbreviations: β_2GPI, β-2 glycoprotein I; CD, cluster of differentiation molecule; FcγR1, Fc gamma receptor; MHCII, major-histocompatibility complex II; oxLDL, oxidized low-density lipoprotein; ICAM-1, intercellular adhesion molecule-1; IL, interleukin; TCR, T cell receptor; TNF-α, tumor necrosis factor α; VCAM-1, vascular cell adhesion molecule-1.

been further detected in the wall of large arteries in the vicinity of CD4$^+$ T cell infiltrates. This supports the assumption that β_2GPI may serve as a target for an autoimmune reaction that could promote lesion progression.[87] In addition, macrophages and endothelial cells bind to β_2GPI during the atherosclerotic process. In this regard, aCL antibodies can induce monocyte adherence to endothelial cells, which is mediated by adhesion molecules such as ICAM-1, vascular cell adhesion molecule-1 (VCAM-1), and E-selectin. Thus, aCL might promote AT by attracting monocytes into the vessel wall. Moreover, various studies have shown a correlation between serum levels of aCL and anti-β2GPI antibodies and the incidence and severity of acute coronary syndrome, myocardial infarction (MI), and stroke.[88–90] These phenomena are the most pronounced in lupus-associated APS, where traditional and nontraditional risk factors are multiplied and AT occurs prematurely. Regarding clinical and diagnostic aspects of APS-associated atherosclerosis, early endothelial dysfunction and increased carotid intima–media thickness (cIMT) have been observed in APS.[91] Endothelial dysfunction, oxidative stress, increase in cell adhesion molecules, and platelet activation are common findings in both diseases. In addition, macrophages, dendritic cells, T cell activation, and CD40–CD40 ligand interaction are pathogenic mechanisms that occur in both AT and APS.[90,92]

Oxidative stress is an important component in the development of atherosclerosis, and evidence of enhanced oxidative stress exists in APS. In a nonlupus murine model, it was recently evaluated whether aCLs could affect oxidant/antioxidant balance as an early biochemical step of APS.[93] That study demonstrated that aCLs are associated with the decreased paraoxonase (PON) activity and reduced nitric oxide (NO) that may occur in the preclinical phase of APS. Afterward, Simoncini et al. investigated the role of reactive oxygen species (ROS) in the pro-adhesive state elicited by aPLs and studied ROS-dependent downstream signaling pathways.[94] They also demonstrated that ROS controlled the upregulation of VCAM-1 expression by aPL-IgG–stimulated HUVEC and the increase in THP-1 monocytic cells adhesion. Taken together, this study indicated that the oxidative stress induced by aPL-IgG is a key intracellular event that might contribute to the thrombotic complications of APS by controlling the endothelial adhesive phenotype.

More recently, López-Pedrera et al. investigated mitochondrial membrane integrity and various parameters of oxidative stress and antioxidant status in peripheral leukocytes from patients with APS, as well as their association with the procoagulant state characteristic of these patients.[95] Cellular oxidative stress, in terms of peroxides and anion superoxide production, was found to be notably increased in monocytes and neutrophils of APS patients versus healthy donors. A significantly higher percentage of circulating monocytes and neutrophils of APS patients contained depolarized mitochondria. Furthermore, mitochondrial membrane potential and peroxide levels showed significant negative and positive correlations, respectively, with monocyte cell surface TF expression levels. These data suggested that the redox-sensitive pathway and mitochondrial membrane alterations might play central roles in the elicitation of thrombotic events in APS. In summary, the induction of oxidative stress by aPL-IgG represents a new pathway potentially contributing to the thrombotic complications in APS.

Assays for the detection of anti-β_2GPI antibodies

The anti-β_2GPI assay was originally developed in an ELISA format and has been available since the 1990s.[11,12] Despite considerable efforts to standardize testing for anti-β_2GPI antibodies, there are still discrepancies among investigators with respect to the type of plate used, source, and purity of the β_2GPI antigen, concentration of β_2GPI used to coat the plates, and the ideal orientation of the β_2GPI on the plate surface.[96] Agreement of test results between different laboratories and assays still remains suboptimal, due largely to the variations in these assay components.[12,97] Of particular concern is the lack of any consensus with respect to units of measurement for anti-β_2GPI. These concerns have led to the development of an international task force, and subsequently, the publishing of a consensus paper outlining guidelines and recommendations for the standardized testing of aPLs, including anti-β_2GPI antibodies.[98] Currently, there is also an international collaborative effort to establish standardized units for the testing of anti-β_2GPI antibodies.

Subsequent modifications have been made to anti-β_2GPI assays in an attempt to improve their clinical relevance, and one such modification is the determination of antibodies that have specific reactivity against domain I of β_2GPI. As stated before, domain I of the β_2GPI molecule contains the primary epitope for aPL antibodies, and this is supported by several studies.[14,99,100] Two large studies, including a double-blinded multicenter study, have been conducted to investigate the clinical significance of the detection of antidomain I antibodies and have confirmed that the presence of these antibodies are more strongly associated with thrombosis, predominantly venous, and pregnancy morbidity compared with anti-β_2GPI antibodies with reactivity against other domains.[15,101] However, the causality of antidomain I antibodies has been demonstrated only by the use of animal models, and additional clinical studies are needed.[16] Currently, the antidomain I β_2GPI assay is mainly used in research-based settings, and more prospective and *in vivo* data are needed before the antidomain I assay can be added to international classification criteria. Currently, there are ongoing efforts at several centers worldwide to conduct prospective studies investigating the value of all assays mentioned in the classification criteria for APS.

Abrogating the binding of β₂GPI/anti-β₂GPI to target cells

Variants of β_2GPI lacking domain I (DI) or with point mutations in DI have reduced ability to bind aPLs derived from patients with APS, but the same is not true for changes in the other domains.[99] Anti-β_2GPI binding to DI of β_2GPI, and subsequent binding of anti-β_2GPI/β_2GPI complexes to endothelial cells, monocytes, or platelets, triggers activation.[14,15] Hence, blocking anti-β_2GPI binding to β_2GPI or β_2GPI binding to target cells may be the most specific approach to ameliorate their pathogenic effects without interrupting any important physiologic mechanism. Ioannou *et al.* have developed the first (and, so far, the only) system for expressing DI in bacterial periplasm; the investigators used this system to create a series of site-directed mutations in DI, which showed that two distinct areas of DI are important in binding IgG-aPLs extracted from the blood of APS patients.[99,102] These regions were aspartic acid residues at positions 8 and 9 (D8–D9) and the region between arginines at 39 and 43 (R39–R43).[101] In particular, they found that the variant in which D8 and D9 were mutated to serine and glycine, respectively (D8S, D9G), bound more strongly than wild-type

DI to all eight human aPL samples tested. In a recent study, Ioannou *et al.* also showed that soluble recombinant domain I of β_2GPI abrogates, in a dose-dependent fashion, the *in vitro* and *in vivo* effects of anti-β_2GPI.[16] Both DI and DI (D8S,D9G) inhibited this aPL-induced enhancement of thrombosis in a dose-dependent manner, and DI (D8S,D9G) was a more potent inhibitor than DI, underscoring the possibility of utilizing decoy peptides that are part of β_2GPI to abrogate the binding of pathogenic aPLs to target cells in the treatment of APS patients.[16] Human studies are needed to establish the safety and efficacy of such treatment.

On the other hand, Ostertag *et al.* demonstrated that a 20 amino acid peptide (TIFI) mimics the PLs-binding region in domain V of β_2GPI and significantly decreases thrombus size in IgG-aPL–injected mice by displacing the binding of β_2GPI to target cells. TIFI also inhibited, in a dose-dependent fashion, the binding of fluorescinated β2GPI to endothelial cells, murine macrophages, and trophoblasts *in vitro*.[103] Similar experiments have demonstrated TIFI's ability to cause dose-dependent inhibition of aPL binding to trophoblasts *in vitro*.[104] In the same experiment, aPL-induced growth retardation and fetal loss in pregnant C57BL/6 mice was significantly decreased in mice receiving concurrent TIFI treatment.

Hence, based on *in vitro* and animal studies, it is possible that inhibiting the binding of β_2GPI to the putative receptor proteins on target cells and/or the interaction of anti-β_2GPI to β_2GPI may be effective approaches to ameliorate aPL-mediated effects in APS patients. Clinical studies are urgently needed to confirm these findings.

Conclusion

β_2GPI is the antigen of major importance in APS, and given that it is an abundant human glycoprotein conserved during evolution, it is likely to have a major physiological role that has yet to be determined. Recent experimental evidence has given us insight into the molecular mechanisms that dictate aPL formation and aPL-mediated activation of various cells. It is clear that β_2GPI acts as an important cofactor in these processes, but the details remain incompletely understood. The elucidation of the dynamic structural and functional roles played by β_2GPI in normal human physiological processes will no doubt shed light on those events that lead to the formation of autoantibodies reactive to β_2GPI. Hopefully, this will also give us some insight into how and why some anti-β_2GPI antibodies will cause clinical disease and others will not.

The ultimate goal of determining the precise molecular mechanisms involved in aPL-mediated cellular activation is to guide the development of novel therapeutic agents for use in patients with APS. APS was first characterized almost 30 years ago, yet the approach to management of these patients has remained relatively unchanged. Current therapeutic guidelines center on conventional anticoagulation therapy with heparin, low-dose aspirin (LDA), or warfarin, singly or in combination, depending on the clinical scenario.[105] However, some patients are refractory to therapy or experience severe side effects, and primary prophylaxis in asymptomatic patients persistently positive for aPLs remains a controversial issue.[106] However, in spite of the relatively slow pace of implementing novel therapeutic approaches in managing APS patients, the last few years have produced several excellent clinical studies highlighting the efficacy of new immunomodulatory drugs. We have also seen the development of several international collaborative initiatives dedicated to furthering APS research. This will hopefully give us the push toward the production of meaningful therapeutic guidelines implementing novel immunomodulatory therapies for managing APS patients.

Conflicts of interest

The authors declare no conflicts of interest.

References

1. Harris, E.N. 1987. Syndrome of the black swan. *Br. J. Rheumatol.* **26:** 324–326.
2. Wilson, W.A., A.E. Ghavari, T. Koike, *et al.* 1999. International concensus statement on preliminary classification criteria for definite antiphospholipid syndrome: report of an international workshop. *Arth. Rheum.* **42:** 1309–1311.
3. Miyakis, S., M.D. lockshin, I. Atsumi, *et al.* 2006. International concensus statement on an update of the classification criteria for definite antiphospholipid syndrome (APS). *J. Thromb. Haemost.* **4:** 295–306.
4. McNeil, H.P., R.J. Simpson, C.N. Cherterman, *et al.* 1990. Antiphospholipid antibodies are directed against a complex antigen that includes lipid binding inhibitor of coagulation: β2 glycoprotein I (apolipoprotein H). *Proc. Natl. Acad. Sci. USA* **87:** 4120–4124.
5. Galli, M., P. Comfurius, C. Maassen, *et al.* 1990. Anticardiolipin antibodies (ACA) directed not to cardiolipin but to a plasma protein cofactor. *Lancet* **335:** 1544–1547.
6. Meroni, P.L., E. Raschi, M. Camera, *et al.* 2000. Endothelial activation by aPL: a potential pathogenetic mechanism for the clinical manifestations of the syndrome. *J. Autoimmun.* **15:** 237–240.
7. Urbanus, R.T., R.H. Derksen, P.G. de Groot. 2008. Platelets and the antiphospholipid syndrome. *Lupus* **17:** 888–894.
8. Krone, K.A., K.L. Allen, K.R. McCrae. 2010. Impaired fibrinolysis in the antiphospholipid syndrome. *Curr. Rheumatol. Rep.* **12:** 53–57.
9. Abrahams, V.M. 2009. Mechanisms of antiphospholipid antibody-associated pregnancy complications. *Thromb. Res.* **124:** 521–525.
10. Ames, P.R., I. Antinolfi, A. Ciampa 2008. Primary antiphospholipid syndrome: a low-grade auto-inflammatory disease? *Rheumatology* **47:** 1832–1837.
11. Reber, G., A. Tincani, M. Sanmarco, *et al.* 2004. Proposals for the measurement of anti-β2-glycoprotein I antibodies. Standardization Group of the European Forum on Antiphospholipid Antibodies. *J. Thromb. Haemost.* **2:** 1860–1862.
12. Lakos, G., E.J. Favaloro, E.N. Harris, *et al.* 2012. International consensus guidelines on anticardiolipin and anti-β(2)-glycoprotein I testing: report from the 13th International Congress on Antiphospholipid Antibodies. *Arth. Rheum.* **64:** 1–10.
13. Čučnik, S., T. Kveder, A. Artenjak, *et al.* 2012. Avidity of anti-β2-glycoprotein I antibodies in patients with antiphospholipid syndrome. *Lupus* **21:** 764–765.
14. Iverson, G.M., E.J. Victoria, D.M. Marquis. 1998. Anti-beta2 glycoprotein I (beta2GPI) autoantibodies recognize an epitope on the first domain of beta2GPI. *Proc. Natl. Acad. Sci. USA* **95:** 15542–15546.
15. de Laat, B., V. Pengo, I. Pabinger, *et al.* 2009. The association between circulating antibodies against domain I of beta2-glycoprotein I and thrombosis: an international multicenter study. *J. Thromb. Haemost.* **7:** 1767–1773.
16. Ioannou, Y., Z. Romay-Penabad, C. Pericleous, *et al.* 2009. In vivo inhibition of antiphospholipid antibody-induced pathogenicity utilizing the antigenic target peptide domain I of beta2-glycoprotein I: proof of concept. *J. Thromb. Haemost.* **7:** 833–842.
17. Lozier, J., N. Takahashi, F.W. Putman. 1991. Complete amino acid sequence of human plasma β2-glycoprotein I. Molecular cloning and mammalian expression of human beta 2 glycoprotein I cDNA. *Proc. Natl. Acad. Sci. USA* **81:** 3640–3644.
18. Kristensen, T., I. Schousboe, E. Boel, *et al.* 1991. Molecular cloning and mammalian expression of human beta 2-glycoprotein I cDNA. *FEBS Lett.* **289:** 183–186.
19. Bouma, B., P.G. de Groot, J.M.H. van der Elsen, *et al.* 1999. Adhesion mechanism of human β2-glycoprotein I to phospholipids based on its crystal structure. *EMBO J.* **18:** 5166–5174.
20. Sheng, Y., D.A. Kandiah, S.A. Krilis. 1998. Anti-beta 2-glycoprotein I autoantibodies from patients with the "antiphospholipid" syndrome bind to beta 2-glycoprotein I with low affinity: dimerization of beta 2-glycoprotein I induces a significant increase in anti-beta 2-glycoprotein I antibody affinity. *J. Immunol.* **161:** 2038–2043.

21. Jankowski, M., I. Vreys, C. Wittevrongel, *et al.* 2003. Thrombogenicity of beta 2-glycoprotein I-dependent antiphospholipid antibodies in a photochemically induced thrombosis model in the hamster. *Blood* **101:** 157–162.

22. Willis, R., E.N. Harris, S.S. Pierangeli. 2012. Pathogenesis of the antiphospholipid syndrome. *Semin. Thromb. Hemost.* **38:** 305–321.

23. Rioche, M., R. Masseyeff. 1974. Synthesis of plasma beta 2 glycoprotein I by human hepatoma cells in tissue culture. *Biomedicine* **21:** 420–423.

24. Lin, F., R. Murphy, B. White, *et al.* 2006. Circulating levels of β2-glycoprotein I in thrombotic disorders and in inflammation. *Lupus* **15:** 87–93.

25. Schwartzenbacher, R., K. Zeth, K. Diederichs, *et al.* 1999. Crystal structure of human β2-glycoprotein I: implications for phospholipid binding and the antiphospholipid syndrome. *EMBO J.* **18:** 6228–6231.

26. de Laat, B., R.H.W.M. Derksen, *et al.* 2006. Pathogenic anti-β2-glycoprotein I antibodies recognize domain I of β2-glycoprotein I only after a conformational change. *Blood* **107:** 1916–1924.

27. Agar, C., G.M. van Os, M. Morgelin, *et al.* 2010. Beta2-Glycoprotein I can exist in two conformations: implications for ourunderstanding of the antiphospholipid syndrome. *Blood* **116:** 1336–1343.

28. Pennings, M.T.T., M. van Lummel, R.H.W.M. Derksen, *et al.* 2006. Interaction of β2-glycoprotein I with members of the low density lipoprotein receptor family. *J. Thromb. Haemost.* **4:** 1680–1690.

29. Haupt, H., H.G. Schwick, K. Storiko. 1968. On a hereditary beta-2-glycoprotein I deficiency. *Humangenetik* **5:** 291–293.

30. Schousboe, I., I. Beta 2-Glycoprotein. 1985. A plasma inhibitor of the contact activation of the intrinsic blood coagulation pathway. *Blood* **66:** 1086–1091.

31. Agar, C., P.G. de Groot, M. Morgelin, *et al.* 2011. β2-glycoprotein I: a novel component of innate immunity. *Blood.* **117:** 6939–6947.

32. Gharavi, A.E., L.R. Sammaritano, J. Wen, K.B. Elkon. 1992. Induction of antiphospholipid autoantibodies by immunization with beta 2 glycoprotein I (apolipoprotein H). *J. Clin. Invest.* **90:** 1105–1109.

33. Uthman, I.W., A.E. Gharavi. 2002. Viral infections and antiphospholipid antibodies. *Semin. Arth. Rheum.* 31: 256–263.

34. Sène, D., J.C. Piette, P. Cacoub. 2009. Antiphospholipid antibodies, antiphospholipid syndrome and viral infections. *Rev. Med. Interne.* **30:** 135–141.

35. Cruz-Tapias, P., M. Blank, J.M. Anaya, Y. Shoenfeld. 2012. Infections and vaccines in the etiology of antiphospholipid syndrome. *Curr. Opin. Rheumatol.* **24:** 389–393.

36. Gharavi, A.E., S.S. Pierangeli, M. Colden-Stanfield, *et al.* 1999. GDKV-induced antiphospholipid antibodies enhance thrombosis and activate endothelial cells *in vivo* and *in vitro*. *J. Immunol.* **163:** 2922–2927.

37. Gharavi, A.E., S.S. Pierangeli, E.E. Gharavi, *et al.* 1998. Thrombogenic properties of antiphospholipid antibodies do not depend on their binding to beta2 glycoprotein 1 (beta2GP1) alone. *Lupus* **7:** 341–346.

38. Gharavi, E.E., H. Chaimovich, E. Cucurull, *et al.* 1999. Induction of antiphospholipid antibodies by immunization with synthetic viral and bacterial peptides. *Lupus* **8:** 449–455.

39. Gharavi, A.E., S.S. Pierangeli, R.G. Espinola, *et al.* 2002. Antiphospholipid antibodies induced in mice by immunization with a cytomegalovirus-derived peptide cause thrombosis and activation of endothelial cells *in vivo*. *Arth. Rheum.* **46:** 545–552.

40. Gharavi, A.E., M. Vega-Ostertag, R.G. Espinola, *et al.* 2004. Intrauterine fetal death in mice caused by cytomegalovirus-derived peptide induced aPL antibodies. *Lupus* **13:** 17–23.

41. Blank, M., I. Krause, M. Fridkin, *et al.* 2002. Bacterial induction of autoantibodies to beta2-glycoprotein-I accounts for the infectious etiology of antiphospholipid syndrome. *J. Clin. Invest.* **109:** 797–804.

42. Pierangeli, S.S., M. Blank, X. Liu, *et al.* 2004. A peptide that shares similarity with bacterial antigens reverses thrombogenic properties of antiphospholipid antibodies *in vivo*. *J. Autoimmun.* **22:** 217–225.

43. de Laat, B., M. van Berkel, R.T. Urbanus, *et al.* 2011. Immune responses against domain I of β(2)-glycoprotein I are driven by conformational changes: domain I of β(2)-glycoprotein I harbors a cryptic immunogenic epitope. *Arth. Rheum.* **63:** 3960–3968.

44. Van Os, G.M., J.C. Meijers, C. Agar, *et al.* 2011. Induction of anti-β(2)-glycoprotein I autoantibodies in mice by protein H of Streptococcus pyogenes. *J. Thromb. Haemost.* **9:** 2447–2456.

45. Rauch, J., M. Dieudé, R. Subang, J.S. Levine. 2010. The dual role of innate immunity in the antiphospholipid syndrome. *Lupus* **19:** 347–353.

46. Aguilar-Valenzuela, R., K. Nickerson, Z. Romay-Penabad, *et al.* 2011. Involvement of TLR7 and TLR9 in the production of antiphospholipid antibodies. *Arth. Rheum.* **63:** s281 (abstract 723).

47. Ioannou, Y., J.Y. Zhang, F.H. Passam, *et al.* 2010. Naturally occurring free thiols within beta 2-glycoprotein I *in vivo*: nitrosylation, redox modification by endothelial cells, and regulation of oxidative stress-induced cell injury. *Blood* **116:** 1961–1970.

48. Passam, F.H., B. Giannakopoulos, P. Mirarabshahi, S.A. Krilis. 2011. Molecular pathophysiology of the antiphospholipid syndrome: the role of oxidative post-translational modification of beta 2 glycoprotein I. *J. Thromb. Haemost.* **9** (Suppl 1): 275–282.

49. Pierangeli, S.S., X. Liu, J.H. Barker, *et al.* 1995. Induction of thrombosis in a mouse model by IgG, IgM and IgA immunoglobulins from patients with the Antiphospholipid Syndrome. *Thromb. Haemost.* **74:** 1361–1367.

50. Fischetti, F., P. Durigutto, V. Pellis, *et al.* 2005. Thrombus formation induced by antibodies to beta2-glycoprotein I is complement dependent and requires a priming factor. *Blood.* **106:** 2340–2346. Epub 2005 Jun 14.

51. Arad, A., V. Proulle, R.A. Furie, *et al.* 2011. β-Glycoprotein-1 autoantibodies from patients with antiphospholipid syndrome are sufficient to potentiate arterial thrombus formation in a mouse model. *Blood* **117:** 3453–3459. Epub 2011 Jan 18.

52. Erkan, D., M.D Lockshin. 2010. Non-criteria manifestations of antiphospholipid syndrome. *Lupus* **19:** 424–427.

53. Pierangeli, S.S., M. Colden-Stanfield, X. Liu, *et al.* 1999. Antiphospholipid antibodies from antiphospholipid syndrome patients activate endothelial cells *in vitro* and *in vivo*. *Circulation* **99:** 1997–2002.

54. Cuadrado, M.J., P. Buendía, F. Velasco, *et al.* 2006. Vascular endothelial growth factor expression in monocytes from patients with primary antiphospholipid syndrome. *J. Thromb. Haemost.* **4:** 2461–2469.

55. Forastiero, R., M. Martinuzzo, L.O. Carreras, J. Maclouf. 1998. Anti-beta2 glycoprotein I antibodies and platelet activation in patients with antiphospholipid antibodies: association with increased excretion of platelet-derived thromboxane urinary metabolites. *Thromb. Haemost.* **79:** 42–45.

56. Satta, N., E.K. Kruithof, C. Fickentscher, *et al.* 2011. Toll-like receptor 2 mediates the activation of human monocytes and endothelial cells by antiphospholipid antibodies. *Blood* **117:** 5523–5531.

57. Raschi, E., C. Testoni, D. Bosisio, *et al.* 2003. Role of the MyD88 transduction signaling pathway in endothelial activation by antiphospholipid antibodies. *Blood.* **101:** 3495–3500.

58. Prinz, N., N. Clemens, D. Strand, *et al.* 2011. Antiphospholipid antibodies induce translocation of TLR7 and TLR8 to the endosome in human monocytes and plasmacytoid dendritic cells. *Blood* **118:** 2322–2332.

59. Romay-Penabad, Z., M.G. Montiel-Manzano, T. Shilagard, *et al.* 2009. Annexin A2 is involved in antiphospholipid antibody-mediated pathogenic effects *in vitro* and *in vivo*. *Blood* **114:** 3074–3083.

60. Urbanus, R.T., M.T. Pennings, R.H. Derksen, P.G. de Groot. 2008. Platelet activation by dimeric beta2-glycoprotein I requires signaling via both glycoprotein Ibalpha and apolipoprotein E receptor 2'. *J. Thromb. Haemost.* **6:** 1405–1412.

61. Romay-Penabad, Z., R. Aguilar-Valenzuela, R.T. Urbanus, *et al.* 2011. Apolipoprotein E receptor 2' is involved in the thrombotic complications in a murine model of the antiphospholipid syndrome. *Blood* **117:** 1408–1414.

62. Allen, K.L., F.V. Fonseca, V. Betapudi, *et al.* 2012. A novel pathway for human endothelial cell activation by antiphospholipid/anti-β2 glycoprotein I antibodies. *Blood* **119:** 884–893.

63. Pierangeli, S.S., M. Vega-Ostertag, E.N. Harris. 2004. Intracellular signaling triggered by antiphospholipid antibodies in platelets and endothelial cells: a pathway to targeted therapies. *Thromb. Res.* **114:** 467–476.

64. Vega-Ostertag, M.E., D.E. Ferrara, Z. Romay-Penabad, *et al.* 2007. Role of p38 mitogen-activated protein kinase in antiphospholipid antibody-mediated thrombosis and endothelial cell activation. *J. Thromb. Haemost.* **5:** 1828–1834.

65. Romay-Penabad, Z., A.L. Carrera-Marin, N. Mackman, S. Pierangeli. 2011. Pathogenic effects of antiphospholipid antibodies are ameliorated in tissue factor deficient mice. *Arth. Rheum.* **63:** s5 (abstract 13).

66. Pierangeli, S.S., M.E. Vega-Ostertag, E. Raschi, *et al.* 2007. Toll-like receptor and antiphospholipid mediated thrombosis: *in vivo* studies. *Ann. Rheum. Dis.* **66:** 1327–1333.

67. Mulla, M.J., J.J. Brosens, L.W. Chamley, *et al.* 2009. Antiphospholipid antibodies induce a pro-inflammatory response in first trimester trophoblast via the TLR4/MyD88 pathway. *Am. J. Reprod. Immunol.* **62:** 96–111.

68. Sorice, M., A. Longo, A. Capozzi, *et al.* 2007. Anti-beta2-glycoprotein I antibodies induce monocyte release of tumor necrosis factor alpha and tissue factor by signal transduction pathways involving lipid rafts. *Arth. Rheum.* **56:** 2687–2697.

69. Raschi, E., V. Broggini, C. Grossi, *et al.* 2009. Mechanisms of action of antiphospholipid antibodies. Handbook of systemic autoimmune diseases. *Antiphosphol. Synd. Sys. Autoimmun. Dis.* **10:** 55–67.

70. Kornberg, A., M. Blank, S. Kaufman, Y. Shoenfeld. 1994. Induction of tissue factor-like activity in monocytes by anti-cardiolipin antibodies. *J. Immunol.* **153:** 1328–1332.

71. Reverter, J.C., D. Tàssies, J. Font, *et al.* 1998. Effects of human monoclonal anticardiolipin antibodies on platelet function and on tissue factor expression on monocytes. *Arth. Rheum.* **41:** 1420–1427.

72. Amengual, O., T. Atsumi, M.A. Khamashta, G.R. Hughes. 1998. The role of the tissue factor pathway in the hypercoagulable state in patients with the antiphospholipid syndrome. *Thromb. Haemost.* **79:** 276–281.

73. López-Pedrera, C., P. Buendía, M.J. Cuadrado, *et al.* 2006. Antiphospholipid antibodies from patients with the antiphospholipid syndrome induce monocyte tissue factor expression through the simultaneous activation of NF-kappaB/Rel proteins via the p38 mitogen-activated protein kinase pathway, and of the MEK-1/ERK pathway. *Arth. Rheum.* **54:** 301–311.

74. Zhou, H., Y. Yan, G. Xu, *et al.* 2009. Annexin A2 mediates anti-beta 2 GPI/beta 2 GPI-induced tissue factor expression on monocytes. *Int. J. Mol. Med.* **24:** 557–562.

75. Zhou, H., Y. Yan, G. Xu, *et al.* 2011. Toll-like receptor (TLR)-4 mediates anti-β2GPI/β2GPI-induced tissue factor expression in THP-1 cells. *Clin. Exp. Immunol.* **163:** 189–198.

76. Shi, T., Giannakopoulos, B., X. Yan, *et al.* 2006. Anti-beta2-glycoprotein I antibodies in complex with beta2-glycoprotein I can activate platelets in a dysregulated manner via glycoprotein Ib-IX-V. *Arth. Rheum.* **54:** 2558–2567.

77. Lutters, B.C., R.H. Derksen, W.L. Tekelenburg, *et al.* 2003. Dimers of beta 2-glycoprotein I increase platelet deposition to collagen via interaction with phospholipids and the apolipoprotein E receptor 2'. *J. Biol. Chem.* **278:** 33831–33838.

78. van Lummel, M., M.T. Pennings, R.H. Derksen, *et al.* 2005, The binding site in beta2-glycoprotein I for ApoER2' on platelets is located in domain V. *J. Biol. Chem.* **280:** 36729–36736.

79. Sikara, M.P., J.G. Routsias, M. Samiotaki, *et al.* 2010. beta2 Glycoprotein I (beta2GPI) binds platelet factor 4 (PF4): implications for the pathogenesis of antiphospholipid syndrome. *Blood* **115:** 713–723.

80. Hammel, M., R. Schwarzenbacher, A. Gries, *et al.* 2001. Mechanism of the interaction of beta(2)-glycoprotein I

with negatively charged phospholipid membranes. *Biochemistry* **40**: 14173–14181.

81. Lee, C.J., A. De Biasio, N. Beglova. 2010. Mode of interaction between beta2GPI and lipoprotein receptors suggests mutually exclusive binding of beta2GPI to the receptors and anionic phospholipids. *Structure* **18**: 366–376.

82. Lambrianides, A., C. Carroll, C. Pericleous, *et al.* 2007. Differential clinical manifestations of the antiphospholipid syndrome may be predicted by different intracellular signalling pathways. *Arth. Rheum.* **56**: S533.

83. Carroll, T.Y., M.J. Mulla, C.S. Han, *et al.* 2011. Modulation of trophoblast angiogenic factor secretion by antiphospholipid antibodies is not reversed by Heparin. *Am. J. Reprod. Immunol.* **66**: 286–296.

84. Soltesz, P., K. Veres, G. Lakos, *et al.* 2003. Evaluation of clinical and laboratory features of antiphospholipid syndrome: a retrospective study of 637 patients. *Lupus* **12**: 302–307.

85. Jimenez, S., M.A. García-Criado, D. Tassies, *et al.* Preclinical vascular disease in systemic lupus erythematosus and primary antiphospholipid syndrome. *Rheumatology* **44**: 756–761.

86. Hasunuma, Y., E. Matsuura, Z. Makita, *et al.* 1997. Involvement of β2-glycoprotein I and anticardiolipin antibodies in oxidatively modified low-density lipoprotein uptake by macrophages. *Clin. Exp. Immunol.* **107**: 569–573.

87. George, J., D. Harats, B. Gilburd, *et al.* 1999. Immunolocalization of β2-glycoprotein I (apolipoprotein H) to human atherosclerotic plaques: potential implications for lesion progression. *Circulation* **99**: 2227–2230.

88. Shoenfeld, Y., Y. Sherer, J. George, D. Harats. 2000. Autoantibodies associated with atherosclerosis. *Ann. Med.* **32**(Suppl. I): 37–40.

89. Vaarala, O. 1996. Antiphospholipid antibodies and atherosclerosis. *Lupus* **5**: 442–447.

90. Veres, K., G. Lakos, A. Kerenyi, *et al.* 2004. Antiphospholipid antibodies in acute coronary syndrome. *Lupus* **13**: 423–427.

91. Shoenfeld, Y., R. Gerli, A. Doria, *et al.* 2005. Accelerated atherosclerosis in autoimmune rheumatic diseases. *Circulation* **112**: 3337–3347.

92. Shoenfeld, Y., Y. Sherer, J. George, D. Harats. 2000. Autoantibodies associated with atherosclerosis. *Ann. Med.* **32**: 37–40.

93. Delgado-Alves, J., L.J. Mason, P.R. Ames, *et al.* 2005. Antiphospholipid antibodies are associated with enhanced oxidative stress, decreased plasma nitric oxide and paraoxonase activity in an experimental mouse model. *Rheumatology* **44**: 1238–1244.

94. Simoncini, S., C. Sapet, L. Camoin-Jau, *et al.* 2005. Role of reactive oxygen species and p38 MAPK in the induction of the pro-adhesive endothelial state mediated by IgG from patients with anti-phospholipid syndrome. *Int. Immunol.* **17**: 489–500.

95. Lopez-Pedrera, C.H., P. Ruiz-Limon, M.A. Aguirre, *et al.* 2009. Oxidative stress and mitochondrial membrane potential in circulating leucocytes from antiphospholipid syndrome patients: key intracellular events in thrombosis development [abstract]. *Arth. Rheum.* **60**(Suppl10): 1272.

96. Iverson, G.M., E. Matsuura, E.J. Victoria, *et al.* 2002. The orientation of beta2GPI on the plate is important for the binding of anti-beta2GPI autoantibodies by ELISA. *J. Autoimmun.* **18**: 289–297.

97. Kaplan, V., D. Erkan, W. Derksen, *et al.* 2004. Real world experience with antiphospholipid antibodies (APL): how useful is anti-β2glycoprotein (β2GPI) test? *Arth. Rheum.* **50**: S67 [abstract].

98. Pierangeli, S.S., E.J. Favaloro, G. Lakos, *et al.* 2012. Standards and reference materials for the anticardiolipin and anti-β2glycoprotein I assays: a report of recommendations from the APL Task Force at the 13th International Congress on Antiphospholipid Antibodies. *Clin. Chim. Acta* **413**: 358–360.

99. Iverson, G.M., S. Reddel, E.J. Victoria, *et al.* 2002. Use of single point mutations in domain I of beta 2-glycoprotein I to determine fine antigenic specificity of antiphospholipid autoantibodies. *J. Immunol.* **169**: 7097–7103.

100. Ioannou, Y., C. Pericleous, I. Giles, *et al.* 2007. Binding of antiphospholipid antibodies to discontinuous epitopes on domain I of human beta(2)-glycoprotein I: mutation studies including residues R39 to R43. *Arth. Rheum.* **56**: 280–290.

101. de Laat, B., R.H. Derksen, R.T. Urbanus, P.G. de Groot. 2005. IgG antibodies that recognize epitope Gly40-Arg43 in domain I of beta 2-glycoprotein I cause LAC, and their presence correlates strongly with thrombosis. *Blood* **105**: 1540–1545.

102. Ioannou, Y., I. Giles, A. Lambrianides, *et al.* 2006. A novel expression system of domain I of human beta2 glycoprotein I in Escherichia coli. *BMC Biotechnol.* **6**: 8.

103. Ostertag, M.V., X. Liu, V. Henderson, S.S. Pierangeli. 2006. A peptide that mimics the Vth region of beta-2-glycoprotein I reverses antiphospholipid-mediated thrombosis in mice. *Lupus* **15**: 358–365.

104. de la Torre, Y.M., F. Pregnolato, F. D'Amelio, *et al.* 2012. Anti-phospholipid induced murine fetal loss: novel protective effect of a peptide targeting the β2 glycoprotein I phospholipid-binding site. Implications for human fetal loss. *J. Autoimmun.* **38**: J209–J215.

105. Ruiz-Irastorza, G., M.J. Cuadrado, I. Ruiz-Arruza, *et al.* 2011. Evidence-based recommendations for the prevention and long-term management of thrombosis in antiphospholipid antibody-positive patients: report of a task force at the 13th International Congress on antiphospholipid antibodies. *Lupus* **20**: 206–218.

106. Erkan, D., M. Harrison, R. Levy, *et al.* 2007. Aspirin for primary thrombosis prevention in the antiphospholipid syndrome: a randomized, double-blind, placebo-controlled trial in asymptomatic antiphospholipid antibody-positive individuals. *Arth. Rheum.* **56**: 2382–2391.

Ann. N.Y. Acad. Sci. ISSN 0077-8923

ANNALS OF THE NEW YORK ACADEMY OF SCIENCES
Issue: *The Year in Immunology*

Getting away with murder: how does the BCL-2 family of proteins kill with immunity?

Thibaud T. Renault[1,3] and Jerry E. Chipuk[1,2,3,4]

[1]Department of Oncological Sciences, [2]Department of Dermatology, [3]The Tisch Cancer Institute, [4]The Graduate School of Biological Sciences, Mount Sinai School of Medicine, New York, New York

Address for correspondence: Jerry Edward Chipuk, Ph.D., Department of Oncological Sciences, Mount Sinai School of Medicine, One Gustave L. Levy Place, Box 1130, New York, New York. jerry.chipuk@mssm.edu

The adult human body produces approximately one million white blood cells every second. However, only a small fraction of the cells will survive because the majority is eliminated through a genetically controlled form of cell death known as apoptosis. This review places into perspective recent studies pertaining to the BCL-2 family of proteins as critical regulators of the development and function of the immune system, with particular attention on B cell and T cell biology. Here we discuss how elegant murine model systems have revealed the major contributions of the BCL-2 family in establishing an effective immune system. Moreover, we highlight some key regulatory pathways that influence the expression, function, and stability of individual BCL-2 family members, and discuss their role in immunity. From lethal mechanisms to more gentle ones, the final portion of the review discusses the nonapoptotic functions of the BCL-2 family and how they pertain to the control of immunity.

Keywords: apoptosis; BCL-2 family; immunity; mitochondria

Introduction

Apoptosis, also known as type I programmed cell death, plays a critical role in a wide range of tissue functions and occurs during embryonic development to establish the architecture and function of tissues and organs.[1] Postdevelopmental apoptosis is also required for the maintenance of homeostasis, which involves, among other things, the control of immunity. Importantly, two distinct signaling cascades engage apoptosis: the extrinsic pathway, which responds to the activation of the surface death receptors, and the intrinsic pathway, triggered by cellular stresses. Although the BCL-2 (B cell chronic lymphocytic leukemia (CLL)/lymphoma-2) family mainly regulates the intrinsic pathway, evidence of regulatory crosstalk between the pathways has been described following death receptor ligation. A detailed overview of the extrinsic and intrinsic apoptotic pathways is presented in Figure 1.

Apoptosis plays a critical role in both the development of immune cells and the execution of an immune response. Throughout the development and maturation of immune cells, many progenitors are produced but not all are suitable candidates to participate in immunity, and apoptosis is required to fulfill a highly selective triage—we will discuss these pathways in the following sections. Furthermore, during an adaptive immune response, a rapid increase within an immune cell population is required to oppose an invading pathogen. Once the pathogen is recognized and eliminated, clearance of the expanded immune cell population occurs through apoptosis, leaving a few remaining cells to ensure durable future responses.[2] Indeed, we will discuss the mechanisms that control the clearance of these dynamic cellular populations.

T cells and B cells are lymphocytes, white blood cells that participate in the adaptive immune response. T cells mediate the cellular immune response (i.e., production of cytotoxic T cells, release of cytokines, antigen presentation, activation of macrophages and natural killer cells), and B cells mediate the humoral immune response (i.e., production of antibodies).[3] Although acting through different mechanisms, T cells and B cells share a

doi: 10.1111/nyas.12045

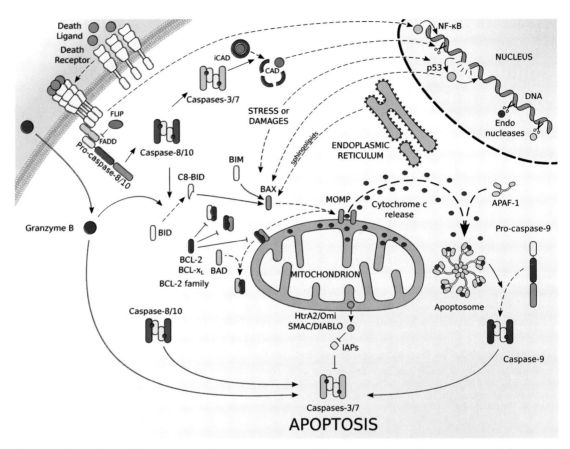

Figure 1. The major signaling pathways leading to cellular apoptosis. The extrinsic pathway of apoptosis (upper left corner) is engaged by plasma membrane–associated death receptors belonging to the TNF-R (tumor necrosis factor receptor) superfamily (e.g., TNF-R1/2, CD95/FAS). Upon engagement of these receptors by their respective ligands (e.g., TNF-α, FASL), conformation changes within the trimerized receptor/ligand complexes recruits adaptor proteins (e.g., FADD) and caspase-8 (and/or caspase-10 in humans, represented in blue) to assemble a death-inducing signaling complex, referred to as the *DISC*. Assembly of the DISC promotes caspase-8 activation; cleavage and activation of executioner caspase-3, caspase-6, or caspase-7 (represented in green); and cell death.[165] The intrinsic pathway (also called the mitochondrial pathway of apoptosis) responds to cellular stresses like DNA damage (through p53), viral infection, protein misfolding, and oxidative stress. These signals converge to activate the proapoptotic proteins of the BCL-2 family. Proapoptotic effectors (e.g., BAX, in blue) are able to target mitochondria and induce mitochondrial outer membrane permeabilization (MOMP), in which numerous proapoptotic proteins of the intermembrane space (e.g., cytochrome c, the second mitochondrial-derived activator of caspases SMAC/DIABLO, and HtrA2/Omi) are released into the cytosol. Direct activator BH3-only proteins (e.g., BID and BIM, in yellow) and other signals (e.g., p53 or sphingolipids from the ER) facilitate the activation of BAX and BAK. Sensitizers/derepressors (e.g., BAD and Noxa, in green) interact with the antiapoptotic members (e.g., BCL-2 and BCL-xL, in red) to lower the cell death threshold. Once in the cytosol, cytochrome c interacts with the adaptor protein apoptotic protease activating factor 1 (APAF-1) to form the apoptosome, which triggers the recruitment and the activation of the caspase-9 (represented in purple). Inhibitors of apoptosis (IAPs) inhibit caspase activation, and SMAC/DIABLO relieves this inhibition. Once initiator caspases (e.g., caspase-8 and caspase-9) are activated, they trigger downstream activation of effector caspase-3 and caspase-7, which cleave numerous cellular substrates, including the inhibitor to the caspase-activated DNAse (iCAD). In addition, granzyme B, which is released by cytotoxic T cells, can also directly trigger effector caspase activation to promote cell death. The extrinsic pathway can also engage the intrinsic pathway via caspase-8–mediated cleavage of BID (in yellow) to amplify proapoptotic signaling.

common feature: they are able to specifically recognize antigens on pathogens or invading cells. This is achieved by the generation of specialized receptors located on the plasma membrane of the lymphocyte that bind to an antigen and trigger an immune response.[4] The generation of these receptors is a complex process, as the receptors must recognize exogenous antigens but not self-antigens.[5]

Because of this requirement, the initial number of lymphocytes far exceeds the actual number of mature cells as unreactive and autoreactive cells are eliminated by apoptosis, as described in the following paragraph.

Looking closer at the T cell maturation process reveals the requirement for both apoptosis and survival mechanisms to modulate cell populations and fulfill their selection. In the early stages of thymocyte development (double negative stage, or $CD4^-CD8^-$), the presence of survival signals (e.g., the cytokine IL-7) is needed to prevent apoptosis. These signals control both the population of progenitors and T cell receptor (TCR) differentiation.[6] Later, thymocytes undergo the first step of selection in the thymus cortex by binding their TCR to major histocompatibility complex (MHC) molecules of the surrounding epithelial cells. Cells which fail to interact do not receive the signals required for their survival (e.g., the expression of antiapoptotic proteins) and are therefore eliminated.[7] This process, termed positive selection, is necessary to ensure that T cells will be able to further participate in the immune response. In contrast, T cells bearing receptors that have too high affinity for MHC are dangerous for an organism as they have the potential to trigger the elimination of cells in healthy, functional tissues. Consequently, these highly reactive cells are also eliminated by apoptosis. This constitutes the negative selection process. Similarly, B cell development and maturation involves positive and negative selection; and the early B cell populations are also dependent on survival cytokines such as IL-7.[8] However, the development of B cells continues in the bone marrow and the selection signals are received through a different class of receptors, the B cell receptors (BCR).[9]

Independent of the death signal, apoptotic cells are eliminated through regulated cellular disassembly and engulfment mechanisms that prevent inflammation-induced stress of the local environment. Common cellular hallmarks associated with apoptosis include caspase (cysteine-dependent aspartate-directed proteases) activation, and subsequent DNA cleavage, chromatin condensation, and cellular contraction.[10] In parallel, apoptotic cells externalize phosphatidylserine on the plasma membrane in a caspase-dependent manner, which contributes to an "eat me signal" for phagocytic cells to recognize and eliminate the stressed cell; there-

fore preserving tissue integrity from the dumping of cellular contents into the environment leading to inflammation.[11]

Next, we will discuss the BCL-2 family in the specific context of immune cell development and function. We will first provide a detailed introduction into the structures, functions, and mechanisms of the BCL-2 family members, and then bring into focus their control of the immune system, much of which has been identified by animal models.

The BCL-2 family

BCL-2, the founding member of the family, was identified in human B cell follicular lymphoma in which the chromosomal translocation t(14;18)(q32;q21) induces BCL-2 gene deregulation and overexpression.[12] Soon after its identification, the role of BCL-2 was linked to B cell tumorigenesis using a murine model of follicular B cell lymphoma. In this model, oncogenic *c-myc* is overexpressed using Eμ, the immunoglobulin heavy chain enhancer (Eμ-*myc*). Although Eμ-*myc* animals develop lymphoma within a few months, the presence of transgenic *bcl-2* markedly decreased tumor-free survival.[13] The mechanism behind this observation is that *c-myc* promotes both prosurvival and prodeath signals and the presence of transgenic *bcl-2* allows for the silencing of the prodeath signal to promote rapid both transformation and apoptotic resistance of the precursor B cells. The Eμ-*myc* model has been used extensively in the BCL-2 family literature, and further studies indicate that the proapoptotic signal induced by Eμ-*myc* is the transcriptional induction of *bim*.[14,15] Interestingly, BCL-2 was the first oncogene identified that exerted its tumor promoting function by inhibiting proapoptotic signaling,[13] rather than directly promoting cellular proliferation.[16]

After the initial studies with BCL-2, nearly all the other members of the BCL-2 family were identified and defined based on their shared function, conserved alpha (α) helical BCL-2 homology (BH) domain composition, and/or structural similarities (see Fig. 2). Based on these functional and structural homologies, the BCL-2 family was subdivided into two functional groups: the antiapoptotic and the proapoptotic proteins.

The antiapoptotic group comprises (listed by date of identification) BCL-2, BCL-xL (BCL2L1

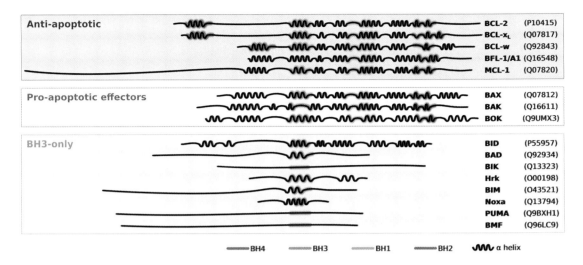

Figure 2. The BCL-2 family: primary structure, domains, and hierarchy. The antiapoptotic members of the BCL-2 family are represented in the red frame. The proapotic effectors and the BH3-only are in the blue and green frames, respectively. The BCL-2 homology (BH) domains and the secondary structure (α helices) are represented for each member, and the UniProt[166] identifier is indicated between parentheses. Antiapoptotics and proapotic effectors have up to four BH domains. The BH1–3 domains (in purple and blue) are spatially close to each other and form a hydrophobic groove that is important for the interaction with the members of the family. Most of the BH3-only proteins are intrinsically unstructured in solution and acquire a secondary structure upon interaction with other members of the family.[167,168] An exception is BID, which is phylogenically[169] and structurally[169,170] most similar to the folded members than to the other BH3-only proteins and natively structured.

long isoform), BCL-w (BCL2L2), MCL-1 (myeloid cell leukemia-1, BCL2L3), and Bfl-1/A1 (BCL2L5). These members share up to four BH domains and a carboxyl terminal transmembrane domain (except for A1) and, in general, are localized to the outer mitochondrial membrane (OMM). Importantly, all the antiapoptotic proteins share a structural fold that is composed of five or six α helices that span the BH1–3 domains. This structural fold forms a hydrophobic groove that is primarily responsible for interacting with proapoptotic members of the BCL-2 family. In the majority of cells, overexpression of individual antiapoptotic BCL-2 proteins suppresses proapoptotic signaling by directly sequestering proapoptotic BCL-2 members;[17] this is frequently associated with resistance to apoptosis, and can lead to immune disorders and tumorigenesis.[18]

The proapoptotic group is further subdivided in two classes of proteins based on their structure and associated function. Members of the first class, the proapoptotic effector proteins, for example, BAX (BCL-2 associated X protein) and BAK (BCL-2 antagonist killer 1), are composed of three BH domains (BH1–3) and oligomerize into proteolipid pores within the OMM. The formation of these pores and the subsequent release of proteins from the mitochondrial intermembrane space[19,20] leads to mitochondrial outer membrane permeabilization (MOMP), which is considered to be the most significant biochemical event in the initiation of the mitochondrial pathway of apoptosis. The diverse signaling pathways that lead to MOMP, along with the extraordinary number of regulatory mechanisms, cannot be summarized here; but it should be kept in mind that BAK- and/or BAX-dependent MOMP is often defined as the point of no return in the cellular commitment to apoptosis.[21] In order for BAK and BAX to form pores within the OMM, BAK and BAX must undergo activation, which is often initiated by interactions with a subset of BH3-only proteins in a particular lipid environment.[22,23] In brief, activation is also associated with conformational rearrangements within monomeric species of BAK and BAX that cause stable association and insertion into the OMM, along with oligomerization at the OMM (although BOK (BCL-2 ovarian killer) is often considered to be an effector protein, there is minimal biochemical evidence directly implicating BOK in MOMP).[24]

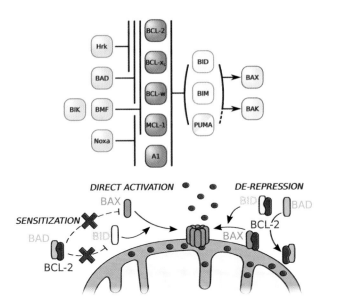

Figure 3. Interactions and mechanisms of the BH3-only proteins. BH3-only proteins are subdivided in two groups. Sensitizers (in green) selectively interact with antiapoptotic BCL-2 proteins (in red); as an example, BAD binds to BCL-2, BCL-x_L, and BCL-w, whereas Noxa binds to MCL-1 and A1. By binding to the antiapoptotic BCL-2 proteins, sensitizers prevent the sequestration of the proapoptotics and prime for BAX/BAK activation. Direct activators (in yellow) have a broad interaction range within the BCL-2 family. They are able to interact directly with and activate BAX and BAK to induce MOMP. On the other hand they can also counteract the antiapoptotics. When proapoptotics are sequestered by antiapoptotics, derepressor BH3-only proteins are able to disrupt these complexes. BID and BIM are well-characterized direct activator BH3-only proteins;[171,172] however, the role of PUMA as direct activator remains controversial.[173–175] Lines with stops and arrows indicate an inhibition and an activation, respectively.

The second class of proapoptotic BCL-2 family members comprises proteins sharing only the BH3 domain and is referred to as the *BH3-only proteins*. Examples of this class include BAD (BCL-2 antagonist of cell death), BID (BH3 interacting-domain death agonist), BIK (BCL-2 interacting killer), BIM (BCL-2 interacting mediator of cell death), BMF (BCL-2 modifying factor), Hrk (Harakiri), Noxa, and PUMA (p53 upregulated mediator of apoptosis). The BH3-only proteins have key functions to directly bind and regulate both the antiapoptotic and proapoptotic effector proteins; their mechanisms of action are summarized in Figure 3. Each BH3-only protein demonstrates a unique set of interactions within the BCL-2 family, and these interactions reveal each BH3-only protein's contribution to BAK/BAK activation and apoptosis. A detailed description of these interactions and subsequent consequences are also presented in Figure 3.

It is important to note that the majority of interactions within the BCL-2 family occur mainly through direct binding of the BH3 domain of one protein into the hydrophobic groove formed by the BH1–3 domains of the partner (e.g., the BIM BH3

domain binding into the groove of BCL-2).[25] These interactions are the classical protein–protein interactions that establish the cellular apoptotic threshold through sensitization and derepression mechanisms (Fig. 3).

Recently, a new set of interactions has been described that leads to BIM-mediated direct activation of BAX. A helical version of the BIM BH3 domain peptide has been shown to directly interact with the $\alpha 1$ and $\alpha 2$ helices of BAX, which, relative to the BAX hydrophobic groove, are located on the opposite side of the protein.[26] This observation revealed a major development in the study of the role of the BH3-only proteins, especially because BIM is considered one of the most important potent and critical among the BH3-only proteins; these features of BIM will be expanded upon in several upcoming sections.

The final class of interactions within the BCL-2 family is the homo-oligomerization of the effector proteins, which is required for pore formation leading to MOMP. Homo-oligomerization of BAX was shown to be dependent not on only on the BH3 domain but also on the BH1 domain,[27] and BAK homo-oligomerization similarly involves

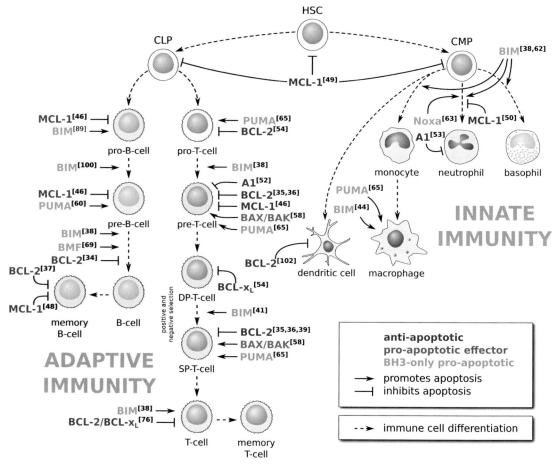

Figure 4. The BCL-2 family in hematopoiesis. The proteins of the BCL-2 family contribute to numerous steps of both innate and adaptive immune system development. The adaptive immune system originates from common lymphoid progenitors (CLP) and comprises B cells and T cells. The BCL-2 family is a critical regulator of most of the lymphocyte differentiation stages (e.g., the positive and negative selections, in which double positive (DP) cells are maturated in single positive (SP) cells, or the differentiation into memory lymphocytes). The innate immune system originates from common myeloid progenitors (CMP) and, similarly, differentiation of the myeloid cells is controlled by the BCL-2 family. Numbers in brackets refer to the reference list.

both the BH3 domain and a region close to the BH1 domain (i.e., α6 helix).[28,29] Directed mutagenesis in the BH1–3 domains is often used as a tool to examine the importance of these interactions;[30,31] in hematopoietic malignancies, spontaneous mutations within the BAX BH1 and BH3 domains are described to promote apoptotic resistance.[32]

With the above summary of definitions, basic interactions, and apoptotic functions of the individual members of the BCL-2 family, we will now present recent mouse models that highlight a role for these proteins in the immune system. In particular, we will focus on the contribution of the BCL-2 proteins in the development and function of lymphocytes.

To aid in summarizing this significant literature, Figure 4 recapitulates some of the major checkpoints regulated by the BCL-2 family. Toward the end of the discussion, we will also touch upon the nonapoptotic functions of the BCL-2 family in regulating immune responses.

What have we learned using mouse models?

BCL-2

The first member of the BCL-2 family to be intensively studied in murine models of immunity and cancer was BCL-2. Early observations reported that BCL-2 overexpression enhanced the survival of

T cells,[33] and when introduced into the Eμ-*myc* background (described previously), BCL-2 promoted enhanced survival of B cells.[34] Furthermore, transgenic *bcl-2* caused an amplification of an IgM and IgG antibody-driven immune response and sensitized the mice to an autolymphoproliferative syndrome phenotype.[34]

Further observations describe that despite completing their development, $bcl2^{-/-}$ mice display several defects, including smaller size, polycystic kidneys, and smaller thymus, because of an increase in apoptosis. The $bcl2^{-/-}$ mice have an impaired development of the immune system and display an abnormal cellularity: the number of double positive ($CD4^+CD8^+$) and single positive ($CD4^+$ or $CD8^+$) T cells are reduced, whereas the number of double negative cells ($CD4^-CD8^-$) is increased.[35] This was confirmed by studying BCL-2 expression levels over time. As described in the introduction, the maturation of T cells requires the population to be dynamic in number because of proliferation, selection and apoptosis. It has been demonstrated that the expression levels of BCL-2 varies accordingly. As an example, BCL-2 is expressed in double negative cells and decreases as they mature into double positive cells; finally, T cells begin to express BCL-2 again when they reach the single positive stage.[36] Another critical role of BCL-2 was discovered in the maintenance of memory B cells. Memory B cells are produced following the interaction with an antigen and constitute a mechanism of adaptation that allows for a more efficient responses to reencounter with antigen. Mice overexpressing Bcl-2 display greater secondary immune responses and extended survival of memory B cells.[37]

BIM

BIM plays a critical role during hematopoiesis and the *in vivo* function of this protein has received the most attention among the proapoptotic BCL-2 members. Notably, BIM participates in the elimination of autoreactive lymphocytes.

Lymphoid cells derived from *bim* deficient mice display resistance to numerous inducers of the mitochondrial pathway of apoptosis (e.g., γ-irradiation and dexamethasone), which results in an increase of both lymphoid and myeloid cells *in vivo*.[38] As previously described, $bcl2^{-/-}$ mice show a dramatic decrease of T cells and B cells;[35,39] eliminating *bim* in the $bcl2^{-/-}$ background, however, restores the

wild-type phenotype.[40] Furthermore, thymocytes derived from *bim* deficient animals have been to be resistant to proapoptotic signaling via TCR–CD3 stimulation during negative selection;[41] a similar negative selection phenotype was observed in B cells. These observations demonstrate the critical role for the proapoptotic function of BIM in the selection of non autoreactive lymphocytes, and implicate BIM in the regulation of autoimmune diseases.[38] Although the above data suggest that the proapoptotic function of BIM is required for numerous aspects of immune system development, the molecular mechanisms directly impacted by *bim* expression remained undefined. Is BIM required to cause the direct activation of BAK/BAX or is the inhibitory affect of BIM on numerous antiapoptotic BCL-2 family members sufficient to promote proper T cell and B cell development and function?

To begin to address this question an elegant study made use of genetically altered mice in which the BH3 domain of BIM was replaced with the BH3 domains of other BH3-only members displaying different biochemical activities (i.e., BAD, Noxa, and PUMA). For example, the BIM BH3 domain sequence was genetically replaced with the BAD BH3 domain to generate a chimeric protein that was under the regulation of the endogenous *bim* promoter and subject to posttranslational control of the BIM protein; this allowed for the normal expression and regulation of the BIM[BAD] chimera, yet afforded the specific evaluation of the BAD BH3 domain in the context of the BIM protein backbone within a cell. The results were intriguing: all the chimeric BIM mutants were less efficient in triggering cell death compared with wild-type BIM, resulting in increased lymphocyte (e.g., thymocytes and B cells) numbers and splenomegaly. The combination of BIM[BAD] and BIM[Noxa] alleles, which together target the entire antiapoptotic BCL-2 repertoire, only partially restored the wild-type phenotype, demonstrating that the function of BIM *in vivo* extends beyond the inhibition of antiapoptotic BCL-2 proteins (similar results were also obtained with the BIM[PUMA] mutant).[42] Interestingly, when expressed in an Eμ-*myc* background, the BIM[BAD] or BIM[Noxa] mutants accelerated the rate of lymphomagenesis either because of incomplete inhibition of the antiapoptotic proteins or a failure to activate BAK/BAX. In contrast, the BIM[PUMA] animals displayed no additional susceptibility to the disease, suggesting that the various biochemical activities of BIM may be differentially utilized in developmental verses oncogenic signaling environments.[43]

The role of *bim* is not restricted to B cells and T cells in the immune system, as the mechanism by which macrophages trigger phagocytosis-induced apoptosis is also dependent on the proapoptotic function of BIM. Subsequent to the phogocytosis of pyrogenic bacteria (e.g., *Escherichia coli*), macrophages are capable of triggering their own death through apoptosis. This pathway, phagocytosis-induced cell death, allows for the clearance of the infected macrophages after the pathogens are removed from the site of infection. Data support that BIM function was upregulated by bacteria-induced Toll-like receptor (e.g., through TLR2, TLR4, and TLR9) signaling involving the adaptor protein MyD88 and downstream dephosphorylation and activation of BIM. However, although BIM was required for phagocytosis-induced cell death, it is likely that additional signals are required, as the overexpression of *bim* alone was not sufficient to induce macrophage death.[44]

MCL-1

The requirement for MCL-1 function presents very early during vertebrate development, as *mcl1* deletion is pre-implantation lethal.[45] To overcome this constraint, the *mcl1* gene was flanked with loxP sites allowing for tissue-specific Cre-mediated deletion. The deletion of *mcl1* in lymphocytes using Lck-*Cre* and CD19-*Cre* demonstrated that MCL-1 is required for the development of CD4$^+$CD8$^+$ T cells and pro-B cells, respectively, by directly antagonizing BIM function. Furthermore, IL-7 signaling during B cell development was shown to promote B cell survival by directly inducing the expression of *mcl1*.[46] Similar to *bim* deficiency but to a lesser extent, MCL-1 overexpression also affected the positive selection of thymocytes in several mice models (e.g., the HY-antigen–specific and ovalbumin-specific [OT-I] transgenic TCR mice).[47] In latter steps of B cells maturation, MCL-1 was shown to be required for the formation of germinal centers, specialized immune structures that allow rapid B cells proliferation upon T cell dependent immunization and, among others, the differentiation in memory B cells.[48]

A master regulatory role for MCL-1 function in immunity was also demonstrated in the mainte-

nance of hematopoietic stem cells (HSC). As HSCs are the progenitors of most cells involved in immune responses, a decrease in the number and quality of HSCs directly affects all subsequent lineages. The role of *mcl1* in HSCs was shown by conditional deletion using Mx1-*Cre*, which caused massive apoptosis in HSC progenitors and, subsequently, resulted in a general decrease of derived progenitors (e.g., CLP and CMP, the common lymphoid and myeloid progenitors).[49]

Over the years studies continued to find an important role for *mcl1* in protecting cells from development and stress-induced apoptosis. For example, *in vivo* murine data revealed a major role for *mcl1* in both macrophage and neutrophil survival. Interestingly, the absence of *mcl1* did not directly affect macrophage survival, because of compensatory overexpression of *bcl-2* and *bcl-x*.[50] More recently, in a model of acute myeloid leukemia (AML), resistance to pharmacologic treatment was demonstrated to be dependent on *mcl1* expression inhibiting BIM function; moreover, transformed murine myeloid cells were shown to be sensitive to *ex vivo* culture in the absence of MCL-1 but not of BCL-xL.[51] Likewise, MCL-1 is an important component for the resistance of cancer cells to ABT-737 treatments.[18]

A1 and BCL-xL

Where BCL-2 and MCL-1 regulate multiple steps of HSC survival and lymphocyte maturation, the described roles for BCL-xL and A1 are more restricted.

A1 has been shown to be a target of pre-TCR signaling pathway during the transition from double-negative to single-positive T cell maturation; for example, after signaling through the pre-TCR, *a1* transcription increases, which leads to decreased activation of caspase-3 in thymocytes. This mechanism correlates with the observed increase of *a1* expression in a subset of T cell leukemia patients with deregulated pre-TCR signaling.[52] A1 has also been shown to be important for the maintenance of neutrophils, and *a1* deficient mice have high rates of spontaneous neutrophil apoptosis.[53] Despite the fact that no proapoptotic BH3-only proteins have been identified as A1 antagonists in this study, one can assume that BIM and Noxa can play this role.

For BCL-xL, the loss of expression in thymocytes was shown to decrease the differentiation of CD4$^-$CD8$^-$ to CD4$^+$CD8$^+$ cells, whereas sustained *bcl-x* expression was observed during the double-positive stage, and was inversely correlated with BCL-2 expression (as reported previously[36]), suggesting a specialized role for BCL-xL in this particular step of T cell differentiation.[54]

BAX and BAK

In the absence of both *bak* and *bax*, embryos fail to thrive and the phenotype is embryonic lethality, although a few *bak*$^{-/-}$*bax*$^{-/-}$ double knockout mice have been born.[55] Under stress conditions, BAX is often considered the major effector molecule within the mitochondrial pathway of apoptosis (see Renault and Manon for review[56]); however, *bax* is dispensable for mammalian development, as the *bak*$^{-/-}$*bax*$^{-/-}$ phenotype can be rescued by *bak* (and vice versa).[57] Despite having an outwardly normal phenotype, *bax* deficient mice display abnormalities in spermatogenesis and in the development of lymphocytes. *Bax* null mice have an overall higher number of B cells and T cells without a substantial change in the proportion of the different cells, and these cells demonstrated only a mild apoptotic resistance.[57] Double knockout *bak*$^{-/-}$*bax*$^{-/-}$ animals display an increase (three- to 10-fold) in both myeloid and lymphoid cells compared with either single *bak*$^{-/-}$ or *bax*$^{-/-}$ knockouts or with wild-type mice. Similarly, *bak*$^{-/-}$*bax*$^{-/-}$ thymocytes are resistant to γ-irradiation and etoposide-induced apoptosis *in vitro* (both classical inducers of the mitochondrial pathway).[55] A later study reported an important role of BAX and BAK in the selection process of single-positive and double-positive T cells. Interestingly, *bak*$^{-/-}$*bax*$^{-/-}$ T cells displayed a memory phenotype as measured by surface receptor expression (similar as what is observed for T cells from an aged individual), suggesting a regulatory role of BAX and BAK in the turnover, fate, and/or maintenance of T lymphocytes.[58]

The third member of the effector class of proteins BOK has a secondary structure relatively close to that of BAX and BAK; however, little is known about its function. BOK is expressed in a wide range of tissues[24,59] and, to a lesser extent, in myeloid cells.[24] *Bok* deficient mice are viable with no major defects; and genetic removal of *bak* or *bax* does not appear to regulate *bok* expression. Most important, there is no marked difference in survival pathways or apoptotic sensitivity within the immune cell populations in *bok* deficient mice.[24]

Noxa and PUMA

Noxa and PUMA were originally identified as proapoptotic regulators of the p53 tumor suppressor pathway but their roles in cell death have recently expanded into several scenarios. Both proteins are transcriptionally induced following genotoxic stress and under conditions of oncogenic signaling, such as deregulated *c-myc*. Significant effort has been made to determine the biochemical and cellular functions of PUMA because it was demonstrated to play a role in the suppression of *c-myc* driven lymphomagenesis. In the Eμ-*myc* model, the development of lymphoma is not highly penetrant, as overexpression of *c-myc* promotes BIM-mediated apoptosis.

Likewise, it appears that PUMA mediates the apoptotic response to *c-myc*–induced BIM function, as the deletion of a single allele of *puma* was sufficient to induce pre-B cell and B cell lymphomagenesis; this study also demonstrated a contributory role of *noxa*.[60] However, the role of *noxa* may not be directly related to apoptosis, as *noxa* expression has been shown to regulate a form a cell death induced by oncogenes, independent of caspase function.[61] That said, a role for *noxa* in mediating neutrophil survival has been shown for spontaneous and cytokine withdrawal–induced apoptosis.[62] It appears that *noxa* functionally compensates for *bim* loss to promote apoptosis. Furthermore, the combined deletion of *bim* and *noxa* has been shown to result in a complete inhibition of apoptosis under these conditions.[63]

The role of *puma* in numerous immune cell subtypes has been expanded in recent years by further examination of the puma-null mouse model. PUMA was also shown to promote apoptosis of mast cells[64] in response to DNA damage and to regulate the number of macrophages.[65] In both cases, PUMA was shown to cooperate with BIM to induce cell death. For example, *bim*$^{-/-}$ *puma*$^{-/-}$ deficient animals, but not *bim* or *puma* single knockout animals, presented abnormal macrophage cellularity. A functional redundancy for the role of BIM and PUMA was demonstrated using primary myeloid cells in culture: the deletion of *bim* and *puma* resulted in strong apoptotic resistance upon cytokine withdrawal or ionizing radiation.[64] However, when *in vivo* depletion of the myeloid populations was performed by carboplatin or γ-irradiation treatment, a nonoverlapping function of BIM and PUMA was revealed. Puma-deficient animals survived whereas most *bim*-deficient animals died within two weeks.[64] The role of PUMA to synergize with BIM in lymphocytes was shown in an additional model: although the deletion of *puma* alone did not alter the development of B cells and T cells, and *puma* deficient animals are indistinguishable from wild-type animals,[66] the combination of *bim* and *puma* deletion demonstrated a role of PUMA in the generation of T cells, in particular, during the steps of double-negative and single-positive cells. The *bim*$^{-/-}$ *puma*$^{-/-}$ knockout animals displayed an accumulation of immature thymocytes *in vivo* and a resistance to apoptosis in culture.[65] Recently, the cooperation between BIM and PUMA to eliminate auto-reactive T cells was confirmed in a mouse model of thymocyte deletion by peripheral neoantigens.[67] In this model, the combined deletion of *bim* and *puma*, but not in either single knockout, impaired the elimination of autoreactive T cells and led to autoimmune reactions in various organs.[67]

Recently, the fate of self-reactive T cells was examined in animals deprived of either BH3-only proteins (i.e., BIM or PUMA) or effector members (i.e., BAX and BAK). The deletion of proapoptotic members of the BCL-2 family constitutes a model for auto-immunity by allowing the self-reactive T cells to escape thymic deletion. Animals deleted of *bim*, *puma,* or *bax* and *bak* presented with high levels of cells with self-reactive TCRs. However, self-reactive TCR positive cells also demonstrated an enhanced expression of Foxp3$^+$ (Forkhead box p3), a gene involved in self-tolerance, and a decreased response to TCR engagement. Thus, it appears that overexpression of Foxp3$^+$ could be a mechanism of adaptation to limit the aggressiveness of self-reactive T cells escaping the control exerted by the BCL-2 family.[68]

BMF

Although dispensable for embryonic development, the BH3-only protein BMF has been shown to be involved in the maturation of B cells but has little affect on the normal development of T cells.[69] The most dramatic phenotype in *bmf*$^{-/-}$ mice is a significant increase of pre-B cells and mature B cells. Likewise, recent work showed that the combined loss of *bad* and *bmf* has a limited impact on the number of B cells and on spontaneous apoptosis in thymocytes deprived of glucose. This phenotype may be reconciled as because of BMF, which is suggested to only establish the apoptotic threshold in cells; for example, BMF has been shown to cooperate with BIM in glucocorticoid-induced apoptosis in acute lymphoblastic leukemias.[70] This cooperation suggests a role for BMF that is similar to the one of BAD, which is a derepressor/sensitizer BH3-only function. Despite the *bmf*$^{-/-}$ animals having no developmental phenotypes in T cells, the animals were shown to be more susceptible to lymphomagenesis upon γ-irradiation.[69] Furthermore, analysis of *bad*$^{-/-}$*bmf*$^{-/-}$ double knockouts revealed an increased susceptibility for spontaneous tumors (non-Hodgkin lymphomas, carcinomas, and lymphomas) and reduced life span.[71] This last example recalls, as for BOK, that not all the members of the BCL-2 family have an absolute role in all apoptotic events, and that original mechanisms and functions may remain to be discovered.

As described throughout the previous section, members of the BCL-2 family control both the development and function of numerous cell types within the immune system, as well as the majority of control centers on setting the cellular threshold leading to apoptosis. The next part of the discussion focuses on how transcriptional and posttranscriptional events regulate the function of individual proteins with the BCL-2 family, and how these events directly affect apoptosis and subsequently, the immune system.

Keeping the BCL-2 family proteins under control

In the early years of the BCL-2 family literature the majority of efforts focused on understanding how the protein–protein interactions within the family directly affected the balance between life and death. More recently, the mechanisms of regulation within the BCL-2 family have greatly broadened to include numerous points of transcriptional and posttranslational control that directly influence immune function, including transcriptional regulation via transcription factors, alternative splicing, miRNAs, and mRNA stability. In addition, several posttranslational effects directly dictate protein–protein interactions, MOMP, and cellular responses.

Transcription factors

Numerous transcription factors regulate the expression of genes encoding the BCL-2 family, and we will highlight just a few recent examples. Several studies show that NF-κB promotes cell survival and plays an important role in the development of lymphocytes[72] and immune response.[73] This may be explained by NF-κB–dependent upregulation of *bcl-2*, *bcl-x*, and *a1*, along with decreasing expression of *bax*.[74] The transcriptional regulation of multiple BCL-2 family members by NF-κB has been shown to promote the survival of mature B cells, pre-T cells,[75] or T cells[76] upon TCR engagement.

The transcriptional activity of p53 also regulates the expression of numerous BCL-2 family members. In multiple model systems, the proapoptotic activity of p53 has been shown to be related to the transcriptional increases in *bax*,[77] *noxa*,[78] *puma*,[79] *bik*,[80] and *bid*[81] expression, along with repression of antiapoptotic target genes like *bcl-2*.[82] In addition to direct transcriptional regulation of apoptosis, the p53 protein has been shown to regulate the BCL-2 family proteins in a transcription-independent manner by direct interaction with BAX,[83] BAK,[84] BCL-2, and BCL-xL.[85] As an example of the control of p53 on the BCL-2 family in immunity, a recent study has shown that p53 is a critical checkpoint in the development of thymocytes. In mice deficient for Rpl22, a ribosomal protein required for the transition of CD4$^-$CD8$^-$ T cells to CD4$^+$CD8$^+$ stage, p53 is stabilized and induces *puma*, *bim*, *bax*, and *noxa* and thereby triggers premature apoptosis and blocks the development of CD4$^+$CD8$^+$ T cells. The death of CD4$^+$CD8$^+$ T cells was shown to be dependent on *bim* and *puma*, as gene silencing of the latter was sufficient to inhibit apoptosis leading to the restoration of CD4$^+$CD8$^+$ T cells development.[86]

As we discussed earlier, deregulated *c-myc* can promote apoptosis, and it is suggested that *c-myc* leads to the expression of numerous proapoptotic genes, including *bax*[87] and *bim*;[14] *c-myc* also decreases the apoptotic threshold by negatively regulating the expression of *bcl-2* and *bcl-x*.[88] Furthermore, the concomitant activation of *c-myc* with transgenic *bcl-2* (thereby preventing the suppression of BCL-2 function) is sufficient to promote lymphomagenesis in the Eμ-*myc* mice.[88] Likewise, the most critical proapoptotic protein responsible for the suppression of B cell lymphomagenesis is *bim*, and numerous studies provide evidence that *c-myc*–induced *bim* expression acts as a tumor suppressor and protects Eμ-*myc* mice against lymphomagenesis.[14] The transcription of *bim* was also shown to be upregulated by the forkhead transcription factor FKHR-L1, leading to apoptosis following cytokine withdrawal in the BaF3 pro-B cell model.[89] Recently, the Zinc-finger protein ASCIZ (Ataxia telangiectasia mutated substrate Chk2-interacting Zn^{2+} finger protein) was shown to regulate the survival of B cells by the upregulation of *dynll1* (dynein light chain 1), a protein of the microtubules cytoskeleton. As this will be described further, BIM can associate with microtubules, thus higher levels of DYNLL1 may contribute to the active sequestration of BIM and thus to the inhibition of apoptosis.[90] Finally, the regulation of *mcl1* expression by numerous pathways including JAK/STAT, HIF-1α, and NF-κB was also demonstrated to influence the life span of multiple cell types, including neutrophils[91] and B cells.[92] As we will continue to explore, the BCL-2 family is regulated by multiple signaling pathways and transcriptional regulators, so the fate of individual cells is often determined by the overall cellular and signaling environment rather than one particular event.

Alternative splicing

Regarding proapoptotic BH3-only protein signaling, the alternative spliced forms of BIM have received the most attention. The presence of multiple BIM isoforms in cells is a commonly observed phenotype, and early data in the BIM literature identified that the different BIM isoforms demonstrate various potencies in proapoptotic function. As an example, the shortest isoform of BIM, BIM$_S$, is expressed preferentially upon IL-3 withdrawal and was more potent to mediate cell death.[93] Nineteen BIM isoforms have been described and are organized in six groups: BIM$_S$, BIM$_L$, BIM$_{EL}$, BIM$_D$, BIM$_{Dd}$, and BIM$_{EDd}$.[94,95] The alternative splicing of *bim* mRNA is believed to be a critical mechanism of its regulation, as it determines the presence of a dynein-binding domain in the protein and thus its interaction with the microtubules (N.B., this interaction is also dependant on BIM phosphorylation). Because the short isoforms of BIM are lacking this regulatory domain and are not actively sequestered, they appear to be more efficient apoptotic inducers than the longer isoforms.

As suggested earlier, other members of the BCL-2 family demonstrate alternative splicing, such as BCL-xL/BCL-xS,[96] BAX-α/BAX-β,[97] and PUMA-α/PUMA-β.[79] Although certain isoforms are biochemically classified as antiapoptotic and proapoptotic—which is the case for BCL-xL and BCL-xS, respectively—the isoforms of BAX, PUMA, and BID appear to be functionally equivalent, although they demonstrate potentially unique expression and posttranslational mechanisms that may contribute to altered immune response; but this is still not well explored.

mRNA regulation

Nucleolin, a member of the ribonucleoprotein-containing family has been identified as a binding partner of bcl-2 mRNA, promoting its stabilization and BCL-2 protein expression. Nucleolin and BCL-2 upregulation (mRNA and protein) have been hypothesized to be a critical feature in CLL; silencing of nucleolin decreased bcl-2 mRNA stability and subsequent BCL-2 protein levels leads to enhanced proapoptotic BCL-2 family function, which is likely to be BIM-dependent.[98] Several miR-NAs have been implicated in the regulation of the BCL-2 family. MiR-17~92 regulates the development of pro-B cells to pre-B cells by targeting bim mRNA and promoting cell survival (e.g., during the development of pro-B cells to pre-B cells). MiR-17~92 deficient mice possess significantly higher BIM levels that result lethality of the developing B cell repertoire and of the heart and lungs.[99] Bcl-2 mRNA has also been described as the target of two miRNAs, miR-15 and miR-16, the downregulation of which has been hypothesized to play a role in the development of CLL.[100] This hypothesis was supported by high-throughput profiling of genes involved in CLL, which revealed downregulation of miR-15 and miR-16, and subsequent upregulation of bcl-2 and mcl1.[101] Another microRNA, miR-21, often implicated in cancer, is also described to be upregulated following the Bacillus Calmette-Guerin vaccine for tuberculosis, which is associated with bcl-2 mRNA decreases and apoptosis in dendritic cells.[102]

An extensive literature describes the role of miR-NAs in immune system development and function[103] and in the regulation of the BCL-2 family.[104] However, not much is currently understood about how these pathways overlap.

Phosphorylation and ubiquitinylation

Phosphorylation and ubiquitinylation are the most commonly described posttranslational modification pathways affecting the BCL-2 family. The antiapoptotic protein BCL-2 possesses multiple residues within a flexible loop region between the BH4 and BH3 domains that are capable of undergoing phosphorylation. One consequence of phosphorylation is enhanced antiapoptotic function, as demonstrated by the phosphorylation of serine 70 by ERK1/2, which is described to promote BCL-2/BAX interactions in myeloid cells during IL-3 signaling.[105] Multisite phosphorylation of BCL-2 has also been described (e.g., serine 70, serine 87, and threonine 69) in human T cells and in murine B cells that was suggested to weaken BCL-2's antiapoptotic function.[106] However, contrasting results were obtained using hematopoietic NSF/N1.H7 cells in which BCL-2 phosphorylation on the same sites resulted in sustained antiapoptotic activity.[107] The phosphorylation of BCL-2 on serine 87 by ERK1/2 has also been implicated in BCL-2 stability, as mutation of this site resulted in ubiquitin-dependant proteasomal degradation.[108,109] More recently, the role of BCL-2 phosphorylation has also been shown to be required for the hematopoietic differentiation of a murine embryonic stem cell line.[110]

As described previously, the BH3-only protein BIM has numerous critical roles in lymphocytes maturation and is functionally regulated by phosphorylation. Notably, the phosphorylation of serine 69 by ERK1/2 has been well characterized as a trigger of BIM_{EL} ubiquitinylation and subsequent degradation by the proteasome.[111,112] This mechanism was implicated in the survival of anti-CD3/CD28 stimulated T cells and anti-IgM stimulated B cells.[113] Although this feature of cell survival through BIM phosphorylation appears to be important in the normal maintenance of lymphocytes, a recent clinical study implicates BIM phosphorylation in the progression of CLL.[114]

BAD is an additional example of a BH3-only protein that undergoes extensive regulation by phosphorylation. Murine BAD possesses three serines at positions 112, 136, and 155, and their phosphorylation leads to the inhibition of BAD activity. Serine 155 is located within the BH3 domain and its phosphorylation by cAMP-dependant kinase,[115] PKA,[116,117] or RSK1[117] promotes an association with BCL-xL. Serines 112 and 136 are located on the opposite face of the protein; upon phosphorylation of serine 112 by RSK1[117] and PKA[118] or of serine 136 by Akt,[119] BAD was shown to associate with 14–3-3, leading to a decrease in BAD activity.

Other posttranslational modifications

Cleavage is another common mechanism of regulating BCL-2 family function. The canonical example is the 22 kDa cytosolic BH3-only protein BID. When a cell receives a death signal through the TNF receptors or CD95/FAS, caspase-8 is activated and cleaves BID at aspartate 60.[120] After cleavage, the amino terminal fragment (p7) remains associated with the carboxyl terminal fragment (p15)[121] until the protein interacts with the mitochondrial outer membrane and the complex dissociates.[122] The removal of the p7 fragment renders the BH3 domain of BID accessible to interact with BAK and BAX, leading to their activation and apoptosis.

The cleavage and activation of BID constitutes a crossroad of different cell death pathways, as other proteases are also able to cleave BID in the same region (Fig. 1). Calpains and cathepsins, lysosomal proteases involved in necrosis and apoptosis.[123] target the glycine 70[124] and arginine 65 and arginine 71,[125,126] respectively. Granzyme B, an effector protease released by cytotoxic T cells and natural killer cells, targets aspartate 75.[127] One further posttranslational modification of BID, N-myristoylation, has been proposed to regulate the cellular localization of BID. N-myristoylation is the addition of a myristoyl group on the N-terminal glycine of a protein, and if often implicated in targeting proteins to membranes. Only the caspase-8–cleaved form of BID, with an exposed glycine 61, can undergo N-myristoylation, and as expected, this modification results in mitochondrial targeting of p15-BID.[121] Importantly, however, the mitochondrial localization of BID should not be considered a pro-apoptotic signal that is sufficient to kill a cell. In order for cell death to proceed, membrane-targeted BID must still directly activate BAK and/or BAX to promote MOMP and apoptosis.

In B cell lymphomas, MCL-1 overexpression is often associated with increased risk of cancer development and chemoresistance; experimentally, this has been reproduced using the Eμ-*myc* model.[128] A dependency for MCL-1 expression in cells derived from B cell lymphoma has been demonstrated with antisense oligonucleotides targeting *mcl-1* mRNA, which leads to decreased protein expression–induced spontaneous apoptotis.[129] In parallel studies, cisplatin treatment of MCL-1–dependent B cell lymphomas was shown to cause caspase-dependent cleavage of MCL-1. Mechanistically, MCL-1 cleavage resulted in the loss of its proapoptotic function, and the authors suggested that cleavage converted MCL-1 into a proapoptotic molecule, which was sufficient to restore apoptosis.[129] The reported MCL-1 cleavage was dependent on caspase-9 and -3 activation, which requires prerequisite engagement of the mitochondrial pathway of apoptosis, and thus must not be seen as an initiating event; it may be speculated that this mechanism would serve as amplification step within the proapoptotic pathway. Similarly, caspase-dependent conversion into a proapoptotic form was reported for BCL-2 and BCL-xL.[130–133]

Finally, the enzyme-independent posttranslational modification deamidation, which relies on a relatively slow spontaneous reaction dependent on the amino acid environment, will be discussed. Asparagine and glutamine undergo deamidation, and it is believed that this event functions as a molecular timer to change a protein's function over long periods of time.[134] BCL-xL is described to be regulated by deamidation in several contexts; indeed, BCL-xL possesses a large unstructured loop between the α1 and α2 helices (see Fig. 2), which contains two asparagines. The deamidation of these asparagines (i.e., the transformation into aspartic acid) is thought to inhibit the antiapoptotic function of BCL-xL by decreasing its affinity to the proapoptotic members of the BCL-2 family, for example, BAX,[135] BIM, and PUMA.[136] This modification has been shown to occur in response to cisplatin or γ-irradiation induced DNA damage in fibroblasts.[135] Because of this resistance, deamidation of BCL-xL and maintenance of its antiapoptotic function could be an important factor leading to resistance to apoptosis and the initiation of transformation. As an example, thymocytes isolated from a mouse model of T cell lymphoma, mediated by the upregulation of the p56[lck] tyrosine kinase on a CD45[−/−] background, present an impaired response to DNA damage because of sustained depletion of BCL-xL deamidation.[137] A very similar resistance mechanism, driven by a loss in BCL-xL deamidation, was observed in primary cells isolated from patients suffering from BCR-ABL and JAK2-dependent chronic myeloid leukemia.[138]

Is the role of the BCL-2 family restricted to apoptosis?

Recent literature has presented increasing evidence for additional, nonapoptotic roles for the BCL-2 family of proteins. In the final part of this review, we discuss how the BCL-2 family of proteins are involved in these processes and their consequences on the regulation of immunity.

Inflammatory responses

For many years it has been suggested that BCL-2 and BCL-xL influence inflammation; as an example, BCL-2 overexpression in immortalized macrophages leads to the inhibition of the pro-inflammatory cytokine IL-1β (which mediates the response to infection), maturation, and secretion.[139] Whether BCL-2 plays a direct role by actively connecting apoptosis to inflammation is still unclear, as BCL-2 binding partners may also regulate these processes. However, an additional study reported a direct role for BCL-2 and BCL-xL on the inhibition of NLRP1, a protein involved in the activation of the pro-inflammatory caspase-1 (i.e, IL-1β converting enzyme, which catalyses the activation of IL-1β). Mechanistically, BCL-2 and BCL-xL were shown to bind NLRP1 through their unstructured loops located between the BH4 and BH3 domains (e.g., residues 71–80 in BCL-2), resulting in the inhibition of ATP binding to NLRP1 and further inhibition of oligomerization-dependent caspase-1 activation.[140]

As mentioned earlier, BCL-2 binding partners may also regulate inflammation, and a recent genome-wide screen for genes regulating NOD1 (nucleotide-binding and oligomerization domain-containing protein (1) signaling led to the identification of BID as critical regulator of inflammation. In an apoptosis-independent manner, BID was shown to participate in NOD2 inflammatory responses by interacting with NOD and the IKK complex in macrophages. BID was further demonstrated to be a required component of the NOD signalosome, as siRNA-induced depletion of BID impaired NF-κB and ERK signaling and downstream production of IL-6.[141]

Autophagy

The BCL-2 family of proteins also regulates autophagy, a catabolic pathway involved in recycling cellular organelles and the degradation of long-lived proteins; importantly, this process can also be triggered during cellular stress and is a contributor to tumorigenesis.[142,143] This function of the BCL-2 family proteins is also thought to be integral part of the immune system regulation via autophagy, as it plays an important role in intracellular pathogen sensing and lymphocyte development and homeostasis (see Kuballa et al.[144]).

It has been speculated that the BCL-2 family directly influences the autophagic machinery through Beclin-1, a BH3 domain–containing protein. Beclin-1 functions to regulate Vps34, a class III PI-3 kinase involved in the formation of autophagosomes, which function to engulf organelles and proteins destined for degradation as well as intracellular viruses. Curiously, viruses that antagonize autophagy, for example, hepatitis B, herpes simplex, and influenza A, often directly target Beclin-1 as resistance mechanism.[144] BCL-2[145,146] and BCL-xL[147] have been shown to interact with and sequester Beclin-1, supposedly inhibiting Beclin-1/Vsp34 interaction, although this hypothesis has been debated.[148] In accordance with a direct role of BCL-2 and BCL-xL on Beclin-1 function, BAD and the BAD-BH3 mimetic molecule ABT-737 have been demonstrated to compete with Beclin-1 for the binding to BCL-2 and BCL-xL to induce autophagic responses.[148] More recently, a different role for BCL-2 and BCL-xL has been reported, showing that the two proteins can stimulate autophagy independently of Beclin-1 and, presumably, through another major regulator of autophagy, Atg7.[149]

Mitochondrial dynamics

Mitochondria are dynamic organelles that undergo fusion and fission, which leads to efficient energy production and maintenance of the mitochondrial genome. Mitochondrial fusion is regulated by large dynamin-like GTPases of the outer (MFN1 and MFN2) and inner mitochondrial membranes (OPA1), and by the fission proteins, DRP-1 and Fis1.[150] Given the localization of several BCL-2 members in the mitochondrial outer membrane, an idea emerged years ago that these proteins could also regulate mitochondrial dynamics (see Martinou and

Youle[151]). In general, the antiapoptotic proteins BCL-2 and BCL-xL seem to regulate mitochondrial fission, yet BAX and BAK seem also to be essential to mitochondrial fusion in healthy cells, potentially by inducing the assembly and activation of MFN-2.[152–154] Similar results were obtained with the antiapoptotic protein BCL-xL, which can interact with MFN-2 and promote mitochondrial fusion.[155] Interestingly, the physiological role of the BCL-2 family on mitochondrial dynamics has been highlighted in several studies using lymphocytes. As an example, the migration of lymphocytes to inflamed tissues requires that these cells become polarized, which has been reported to be dependent on mitochondrial fission. Modulation of the fission/fusion balance by overexpressing or silencing MFN1, OPA1, or DRP-1 was demonstrated to be sufficient to abolish lymphocytes polarization and their subsequent migration.[156] Furthermore, the profusion GTPase DRP-1 has also been implicated in the activation of T cells, as a critical component of TCR assembly.[157]

Metabolism

The role of metabolism in immune responses is beginning to emerge in numerous systems, including T cell activation and B cell lymphomas.[158,159] However, the mechanistic interplay between the BCL-2 family, metabolism, and immunity is still in its infancy. MCL-1 is a master regulator or HSC development and function, and recent studies have demonstrated that MCL-1 may directly influence cellular ATP generation. In many cell types MCL-1 protein is found as both large and small isoforms; the functional differences between these isoforms remained unknown for years. A series of elegant studies have now revealed that the shorter form of MCL-1 can localize to the mitochondrial matrix in a TOM/TIM- (translocase of the outer/inner membrane) dependent manner, leading to enhanced mitochondrial fusion, appropriate structure of inner mitochondrial membrane, and proper assembly of the F_1–F_0 ATP synthase.[160] Similarly, BCL-2 has been suggested to be a regulator of mitochondrial respiration through an interaction with multiple cytochrome c oxidase subunits. Functionally, these interactions lead to increased mitochondrial respiration in untreated conditions, and decreased cellular respiration during oxidative stress.[161] Additional studies have also reported a protective role

for BCL-2 against oxidative stress[162] and cytosolic acidification during ischemia-reperfusion, which may also be due metabolic influences.[163] Furthermore, the BH3-only protein BAD is probably the best-characterized BCL-2 family member regarding its regulation of metabolism, yet BAD's influence on immunity remains unknown. Thus far, BAD has been shown to significantly influence glucose metabolism; the phenotype of BAD-deficient mice contains several metabolic deficiencies because of an impairment of glucose-stimulated insulin secretion. The effect of BAD on glucose metabolism was identified to be dependent upon a direct interaction with glucokinase via the BAD BH3 domain, leading to glucokinase activation.[164]

Summary

The members of the BCL-2 family are critical regulators of immune system development and function. Throughout our discussion, we focused on the apoptotic role for these proteins, but the influence of this family of proteins on numerous cellular pathways, including autophagy, metabolism, organelle function, and signal transduction, greatly broadens our interest and view on the significance of these proteins. Furthermore, the marked regulation of BCL-2 family function by numerous transcriptional and posttranslational pathways suggests that the total cellular signaling environment must be integrated to better understand the influence of BCL-2 proteins on all the pathways in the context of the immune system. Indeed, continuing effort to understand the BCL-2 family promises further insights into the complexity of cellular life and death.

Acknowledgments

We would like to thank everyone in the Chipuk Laboratory for their assistance and support. This work was supported by NIH CA157740 (to J.E.C.), the JJR Foundation (to J.E.C.), the William A. Spivak Fund (to J.E.C.), and the Fridolin Charitable Trust (to J.E.C.). This work was also supported in part by Research Grant 5-FY11–74 from the March of Dimes Foundation (to J.E.C.).

Conflicts of interest

The authors declare no conflicts of interest.

References

1. Meier, P., A. Finch & G. Evan. 2000. Apoptosis in development. *Nature* **407:** 796–801.

2. Sprent, J. & D.F. Tough. 2001. T cell death and memory. *Science* **293:** 245–248.

3. Murphy, K. 2011. Janeway's Immunobiology (Immunobiology: the Immune System). 8th ed. New York: Garland Science.

4. Huse, M. 2009. The T-cell-receptor signaling network. *J. Cell. Sci.* **122**(Pt 9)**:** 1269–1273.

5. Zemlin, M., R.L. Schelonka, K. Bauer & H.W. Schroeder Jr. 2002. Regulation and chance in the ontogeny of B and T cell antigen receptor repertoires. *Immunol. Res.* **26:** 265–278.

6. Opferman, J.T. 2007. Life and death during hematopoietic differentiation. *Curr. Opin. Immunol.* **19:** 497–502.

7. Hernandez, J.B., R.H. Newton & C.M. Walsh. 2010. Life and death in the thymus—cell death signaling during T cell development. *Curr. Opin. Cell. Biol.* **22:** 865–871.

8. Corfe, S.A. & C.J. Paige. 2012. The many roles of IL-7 in B cell development; mediator of survival, proliferation and differentiation. *Semin. Immunol.* **24:** 198–208.

9. Hardy, R.R. & K. Hayakawa. 2001. B cell development pathways. *Annu. Rev. Immunol.* **19:** 595–621.

10. Häcker, G. 2000. The morphology of apoptosis. *Cell. Tissue Res.* **301:** 5–17.

11. Fadok, V.A. 1999. Clearance: the last and often forgotten stage of apoptosis. *J. Mammary Gland. Biol. Neoplasia.* **4:** 203–211.

12. Tsujimoto, Y., J. Cossman, E. Jaffe & C.M. Croce. 1985. Involvement of the bcl-2 gene in human follicular lymphoma. *Science* **228:** 1440–1443.

13. Vaux, D.L., S. Cory & J.M. Adams. 1988. Bcl-2 gene promotes haemopoietic cell survival and cooperates with c-myc to immortalize pre-B cells. *Nature* **335:** 440–442.

14. Egle, A., A.W. Harris, P. Bouillet & S. Cory. 2004. Bim is a suppressor of Myc-induced mouse B cell leukemia. *Proc. Natl. Acad. Sci. U.S.A.* **101:** 6164–6169.

15. Hemann, M.T., A. Bric, J. Teruya-Feldstein, *et al.* 2005. Evasion of the p53 tumour surveillance network by tumour-derived MYC mutants. *Nature* **436:** 807–811.

16. Hipfner, D.R. & S.M. Cohen. 2004. Connecting proliferation and apoptosis in development and disease. *Nat. Rev. Mol. Cell Biol.* **5:** 805–815.

17. Cheng, E.H., M.C. Wei, S. Weiler, *et al.* 2001. BCL-2, BCL-X(L) sequester BH3 domain-only molecules preventing BAX- and BAK-mediated mitochondrial apoptosis. *Mol. Cell* **8:** 705–711.

18. Certo, M., V.D.G. Moore, M. Nishino, *et al.* 2006. Mitochondria primed by death signals determine cellular addiction to antiapoptotic BCL-2 family members. *Cancer Cell* **9:** 351–365.

19. Liu, X., C.N. Kim, J. Yang, *et al.* 1996. Induction of apoptotic program in cell-free extracts: requirement for dATP and cytochrome c. *Cell* **86:** 147–157.

20. Kluck, R.M., E. Bossy-Wetzel, D.R. Green & D.D. Newmeyer. 1997. The release of cytochrome c from mitochondria: a primary site for Bcl-2 regulation of apoptosis. *Science* **275:** 1132–1136.

21. Chipuk, J.E. & D.R. Green. 2008. How do BCL-2 proteins induce mitochondrial outer membrane permeabilization? *Trends Cell Biol.* **18:** 157–164.

22. Kuwana, T., M.R. Mackey, G. Perkins, *et al.* 2002. Bid, Bax, and lipids cooperate to form supramolecular openings in the outer mitochondrial membrane. *Cell* **111:** 331–342.

23. Chipuk, J.E., G.P. McStay, A. Bharti, *et al.* 2012. Sphingolipid Metabolism Cooperates with BAK and BAX to Promote the Mitochondrial Pathway of Apoptosis. *Cell* **148:** 988–1000.

24. Ke, F., A. Voss, J.B. Kerr, *et al.* 2012. BCL-2 family member BOK is widely expressed but its loss has only minimal impact in mice. *Cell Death Differ.* **19:** 915–925.

25. Sattler, M., H. Liang, D. Nettesheim, *et al.* 1997. Structure of Bcl-xL-Bak peptide complex: recognition between regulators of apoptosis. *Science* **275:** 983–986.

26. Gavathiotis, E., M. Suzuki, M.L. Davis, *et al.* 2008. BAX activation is initiated at a novel interaction site. *Nature* **455:** 1076–1081.

27. George, N.M., J.J.D. Evans, X. Luo. 2007. A three-helix homo-oligomerization domain containing BH3 and BH1 is responsible for the apoptotic activity of Bax. *Genes. Dev.* **21:** 1937–1948.

28. Dewson, G., T. Kratina, H.W. Sim, *et al.* 2008. To trigger apoptosis, Bak exposes its BH3 domain and homodimerizes via BH3: groove interactions. *Mol. Cell* **30:** 369–380.

29. Dewson, G., T. Kratina, P. Czabotar, *et al.* 2009. Bak activation for apoptosis involves oligomerization of dimers via their alpha6 helices. *Mol. Cell* **36:** 696–703.

30. Yin, X.M., Z.N. Oltvai & S.J. Korsmeyer. 1994. BH1 and BH2 domains of Bcl-2 are required for inhibition of apoptosis and heterodimerization with Bax. *Nature* **369:** 321–323.

31. Sedlak, T.W., Z.N. Oltvai, E. Yang, *et al.* 1995. Multiple Bcl-2 family members demonstrate selective dimerizations with Bax. *Proc. Natl. Acad. Sci. USA* **92:** 7834–7838.

32. Meijerink, J.P., E.J. Mensink, K. Wang, *et al.* 1998. Hematopoietic malignancies demonstrate loss-of-function mutations of BAX. *Blood* **91:** 2991–2997.

33. Strasser, A., A.W. Harris & S. Cory. 1991. bcl-2 transgene inhibits T cell death and perturbs thymic self-censorship. *Cell* **67:** 889–899.

34. Strasser, A., S. Whittingham, D.L. Vaux, *et al.* 1991. Enforced BCL2 expression in B-lymphoid cells prolongs antibody responses and elicits autoimmune disease. *Proc. Natl. Acad. Sci. USA* **88:** 8661–8665.

35. Veis, D.J., C.M. Sorenson, J.R. Shutter & S.J. Korsmeyer. 1993. Bcl-2-deficient mice demonstrate fulminant lymphoid apoptosis, polycystic kidneys, and hypopigmented hair. *Cell* **75:** 229–240.

36. Veis, D.J., C.L. Sentman, E.A. Bach & S.J. Korsmeyer. 1993. Expression of the Bcl-2 protein in murine and human thymocytes and in peripheral T lymphocytes. *J. Immunol.* **151:** 2546–2554.

37. Nuñez, G., D. Hockenbery, T.J. McDonnell, *et al.* 1991. Bcl-2 maintains B cell memory. *Nature* **353:** 71–73.

38. Bouillet, P., D. Metcalf, D.C. Huang, *et al.* 1999. Proapoptotic Bcl-2 relative Bim required for certain apoptotic

responses, leukocyte homeostasis, and to preclude autoimmunity. *Science* **286:** 1735–1738.

39. Nakayama, K., K. Nakayama, I. Negishi, *et al.* 1993. Disappearance of the lymphoid system in Bcl-2 homozygous mutant chimeric mice. *Science* **261:** 1584–1588.

40. Bouillet, P., S. Cory, L.C. Zhang, *et al.* 2001. Degenerative disorders caused by Bcl-2 deficiency prevented by loss of its BH3-only antagonist Bim. *Dev. Cell* **1:** 645–653.

41. Bouillet, P., J.F. Purton, D.I. Godfrey, *et al.* 2002. BH3-only Bcl-2 family member Bim is required for apoptosis of autoreactive thymocytes. *Nature* **415:** 922–926.

42. Mérino, D., M. Giam, P.D. Hughes, *et al.* 2009. The role of BH3-only protein Bim extends beyond inhibiting Bcl-2–like prosurvival proteins. *J. Cell Biol.* **186:** 355–362.

43. Mérino, D. & P. Bouillet. 2009. The Bcl-2 family in autoimmune and degenerative disorders. *Apoptosis* **14:** 570–583.

44. Kirschnek, S., S. Ying, S.F. Fischer, *et al.* 2005. Phagocytosis-Induced Apoptosis in Macrophages Is Mediated by Up-Regulation and Activation of the Bcl-2 Homology Domain 3-Only Protein Bim. *J. Immunol.* **174:** 671–679.

45. Rinkenberger, J.L., S. Horning, B. Klocke, *et al.* 2000. Mcl-1 deficiency results in peri-implantation embryonic lethality. *Genes. Dev.* **14:** 23–27.

46. Opferman, J.T., A. Letai, C. Beard, *et al.* 2003. Development and maintenance of B and T lymphocytes requires antiapoptotic MCL-1. *Nature* **426:** 671–676.

47. Campbell, K.J., D.H.D. Gray, N. Anstee, *et al.* 2012. Elevated Mcl-1 inhibits thymocyte apoptosis and alters thymic selection. *Cell Death Differ.* **19:** 1962–1971.

48. Vikstrom, I., S. Carotta, K. Lüthje, *et al.* 2010. Mcl-1 is essential for germinal center formation and B cell memory. *Science* **330:** 1095–1099.

49. Opferman, J.T., H. Iwasaki, C.C. Ong, *et al.* 2005. Obligate role of anti-apoptotic MCL-1 in the survival of hematopoietic stem cells. *Science* **307:** 1101–1104.

50. Dzhagalov, I., A.S. John & Y-W. He. 2007. The antiapoptotic protein Mcl-1 is essential for the survival of neutrophils but not macrophages. *Blood* **109:** 1620–1626.

51. Glaser, S.P., E.F. Lee, E. Trounson, *et al.* 2012. Antiapoptotic Mcl-1 is essential for the development and sustained growth of acute myeloid leukemia. *Genes. Dev.* **26:** 120–125.

52. Mandal, M., C. Borowski, T. Palomero, *et al.* 2005. The BCL2A1 gene as a pre–T cell receptor–induced regulator of thymocyte survival. *J. Exp. Med.* **201:** 603–614.

53. Hamasaki, A., F. Sendo, K. Nakayama, *et al.* 1998. Accelerated neutrophil apoptosis in mice lacking A1-a, a subtype of the bcl-2–related A1 gene. *J. Exp. Med.* **188:** 1985–1992.

54. Ma, A., J.C. Pena, B. Chang, *et al.* 1995. Bclx regulates the survival of double-positive thymocytes. *Proc. Natl. Acad. Sci. U.S.A.* **92:** 4763–4767.

55. Lindsten, T., A.J. Ross, A. King, *et al.* 2000. The combined functions of proapoptotic Bcl-2 family members bak and bax are essential for normal development of multiple tissues. *Mol. Cell.* **6:** 1389–1399.

56. Renault, T.T. & S. Manon. 2011. Bax: addressed to kill. *Biochimie* **93:** 1379–1391.

57. Knudson, C.M., K.S. Tung, W.G. Tourtellotte, *et al.* 1995. Bax-deficient mice with lymphoid hyperplasia and male germ cell death. *Science* **270:** 96–99.

58. Rathmell, J.C., T. Lindsten, W-X. Zong, *et al.* 2002. Deficiency in Bak and Bax perturbs thymic selection and lymphoid homeostasis. *Nat. Immunol.* **3:** 932–939.

59. Hsu, S.Y., A. Kaipia, E. McGee, *et al.* 1997. Bok is a proapoptotic Bcl-2 protein with restricted expression in reproductive tissues and heterodimerizes with selective antiapoptotic Bcl-2 family members. *Proc. Natl. Acad. Sci. U.S.A.* **94:** 12401–12406.

60. Michalak, E.M., E.S. Jansen, L. Happo, *et al.* 2009. Puma and to a lesser extent Noxa are suppressors of Myc-induced lymphomagenesis. *Cell Death Differ.* **16:** 684–696.

61. Elgendy, M., C. Sheridan, G. Brumatti & S.J. Martin. 2011. Oncogenic Ras-induced expression of Noxa and Beclin-1 promotes autophagic cell death and limits clonogenic survival. *Mol. Cell* **42:** 23–35.

62. Villunger, A., C. Scott, P. Bouillet & A. Strasser. 2003. Essential role for the BH3-only protein Bim but redundant roles for Bax, Bcl-2, and Bcl-w in the control of granulocyte survival. *Blood* **101:** 2393–2400.

63. Kirschnek, S., J. Vier, S. Gautam, *et al.* 2011. Molecular analysis of neutrophil spontaneous apoptosis reveals a strong role for the pro-apoptotic BH3-only protein Noxa. *Cell Death Differ.* **18:** 1805–1814.

64. Garrison, S.P., D.C. Phillips, J.R. Jeffers, *et al.* 2012. Genetically defining the mechanism of Puma- and Bim-induced apoptosis. *Cell Death Differ.* **19:** 642–649.

65. Erlacher, M., V. Labi, C. Manzl, *et al.* 2006. Puma cooperates with Bim, the rate-limiting BH3-only protein in cell death during lymphocyte development, in apoptosis induction. *J. Exp. Med.* **203:** 2939–2951.

66. Villunger, A., E.M. Michalak, L. Coultas, *et al.* 2003. p53- and drug-induced apoptotic responses mediated by BH3-only proteins puma and noxa. *Science* **302:** 1036–1038.

67. Gray, D.H.D., F. Kupresanin, S.P. Berzins, *et al.* 2012. The BH3-only proteins Bim and Puma cooperate to impose deletional tolerance of organ-specific antigens. *Immunity* **37:** 451–462.

68. Zhan, Y., Y. Zhang, D. Gray, *et al.* 2011. Defects in the Bcl-2-regulated apoptotic pathway lead to preferential increase of CD25 low Foxp3+ anergic CD4+ T cells. *J. Immunol.* **187:** 1566–1577.

69. Labi V, M. Erlacher, S. Kiessling, *et al.* 2008. Loss of the BH3-only protein Bmf impairs B cell homeostasis and accelerates γ irradiation–induced thymic lymphoma development. *J. Exp. Med.* **205:** 641–655.

70. Ploner, C., J. Rainer, H. Niederegger, *et al.* 2008. The BCL2 rheostat in glucocorticoid-induced apoptosis of acute lymphoblastic leukemia. *Leukemia* **22:** 370–377.

71. Baumgartner, F., C. Woess, V. Pedit, *et al.* 2012. Minor cell-death defects but reduced tumor latency in mice lacking the BH3-only proteins Bad and Bmf. Mar 19. DOI: 10.1038/onc.2012.78. [Epub ahead of print].

72. Siebenlist, U., K. Brown & E. Claudio. 2005. Control of lymphocyte development by nuclear factor-kappaB. *Nat. Rev. Immunol.* **5:** 435–445.

73. Hayden, M.S., A.P. West, S. Ghosh. 2006. NF-kappaB and the immune response. *Oncogene* **25:** 6758–6780.

74. Kucharczak, J., M.J. Simmons, Y. Fan & C. Gélinas. 2003. To be, or not to be: NF-kappaB is the answer–role of Rel/NF-kappaB in the regulation of apoptosis. *Oncogene* **22:** 8961–8982.

75. Voll, R.E., E. Jimi, R.J. Phillips, *et al.* 2000. NF-kappa B activation by the pre-T cell receptor serves as a selective survival signal in T lymphocyte development. *Immunity* **13:** 677–689.

76. Zheng, Y., M. Vig, J. Lyons, *et al.* 2003. Combined deficiency of p50 and cRel in CD4+ T cells reveals an essential requirement for nuclear factor κB in regulating mature T cell survival and in vivo function. *J. Exp. Med.* **197:** 861–874.

77. Miyashita, T. & J.C. Reed. 1995. Tumor suppressor p53 is a direct transcriptional activator of the human bax gene. *Cell* **80:** 293–299.

78. Oda, E., R. Ohki, H. Murasawa, *et al.* 2000. Noxa, a BH3-only member of the Bcl-2 family and candidate mediator of p53-induced apoptosis. *Science* **288:** 1053–1058.

79. Nakano, K. & K.H. Vousden. 2001. PUMA, a novel proapoptotic gene, is induced by p53. *Mol. Cell* **7:** 683–694.

80. Mathai, J.P., M. Germain, R.C. Marcellus & G.C. Shore. 2002. Induction and endoplasmic reticulum location of BIK/NBK in response to apoptotic signaling by E1A and p53. *Oncogene* **21:** 2534–2544.

81. Sax, J.K., P. Fei, M.E. Murphy, *et al.* 2002. BID regulation by p53 contributes to chemosensitivity. *Nat. Cell Biol.* **4:** 842–849.

82. Miyashita, T., S. Krajewski, M. Krajewska, *et al.* 1994. Tumor suppressor p53 is a regulator of bcl-2 and bax gene expression in vitro and in vivo. *Oncogene* **9:** 1799–1805.

83. Chipuk, J.E., T. Kuwana, L. Bouchier-Hayes, *et al.* 2004. Direct activation of Bax by p53 mediates mitochondrial membrane permeabilization and apoptosis. *Science* **303:** 1010–1014.

84. Leu, JI-J., P. Dumont, M. Hafey, *et al.* 2004. Mitochondrial p53 activates Bak and causes disruption of a Bak-Mcl1 complex. *Nat. Cell Biol.* **6:** 443–450.

85. Mihara, M., S. Erster, A. Zaika, *et al.* 2003. p53 has a direct apoptogenic role at the mitochondria. *Mol. Cell* **11:** 577–590.

86. Stadanlick, J.E., Z. Zhang, S-Y. Lee, *et al.* 2011. Developmental arrest of T cells in Rpl22-deficient mice is dependent upon multiple p53 effectors. *J. Immunol.* **187:** 664–675.

87. Mitchell, K.O., M.S. Ricci, T. Miyashita, *et al.* 2000. Bax is a transcriptional target and mediator of c-myc-induced apoptosis. *Cancer Res.* **60:** 6318–6325.

88. Eischen, C.M., D. Woo, M.F. Roussel & J.L. Cleveland. 2001. Apoptosis triggered by Myc-induced suppression of Bcl-XL or Bcl-2 is bypassed during lymphomagenesis. *Mol. Cell Biol.* **21:** 5063–5070.

89. Dijkers, P.F., R.H. Medema, J.W. Lammers, *et al.* 2000. Expression of the pro-apoptotic Bcl-2 family member Bim is regulated by the forkhead transcription factor FKHR-L1. *Curr. Biol.* **10:** 1201–1204.

90. Jurado, S., K. Gleeson, K. O'Donnell, *et al.* 2012. The Zinc-finger protein ASCIZ regulates B cell development via DYNLL1 and Bim. *J. Exp. Med.* **209:** 1629–1639.

91. Milot, E. & J.G. Filep. 2011. Regulation of neutrophil survival/apoptosis by Mcl-1. *Sci. World J.* **11:** 1948–1962.

92. Allen, J.C., F. Talab, M. Zuzel, *et al.* 2011. c-Abl regulates Mcl-1 gene expression in chronic lymphocytic leukemia cells. *Blood* **117:** 2414–2422.

93. O'Connor, L., A. Strasser, L.A. O'Reilly, *et al.* 1998. Bim: a novel member of the Bcl-2 family that promotes apoptosis. *EMBO J.* **17:** 384–395.

94. Adachi, M., X. Zhao & K. Imai. 2005. Nomenclature of dynein light chain-linked BH3-only protein Bim isoforms. *Cell Death and Differen.* **12:** 192–193.

95. Liu, L., J. Chen, J. Zhang, *et al.* 2007. Overexpression of BimSs3, the novel isoform of Bim, can trigger cell apoptosis by inducing cytochrome c release from mitochondria. *Acta Biochim. Pol.* **54:** 603–610.

96. Boise, L.H., M. Gonzalez-Garcia, C.E. Postema, *et al.* 1993. Bcl-x, a bcl-2-related gene that functions as a dominant regulator of apoptotic cell death. *Cell* **74:** 597–608.

97. Oltvai, Z.N., C.L. Milliman & S.J. Korsmeyer. 1993. Bcl-2 heterodimerizes in vivo with a conserved homolog, Bax, that accelerates programmed cell death. *Cell* **74:** 609–619.

98. Otake, Y., S. Soundararajan, T.K. Sengupta, *et al.* 2007 Overexpression of nucleolin in chronic lymphocytic leukemia cells induces stabilization of bcl2 mRNA. *Blood* **109:** 3069–3075.

99. Ventura, A., A.G. Young, M.M. Winslow, *et al.* 2008. Targeted deletion reveals essential and overlapping functions of the miR-17~92 family of miRNA clusters. *Cell* **132:** 875–886.

100. Cimmino, A., G.A. Calin, M. Fabbri, *et al.* 2005. miR-15 and miR-16 induce apoptosis by targeting BCL2. *Proc. Natl. Acad. Sci. USA* **102:** 13944–13949.

101. Calin, G.A., A. Cimmino, M. Fabbri, *et al.* 2008. MiR-15a and miR-16–1 cluster functions in human leukemia. *Proc. Natl. Acad. Sci. USA.* **105:** 5166–5171.

102. Wu, Z., H. Lu, J. Sheng & L. Li. 2012. Inductive microRNA-21 impairs anti-mycobacterial responses by targeting IL-12 and Bcl-2. *FEBS Letters* [Internet]. Available from: http://www.sciencedirect.com/science/article/pii/S0014579312004681 [accessed on 23 July 2012].

103. Lindsay, M.A. 2008. microRNAs and the immune response. *Trends Immunol.* **29:** 343–351.

104. Lima, R.T., S. Busacca, G.M. Almeida, *et al.* 2011. MicroRNA regulation of core apoptosis pathways in cancer. *Eur. J. Cancer* **47:** 163–174.

105. Deng, X., P. Ruvolo, B. Carr & W.S. May. 2000. Survival function of ERK1/2 as IL-3-activated, staurosporine-resistant Bcl2 kinases. *Proc. Natl. Acad. Sci. USA* **97:** 1578–1583.

106. Yamamoto, K., H. Ichijo & S.J. Korsmeyer. 1999. BCL-2 is phosphorylated and inactivated by an ASK1/Jun

N-terminal protein kinase pathway normally activated at G2/M. *Mol. Cell Biol.* **19:** 8469–8478.

107. Deng, X., F. Gao, T. Flagg & W.S. May. 2004. Mono- and multisite phosphorylation enhances Bcl2's antiapoptotic function and inhibition of cell cycle entry functions. *Proc. Natl. Acad. Sci. USA* **101:** 153–158.

108. Dimmeler, S., K. Breitschopf, J. Haendeler & A.M. Zeiher. 1999. Dephosphorylation targets Bcl-2 for ubiquitin-dependent degradation: a link between the apoptosome and the proteasome pathway. *J. Exp. Med.* **1189:** 1815–1822.

109. Breitschopf, K., J. Haendeler, P. Malchow, *et al.* 2000. Posttranslational modification of Bcl-2 facilitates its proteasome-dependent degradation: molecular characterization of the involved signaling pathway. *Mol. Cell. Biol.* **20:** 1886–1896.

110. Wang, Y-Y, X. Deng, L. Xu, *et al.* 2008. Bcl2 enhances induced hematopoietic differentiation of murine embryonic stem cells. *Exp. Hematol.* **36:** 128–139.

111. Luciano, F., A. Jacquel, P. Colosetti, *et al.* 2003. Phosphorylation of Bim-EL by Erk1/2 on serine 69 promotes its degradation via the proteasome pathway and regulates its proapoptotic function. *Oncogene* **22:** 6785–6793.

112. Ley, R., K.E. Ewings, K. Hadfield, *et al.* 2004. Extracellular signal-regulated kinases 1/2 are serum-stimulated "BimEL kinases" that bind to the BH3-only protein BimEL causing its phosphorylation and turnover. *J. Biol. Chem.* **279:** 8837–8847.

113. O'Reilly, L.A., E.A. Kruse, H. Puthalakath, *et al.* 2009. MEK/ERK-mediated phosphorylation of bim is required to ensure survival of T and B lymphocytes during mitogenic stimulation. *J. Immunol.* **183:** 261–269.

114. Paterson, A., C.I. Mockridge, J.E. Adams, *et al.* 2012. Mechanisms and clinical significance of BIM phosphorylation in chronic lymphocytic leukemia. *Blood* **119:** 1726–1736.

115. Lizcano, J.M., N. Morrice & P. Cohen. 2000. Regulation of BAD by cAMP-dependent protein kinase is mediated via phosphorylation of a novel site, Ser155. *Biochem. J.* **349**(Pt 2): 547–557.

116. Virdee, K., P.A. Parone & A.M. Tolkovsky. 2000. Phosphorylation of the pro-apoptotic protein BAD on serine 155, a novel site, contributes to cell survival. *Curr. Biol.* **10:** 1151–1154.

117. Tan, Y., M.R. Demeter, H. Ruan & M.J. Comb. 2000. BAD Ser-155 phosphorylation regulates BAD/Bcl-XL interaction and cell survival. *J. Biol. Chem.* **275:** 25865–25869.

118. Harada, H., B. Becknell, M. Wilm, *et al.* 1999. Phosphorylation and inactivation of BAD by mitochondria-anchored protein kinase A. *Mol. Cell* **3:** 413–422.

119. Datta, S.R., H. Dudek, X. Tao, *et al.* 1997. Akt phosphorylation of BAD couples survival signals to the cell-intrinsic death machinery. *Cell* **91:** 231–241.

120. Li, H., H. Zhu, C.J. Xu & J. Yuan. 1998. Cleavage of BID by caspase 8 mediates the mitochondrial damage in the Fas pathway of apoptosis. *Cell* **94:** 491–501.

121. Zha, J., S. Weiler, K.J. Oh, *et al.* 2000. Posttranslational N-myristoylation of BID as a molecular switch for targeting mitochondria and apoptosis. *Science* **290:** 1761–1765.

122. Lovell, J.F., L.P. Billen, S. Bindner, *et al.* 2008. Membrane binding by tBid initiates an ordered series of events culminating in membrane permeabilization by Bax. *Cell* **135:** 1074–1084.

123. Boya, P., K. Andreau, D. Poncet, *et al.* 2003. Lysosomal membrane permeabilization induces cell death in a mitochondrion-dependent fashion. *J. Exp. Med.* **197:** 1323–1334.

124. Chen, M., H. He, S. Zhan, *et al.* 2001. Bid is cleaved by calpain to an active fragment in vitro and during myocardial ischemia/reperfusion. *J. Biol. Chem* **276:** 30724–30728.

125. Stoka, V., B. Turk, S.L. Schendel, *et al.* 2001. Lysosomal protease pathways to apoptosis. Cleavage of bid, not procaspases, is the most likely route. *J. Biol. Chem.* **276:** 3149–31457.

126. Cirman, T., K. Oresić, G.D. Mazovec, *et al.* 2004. Selective disruption of lysosomes in HeLa cells triggers apoptosis mediated by cleavage of Bid by multiple papain-like lysosomal cathepsins. *J. Biol. Chem.* **279:** 3578–3587.

127. Sutton, V.R., J.E. Davis, M. Cancilla, *et al.* 2000. Initiation of apoptosis by granzyme B requires direct cleavage of bid, but not direct granzyme B-mediated caspase activation. *J. Exp. Med.* **192:** 1403–1414.

128. Campbell, K.J., M.L. Bath, M.L. Turner, *et al.* 2010. Elevated Mcl-1 perturbs lymphopoiesis, promotes transformation of hematopoietic stem/progenitor cells, and enhances drug resistance. *Blood* **116:** 3197–3207.

129. Michels, J., J.W. O'Neill, C.L. Dallman, *et al.* 2004. Mcl-1 is required for Akata6 B-lymphoma cell survival and is converted to a cell death molecule by efficient caspase-mediated cleavage. *Oncogene* **23:** 4818–4827.

130. Cheng, E.H., D.G. Kirsch, *et al.* 1997. Conversion of Bcl-2 to a Bax-like death effector by caspases. *Science* **278:** 1966–1968.

131. Clem, R.J., E.H. Cheng, C.L. Karp, *et al.* 1998. Modulation of cell death by Bcl-XL through caspase interaction. *Proc. Natl. Acad. Sci. U.S.A.* **95:** 554–559.

132. Kirsch, D.G., A. Doseff, B.N. Chau, *et al.* 1999. Caspase-3-dependent cleavage of Bcl-2 promotes release of cytochrome c. *J. Biol. Chem.* **274:** 21155–21161.

133. Basañez, G., J. Zhang, B.N. Chau, *et al.* 2001. Pro-apoptotic cleavage products of Bcl-xL form cytochrome c-conducting pores in pure lipid membranes. *J. Biol. Chem.* **276:** 31083–31091.

134. Robinson, N.E. & A.B. Robinson. 2001. Molecular clocks. *Proc. Natl. Acad. Sci. USA* **98:** 944–949.

135. Deverman, B.E., B.L. Cook, S.R. Manson, *et al.* 2002. Bcl-xL deamidation is a critical switch in the regulation of the response to DNA damage. *Cell* **111:** 51–62.

136. Zhao, R., D. Oxley, T.S. Smith, *et al.* 2007. DNA damage-induced Bcl-xL deamidation is mediated by NHE-1 antiport regulated intracellular pH. *PLoS Biol.* **5:** e1.

137. Zhao, R., F.T. Yang, D.R. Alexander. 2004. An oncogenic tyrosine kinase inhibits DNA repair and

DNA-damage-induced Bcl-xL deamidation in T cell transformation. *Cancer Cell* **5**: 37–49.

138. Zhao, R., G.A. Follows, P.A. Beer, *et al.* 2008. Inhibition of the Bcl-xL deamidation pathway in myeloproliferative disorders. *N. Engl. J. Med.* **359**: 2778–2789.

139. Shimada, K., T.R. Crother, J. Karlin, *et al.* 2012. Oxidized mitochondrial DNA activates the NLRP3 inflammasome during apoptosis. *Immunity* **36**: 401–414.

140. Faustin, B., Y. Chen, D. Zhai, *et al.* 2009. Mechanism of Bcl-2 and Bcl-X(L) inhibition of NLRP1 inflammasome: loop domain-dependent suppression of ATP binding and oligomerization. *Proc. Natl. Acad. Sci. U.S.A.* **106**: 3935–3940.

141. Yeretssian, G., R.G. Correa, K. Doiron, *et al.* 2011. Non-apoptotic role of BID in inflammation and innate immunity. *Nature* **474**: 96–99.

142. Guo, J.Y., Chen H-Y, R. Mathew, *et al.* 2011. Activated Ras requires autophagy to maintain oxidative metabolism and tumorigenesis. *Genes. Dev.* **25**: 460–470.

143. Mathew, R. & E. White. 2011. Autophagy in tumorigenesis and energy metabolism: friend by day, foe by night. *Curr. Opin. Genet. Dev.* **21**: 113–119.

144. Kuballa, P., W.M. Nolte, A.B. Castoreno & R.J. Xavier. 2012. Autophagy and the immune system. *Annu. Rev. Immunol.* **30**: 611–646.

145. Liang, X.H., L.K. Kleeman, H.H. Jiang, *et al.* 1998. Protection against fatal Sindbis virus encephalitis by beclin, a novel Bcl-2-interacting protein. *J. Virol.* **72**: 8586–8596.

146. Pattingre, S., A. Tassa, X. Qu, *et al.* 2005. Bcl-2 antiapoptotic proteins inhibit Beclin 1-dependent autophagy. *Cell* **122**: 927–939.

147. Maiuri, M.C., G. Le Toumelin, A. Criollo, *et al.* 2007. Functional and physical interaction between Bcl-X(L) and a BH3-like domain in Beclin-1. *EMBO J.* **26**: 2527–2539.

148. Maiuri, M.C., A. Criollo, E. Tasdemir, *et al.* 2007. BH3-only proteins and BH3 mimetics induce autophagy by competitively disrupting the interaction between Beclin 1 and Bcl-2/Bcl-X(L). *Autophagy* **3**: 374–376.

149. Priault, M., E. Hue, F. Marhuenda, *et al.* 2010. Differential dependence on Beclin 1 for the regulation of pro-survival autophagy by Bcl-2 and Bcl-xL in HCT116 colorectal cancer cells. *PLoS One* **5**: e8755.

150. Okamoto, K. & J.M. Shaw. 2005. Mitochondrial morphology and dynamics in yeast and multicellular eukaryotes. *Annu. Rev. Genet.* **39**: 503–536.

151. Martinou, J-C. & R.J. Youle. 2011. Mitochondria in apoptosis: Bcl-2 family members and mitochondrial dynamics. *Dev. Cell* **21**: 92–101.

152. Karbowski, M., K.L. Norris, M.M. Cleland, *et al.* 2006. Role of Bax and Bak in mitochondrial morphogenesis. *Nature* **443**: 658–662.

153. Cleland, M.M., K.L. Norris, M. Karbowski, *et al.* 2011. Bcl-2 family interaction with the mitochondrial morphogenesis machinery. *Cell Death Differ.* **18**: 235–247.

154. Hoppins, S., F. Edlich, M.M. Cleland, *et al.* 2011. The soluble form of Bax regulates mitochondrial fusion via MFN2 homotypic complexes. *Mol. Cell* **41**: 150–160.

155. Delivani, P., C. Adrain, R.C. Taylor, *et al.* 2006. Role for CED-9 and Egl-1 as regulators of mitochondrial fission and fusion dynamics. *Molecular Cell* **21**: 761–773.

156. Campello, S., R.A. Lacalle, M. Bettella, *et al.* 2006. Orchestration of lymphocyte chemotaxis by mitochondrial dynamics. *J. Exp. Med.* **203**: 2879–2886.

157. Baixauli, F., N.B. Martín-Cófreces, G. Morlino, *et al.* 2011. The mitochondrial fission factor dynamin-related protein 1 modulates T-cell receptor signalling at the immune synapse. *EMBO J.* **30**: 1238–1250.

158. Wang, R., C.P. Dillon, L.Z. Shi, *et al.* 2011. The transcription factor Myc controls metabolic reprogramming upon T lymphocyte activation. *Immunity* **35**: 871–882.

159. Caro, P., A.U. Kishan, E. Norberg, *et al.* 2012. Metabolic signatures uncover distinct targets in molecular subsets of diffuse large B cell lymphoma. *Cancer Cell* **22**: 547–560.

160. Perciavalle, R.M., D.P. Stewart, B. Koss, *et al.* 2012. Anti-apoptotic MCL-1 localizes to the mitochondrial matrix and couples mitochondrial fusion to respiration. *Nat. Cell Biol.* **14**: 575–583.

161. Chen, Z.X. & S. Pervaiz. 2010. Involvement of cytochrome c oxidase subunits Va and Vb in the regulation of cancer cell metabolism by Bcl-2. *Cell Death Differ.* **17**: 408–420.

162. Hockenbery, D.M., Z.N. Oltvai, X-M. Yin, *et al.* 1993. Bcl-2 functions in an antioxidant pathway to prevent apoptosis. *Cell* **75**: 241–251.

163. Imahashi, K., M.D. Schneider, C. Steenbergen & E. Murphy. 2004. Transgenic expression of Bcl-2 modulates energy metabolism, prevents cytosolic acidification during ischemia, and reduces ischemia/reperfusion injury. *Circ. Res.* **95**: 734–741.

164. Danial, N.N., L.D. Walensky, C-Y. Zhang, *et al.* 2008. Dual role of proapoptotic BAD in insulin secretion and beta cell survival. *Nat. Med.* **14**: 144–153.

165. Guicciardi, M.E. & G.J. Gores. 2009. Life and death by death receptors. *FASEB J.* **23**: 1625–1637.

166. The UniProt Consortium. 2011. Reorganizing the protein space at the Universal Protein Resource (UniProt). *Nucleic Acids Res.* **40**: D71–D75.

167. Petros, A.M., D.G. Nettesheim, Y. Wang, *et al.* 2000. Rationale for Bcl-xL/Bad peptide complex formation from structure, mutagenesis, and biophysical studies. *Protein Sci.* **9**: 2528–2534.

168. Hinds, M.G., C. Smits, R. Fredericks-Short, *et al.* 2007. Bim, Bad and Bmf: intrinsically unstructured BH3-only proteins that undergo a localized conformational change upon binding to prosurvival Bcl-2 targets. *Cell Death Differ.* **14**: 128–136.

169. Billen, L.P., A. Shamas-Din & D.W. Andrews. 2009. Bid: a Bax-like BH3 protein. *Oncogene* **27**: S93–S104.

170. Yan, N. & Y. Shi. 2005. Mechanisms of apoptosis through structural biology. *Ann. Rev. Cell Dev. Biol.* **21**: 35–56.

171. Wang, K., X.M. Yin, D.T. Chao, *et al.* 1996. BID: a novel BH3 domain-only death agonist. *Genes. Dev.* **10**: 2859–2869.

172. Eskes, R., S. Desagher, B. Antonsson & J.C. Martinou. 2000. Bid induces the oligomerization and insertion of Bax into

the outer mitochondrial membrane. *Mol. Cell. Biol.* **20:** 929–935.

173. Cartron, P.-F., T. Gallenne, G. Bougras, *et al.* 2004. The first [alpha] helix of Bax plays a necessary role in its ligand-induced activation by the BH3-only proteins Bid and PUMA. *Mol. Cell* **16:** 807–818.

174. Kim, H., H-C. Tu, D. Ren, *et al.* 2009. Stepwise activation of BAX and BAK by tBID, BIM, and PUMA initiates mitochondrial apoptosis. *Mol. Cell* **36:** 487–499.

175. Jabbour, A.M., J.E. Heraud, C.P. Daunt, *et al.* 2009. Puma indirectly activates Bax to cause apoptosis in the absence of Bid or Bim. *Cell Death Differ.* **16:** 555–563.

Ann. N.Y. Acad. Sci. ISSN 0077-8923

ANNALS OF THE NEW YORK ACADEMY OF SCIENCES
Issue: *The Year in Immunology*

Control of inflammatory heart disease by CD4+ T cells

Jobert G. Barin and Daniela Čiháková

The Johns Hopkins University School of Medicine, Department of Pathology, Division of Immunology, Baltimore, Maryland

Address for correspondence: Daniela Čiháková, M.D., Ph.D., The Johns Hopkins University School of Medicine, Ross 648, 720 Rutland Ave., Baltimore, MD 21205. dcihako1@jhmi.edu

This review focuses on autoimmune myocarditis and its sequela, inflammatory dilated cardiomyopathy (DCMI), and the inflammatory and immune mechanisms underlying the pathogenesis of these diseases. Several mouse models of myocarditis and DCMI have improved our knowledge of the pathogenesis of these diseases, informing more general problems of cardiac remodeling and heart failure. CD4+ T cells are critical in driving the pathogenesis of myocarditis. We discuss in detail the role of T helper cell subtypes in the pathogenesis of myocarditis, the biology of T cell–derived effector cytokines, and the participation of other leukocytic effectors in mediating disease pathophysiology. We discuss interactions between these subsets in both suppressive and collaborative fashions. These findings indicate that cardiac inflammatory disease, and autoimmunity in general, may be more diverse in divergent effector mechanisms than has previously been appreciated.

Keywords: myocarditis; CD4+ T cells; Th17 cells; autoimmune disease; cytokines

Myocarditis and inflammatory dilated cardiomyopathy

Inflammation of the myocardium, myocarditis, is a highly heterogeneous disease, with the majority of cases associated with infectious agents, including bacterial, rickettsial, mycotic, protozoan, and viral pathogens.[1] However, in many cases of myocarditis, no infectious or toxic agent can be found to still be active. Evidence shows that this disease is autoimmune in nature, and patients benefit from immunosuppressive therapies.[2,3] The diagnosis of myocarditis is based on the presence of mononuclear infiltration and cardiomyocyte necrosis, using the Dallas criteria.[4–7] The American Heart Association, the American College of Cardiology, and the European Society of Cardiology summarized clinical scenarios when endomyocardial biopsy should be performed, and emphasized the usefulness of biopsy in establishing the diagnosis of myocarditis in certain clinical settings.[8] Based on the character of the heart infiltrate, different types of myocarditis are recognized, such as lymphocytic, borderline, granulomatous, giant cell, and eosinophilic.[9] It has been shown that around 9–16% of patients with myocarditis progress to inflammatory dilated cardiomyopathy (DCMI),[10,11] characterized by chronic left and right ventricular dilatation with normal or reduced left ventricular wall thickness, and impaired contraction. DCMI is the major cause of heart failure in individuals below the age of 40 and a major indication for cardiac transplantation. The 5-year survival rate of patients with DCM is less than 50%.[12]

Experimental myocarditis

Attempts to conclusively identify specific infectious pathogens as triggers of idiopathic myocarditis and DCMI have been largely unsuccessful in fulfilling Koch's postulates (a series of criteria used to determine whether a specific microbe is the cause of a given disease). However, several of these pathogens, viruses in particular, were shown to be associated with the presence of autoreactive T cells and antibodies. To validate a causative relationship between viral infection and the induction of cardiac autoimmunity, infection of experimental animals with these pathogens, including coxsackievirus B3 (CVB3), encephalomyocarditis virus (EMCV), and cytomegalovirus (CMV) to name a few, can result in chronic cardiomyopathy subsequent to the

doi: 10.1111/nyas.12134

Ann. N.Y. Acad. Sci. 1285 (2013) 80–96 © 2013 New York Academy of Sciences.

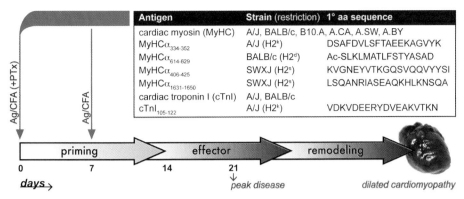

Antigen	Strain (restriction)	1° aa sequence
cardiac myosin (MyHC)	A/J, BALB/c, B10.A, A.CA, A.SW, A.BY	
MyHC$\alpha_{334-352}$	A/J (H2^k)	DSAFDVLSFTAEEKAGVYK
MyHC$\alpha_{614-629}$	BALB/c (H2^d)	Ac-SLKLMATLFSTYASAD
MyHC$\alpha_{406-425}$	SWXJ (H2^s)	KVGNEYVTKGQSVQQVYYSI
MyHC$\alpha_{1631-1650}$	SWXJ (H2^s)	LSQANRIASEAQKHLKNSQA
cardiac troponin I (cTnI)	A/J, BALB/c	
cTnI$_{105-122}$	A/J (H2^k)	VDKVDEERYDVEAKVTKN

Figure 1. Schematic representation of the induction of experimental autoimmune myocarditis (EAM). A subset of inbred mouse strains are susceptible to the induction of myocarditis.[14] Minimal synthetic peptides derived from the sequence of the known autoantigens have been described for some of these strains.[179–182] Antigen (Ag) is delivered with adjuvant, most commonly complete Freund's adjuvant (CFA), with optional pertussis toxin (PTx).[15]

clearance of viremia, depending on the background genetics of the host animal. In spite of these findings, evidence for infectious etiologies is often not apparent during clinical presentation; the presence of antimicrobial antibodies or a nonreplicating virus is not sufficient evidence to prove causation of myocarditis by infection.[13]

A key insight into the pathogenesis of this disease model came from adapting an autoimmunization model of priming with cardiac myosin that had demonstrated that the same strains of inbred mice are susceptible to postviral chronic myocarditis, indicating that the background genetics responsible for both diseases are similar, if not shared (Fig. 1).[14] This experimental autoimmunization model, termed experimental autoimmune myocarditis (EAM), has since served as a key model of autoimmune disease research.[15] EAM is induced by immunizing susceptible mice strains with cardiac myosin or myocarditogenic peptide derived from the α-cardiac myosin heavy chain emulsified in complete Freund's adjuvant (CFA). The disease process of EAM consists of three distinct phases: priming (days 0–10), during which cardiac inflammation is not yet apparent, but autoaggressive responses are being programmed; the effector phase, starting around day 10 when infiltration begins in the heart and peaking at day 21; and finally, DCMI is fully developed around days 60–65 (Fig. 1). By virtue of anatomy, the heart is not sequestered behind immunologic barriers, as is the central nervous system (CNS), retina, gonad, or joint synovium. Like these other models, EAM was shown to be depen-

dent on CD4$^+$ helper T cells. In now classic experiments, Smith et al.[16,17] demonstrated that depletion of CD4$^+$ T cells with monoclonal antibodies abolished the development of EAM. Similarly, transfer of CD4$^+$ T cells was sufficient to transfer EAM from primed donors to naive recipients.[16,17] Employing major histocompatibility complex (MHC) class II tetramer technology, CD4$^+$ T cells specific for cardiac myosin can be detected in the heart following infection CVB3.[18] Thus, CD4$^+$ T cells are both necessary and sufficient for the development of myocarditis. Similar work demonstrated more ambiguous roles for CD8$^+$ T and B cells in the pathogenesis of EAM.[19] It should be underscored that these data should not be taken as evidence that CD8$^+$ T and B cells do not contribute to the pathophysiology of this disease; only that their contributions are not as central or decisive as those mediated by CD4$^+$ T cells. Furthermore, the critical importance of CD4$^+$ T cells immediately implies that a cytokine product of these helper T (Th) cells is an essential mediator of the autoaggressive disease process. What is even more exciting is the notion that a soluble intracellular signaling protein as a key effector of disease would make such a putative candidate cytokine an attractive therapeutic target of newly emergent monoclonal antibody technology.

Th cell subsets and the development of myocarditis, a primer

The functional and phenotypic diversity of CD4$^+$ T cells were first characterized by the seminal work of Mosmann and Coffmann,[20] who demonstrated the segregation of production of interferon γ (IFN-γ) and interleukin (IL)-4 by CD4$^+$ T cells. Most importantly, Mosmann and Coffmann went on to demonstrate that IFN-γ and IL-4–producing CD4$^+$ T cells, subsequently termed Th1 and Th2 cells, conveyed critically different effector mechanisms in host defenses to infection with *Mycobacterium tuberculosis*, resulting in drastically different outcomes.[20] In the decades since, the Th1/Th2 model has come to predominate investigations of immunopathologic disease and host defense to infectious pathogens.

Key to this model was the insight that the development of the Th1 and Th2 programs was mutually antagonistic at a clonal level. Transcription factors have since been cloned that appear to control the lineage commitment programs of these cell subsets, and restrict the development of the alternate program. As discussed below, the diversity of these subsets has gained appreciation in recent years, with important implications for autoimmunity and other inflammatory disorders. However, issues of heterogeneity and plasticity among these subsets have complicated the original, elegant binary logic of the original Th1/Th2 model with respect to clinical application.

Th1 cells: paradoxes of interferon γ and interleukin 12

Originally identified by Mosmann and Coffmann[20] as IFN-γ–producing CD4$^+$ cells, Th1 cells are instructed by the proximal heterodimeric innate cytokine IL12p70 to express the transcription factor T-box expressed in T cells (Tbet), which enables lineage commitment to the Th1 program. Through IFN-γ signaling, Th1 cells are thought to have adapted to the clearance of viral or intracellular bacterial infections by eliciting effector responses from CD8α$^+$ cytotoxic T cells, natural killer (NK) cells, and a classical program of macrophage activation specialized for lysozomal killing of microbes.[20]

In many CD4$^+$-dependent autoimmune diseases and disease models, Th1 cells were prime candidates as the potential culprits. Investigations in animal models and patient cohorts have provided some circumstantial evidence that Th1 cells and IFN-γ mediate pathology in autoimmune disease. For example, IFN-γ has been detected in response to experimental cardiotropic viral infection,[21,22] and importantly, in patients with myocarditis or idiopathic dilated cardiomyopathy.[23,24] Employing IFN-γ as

an antiviral strategy succeeded in suppressing viral replication and subsequent cardiac pathology in infective myocarditis models.[25] A novel humanized nonobese diabetic (NOD)-background strain bearing the class II *DQ8* allele developed spontaneous myocarditis; IFN-γ production was associated with the propensity toward disease incidence in female mice in this model.[26,27] Transgenic mice overexpressing IFN-γ under a hepatic promoter developed chronic myocarditis and cardiomyopathy through upregulation of a potent systemic proinflammatory program, including IL-12 and tumor necrosis factor α (TNF-α).[28,29] In a similar vein, potentiating Th1 responses through treatment with IL-12 in mice resulted in more severe disease,[30,31] or enhanced the transfer of EAM.[32]

The most problematic and paradoxical findings surrounded experimental manipulations of IFN-γ itself in autoimmune settings. Blocking IFN-γ signaling with monoclonal antibodies (mAbs) or ablating IFN-γ signaling using knockout mice resulted in more severe disease in several autoimmune disease models, including the encephalomyelitis model of multiple sclerosis (EAE), and models of rheumatoid arthritis and other diseases.[33,34] Extensive, severe EAM developed in IFN-γ–deficient (*Ifng$^{-/-}$*) (Fig. 2) and IFN-γ receptor 1–deficient (*Ifngr$^{-/-}$*) mice,[30,31,35] in animals treated with anti-IFN-γ mAb,[30] as well as in Tbet-deficient (*Tbx21$^{-/-}$*) mice.[36] Intriguingly, when *Ifng$^{-/-}$* mice were infected with coxsackievirus B3, the chronic postviral myocarditis of these mice was dramatically more severe in a manner that was independent of the antiviral functions of IFN-γ.[37] Importantly, the severe myocarditis of IFN-γ–deficient mice was shown to progress to extreme, fatal cardiopathologic sequelae, including constrictive and dilated cardiomyopathies, accompanied by extensive fibrotic remodeling.[37–39] On the other hand, a number of investigators in various models pointed to disease-protective functions of IFN-γ–driven responses that included apoptogenic control of autoreactive T cells,[40–42] as well as antiproliferative or other suppressive effects on lymphoid and myeloid cells.[37,43–46] How can these conflicting findings and conclusions be resolved? It is entirely likely that IFN-γ (and other cytokines) is capable of exerting both pathogenic and protective effector functions; which of these functions comes to predominate depends on a multitude of contextual

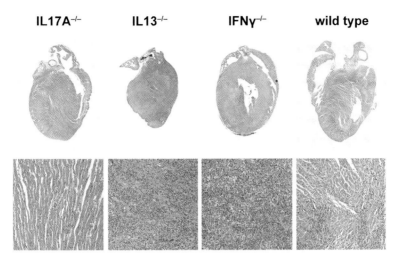

IL17A⁻/⁻   **IL13⁻/⁻**   **IFNγ⁻/⁻**   **wild type**

Figure 2. Representative histopathologic presentation of EAM in BALB/c mice deficient in T cell–derived effector cytokines, at the peak of inflammatory disease on day 21. Sections (5 μm) are H&E stained, at 64× magnification in the right column.

Th2 cells: complexities of IL-4 and IL-13

microenvironmental signals. IFN-γ receptor is nearly ubiquitous in expression; however, different cell signaling targets may induce qualitatively different programs, as discussed below. Other cytokines or costimulatory molecules may modulate IFN-γ signaling in a manner that requires network systems biologic approaches to understand.

Th2 cells: complexities of IL-4 and IL-13

In the original formulation of the Th1/Th2 model, IL-4–producing Th2 cells were responsible for mounting IgE-dependent mast cell responses, and providing B cell help in response to parasitic infection or in atopy. Evidence from the EAM or viral infection models in mice for Th2 involvement has been limited but notable. IL-4 and other Th2-associated cytokines can be detected in the hearts of animals infected with CVB3,[47] as well as in patients with myocarditis or idiopathic cardiomyopathy.[48]

A/J mice develop EAM with a generally more severe baseline than BALB/c animals.[14] Our laboratory reported that EAM in A/J mice bears phenotypic characteristics of a Th2 response, including the presence of eosinophils and giant cells. While blockade of IL-4 diminished the severity of cardiac inflammation in these mice,[49] Il4⁻/⁻ BALB/c mice developed disease comparable to wild-type BALB/c controls, indicating that dependence on IL-4 represents a mechanism of disease variation between these two susceptible strains.[50] We have since ver-

ified this IL-4 dependence of disease in A/J mice, using a null-mutant allele (unpublished observations, J.G. Barin and D. Čiháková). These data further suggest that the extent to which the disease in A/J mice is Th2-driven may facilitate the more severe disease phenotype associated with the A/J background.[14]

In infectious models of cardiac inflammation, IL-4 suppresses antiviral or antibacterial host responses. Administration of recombinant IL-4 improved cardiac function following CVB3 infection.[51] After infection with *Borrelia* spirochetes, IL-4–deficient animals developed severe myocarditis, although this resolves.[52] In a similar vein, despite the commonly held understanding of Th2 responses being important in antiparasitic responses, investigators in chagasic cardiomyopathy reported that *Il4⁻/⁻* mice develop more severe cardiac inflammation in association with superior clearance of *Trypanasoma cruzi*.[53]

While IL-4 may represent the canonical archetype of Th2 cytokines, GATA3, the transcription factor responsible for controlling the Th2 program, drives additional cytokines. *Il13* encodes adjacent to the *Il4* gene in both mouse and human. Transcriptional control of both cytokines is known to be linked by shared enhancers embedded within the Th2 locus.[54,55] IL-13 is believed to exert a substantial portion of effector functions of Th2 cells, due to ubiquitous expression of its receptor.[56]

When EAM was induced in IL-13–deficient animals, they surprisingly developed a robust, severe cardiac inflammation, characterized by fibrosis and progression to dilative function (Fig. 2). Intriguingly, IL-13 is widely understood to exert a fibrogenic program, indicating the importance of an IL-13–independent pathway by which cardiac scarring is controlled. By crossing the $Il13^{-/-}$ onto the $Il4^{-/-}$ background, we further observed that whatever protective effect was exerted by $Il13$ epistatically dominated any pathogenic functions mediated by $Il4$.[50] Importantly, markers of both T and B cell activation were enhanced in $Il13^{-/-}$ mice, in spite of the fact that mouse lymphocytes do not express the receptor for IL-13, pointing to a nonlymphoid signaling target for this protective effect, as discussed below for macrophages.

Regulatory T cells

Since the formulation of the Th1/Th2 model, it has been clear that the binary countersuppression theory did not adequately account for a variety of pathologic or host defense responses.[57] The emergence of a novel subset of immunosuppressive T cells, termed regulatory T (T_{reg}) cells, essentially resurrected theories of suppressor T cells from decades earlier.[58] Central to the resurgence of the T_{reg} cell model in the past decade was the identification of FoxP3 as the transcription factor essential to the regulatory program of T_{reg} cells.[59,60] While investigation into the mechanisms of suppression and ontogeny of these cells continues, the essential role of T_{reg} cells in facilitating tolerance is clear.[61]

FoxP3 expression can be detected in endomyocardial biopsies of patients with dilated cardiomyopathy.[62] A study in recipients of a thymocyte transfer model showed that depletion of T_{reg} cells permitted the spontaneous development of myocarditis.[63] Furthermore, transfer of T_{reg} cells has been shown to limit cardiac inflammation and attenuate viral replication in response to infection with CVB3[64] or T. cruzi.[65] T_{reg} cells also appear to be responsible for the induction of nasal tolerance to autoantigens in a manner that abrogated the progression of CVB3 infection to chronic myocarditis.[66] Similarly, the T_{reg} cell–associated immunoregulatory cytokine IL-10 has a clear role in limiting autoaggressive inflammation in the heart by way of nasal tolerance.[67]

Transgenic expression of the T_{reg} cell–associated cytokine TGF-β in the pancreas protected mice from CVB3-elicited myocarditis.[68] Using gonadectomy, one study showed the testosterone-dependence of T_{reg} cell expansion as a potential underlying basis of sex differences in susceptibility to myocarditis resulting from CVB3 infection.[69] Substantial disagreement surrounds the predictive value of circulating T_{reg} cell proportions for patients with other acute and chronic cardiac pathologies.[70–72]

While these findings, as a whole, point to a general role for T_{reg} cells in maintaining cardiac tolerance, the NOD.DQ8 model of spontaneous cardiac autoimmunity does not show a major role for central thymic selection in the programming of natural T_{reg} cells specific to the heart—perhaps underscoring peripheral mechanisms of tolerance as more important for cardiac immunohomeostasis.[73] Signaling pathways important to the elicitation, activation, or maintenance of T_{reg} cells have an immediate impact upon cardiac autoimmunity. $Ctla4^{-/-}$ mice die at 3–4 weeks of age of a massive lymphoproliferative polyautoimmunity, most notably extensive cardiac inflammation.[74] Similarly, mice deficient in the negative costimulatory receptor PD-1 or its ligand PD-L1 spontaneously develop rapid, fatal cardiac inflammation when the knockout alleles are crossed onto the autoimmunity-prone MRL background.[75–77] Morever, the PD-1 pathway appears to synergize with negative costimulation through the receptor LAG3; when $Lag3^{-/-}$ mice were crossed to PD-1–deficient ($Pdcd1^{-/-}$) mice on the BALB/c background (which do not develop the same spontaneous myocarditis as MRL mice), the resulting double knockout animals developed lethal myocarditis.[78] It should be noted that in spite of these findings in animal models, myocarditis has not been a reported presentation of patients with immune dysregulation, polyendocrinopathy, enteropathy, X-linked (IPEX) syndrome with spontaneous deleterious mutations in FoxP3,[79,80] and may represent a species difference, or perhaps a more nuanced distinction in the specific pathways controlling T_{reg} cell function.

Th17 cells

Myocarditis illustrates only one of the models for which the Th1/Th2 dichotomy was not entirely sufficient to account for disease pathophysiology, particularly with regard to the paradoxical protective functions mediated by IFN-γ. A potential resolution for this problem arrived when a novel subset of effector CD4+ T cells was reported to produce the novel proinflammatory cytokine IL-17A, under the control of coordinate signaling by TGF-β, IL-6, and the IL-12-related innate cytokine IL-23.[81–84] Termed Th17 cells, the independence of this lineage was underscored by the identification of unique transcription factors, particularly retinoid acid receptor–related orphan receptor γ expressed in T cells (RORγt), that enabled the differentiation of these cells.[85]

Seminal to the rapid advances in understanding the Th17 lineage was the finding that IL-23, rather than the related cytokine IL-12, drove autoreactive CNS inflammation in EAE.[86] Roles for Th17 cells have since been investigated in numerous other autoimmune diseases, and other immunopathologic models.[87,88] Similarly, EAM was shown to be dependent on IL-23, rather than IL-12, signaling for the induction of cardiac autoimmunity. This study demonstrated that Th17-polarized CD4+ cells were more effective than Th1 cells at eliciting cardiac immunopathology in recipients of adoptive transfers.[36] Suppressing Th17 differentiation through blocking or preventing IL-6 signaling has been reported to prevent the development of EAM.[89,90] We have recently shown evidence that intrinsic differences in the ability to mount Th17 responses may underlie background genetic differences in the susceptibility of A.SW mice and resistance of B10.S mice to EAM.[91]

If Th17-lineage cells were responsible for the pathophysiology of EAM and other autoimmune diseases, the logical corollary would be that a cytokine product of Th17 cells mediates that effect, and may represent an attractive target amenable to therapeutic intervention. To address the pathophysiologic potential of the archetypal product of these cells, our laboratory elicited EAM in IL-17A–deficient (*Il17a*−/−) mice, and surprisingly found that *Il17a*−/− mice developed inflammatory cardiac infiltration in a manner similar to wild-type control mice (Fig. 2). However, when animals were echocardiographically imaged at late time points of the EAM model, cardiac function was decidedly preserved in *Il17a*−/− mice. This functional protection in *Il17a*−/− animals was accompanied by diminished cardiac fibrosis, as well as expression of fibrotic collagens and metalloproteinases.[92]

These data pointed to a critical role for IL-17 in driving a maladaptive fibrotic and remodeling program in the diseased heart. Similar profibrotic functions of IL-17 signaling have also been reported in a bleomycin-induced model of fibrotic lung injury.[93]

Roles for antipathogen functions of IL-17 and Th17 cells in response to infection with CVB3 or *T. cruzi* have also been reported.[94,95] Evidence for a clinical role for Th17 cells and IL-17 in patients is forthcoming. Detection of cardiac expression of IL-17A and RORγt has been reported from patients with viral myocarditis.[96] Furthermore, lipocalin-2, a signature stress product elicited by IL-17, can be detected in patients with myocarditis.[97] Like other CD4+ T cell lineages, Th17 cells produce other cytokines to varying degrees, including IL-6, IL-17F, IL-22, and granulocyte macrophage colony-stimulating factor (GM-CSF). The role of these other products as effectors of the Th17 inflammatory or remodeling programs continue to be investigated in EAM and other immunopathologic models.

Th9, T_FH, Th22, and beyond

In recent years, the diversity of CD4+ effector programs has been increasingly appreciated, as novel profiles of cytokine production and transcription factor-driven differentiation show discrete effector fates that seem to be independent of the Th1, Th2, Th17, and T_reg cell programs.[98] While many of these models have yet to be applied to cardiac inflammation and autoimmunity in general, it is certain they will be a rapidly evolving field of investigation in the near future.

Among the most intriguing in cardiac immunology are Th9 cells, which produce IL-9 in a manner dependent on TGF-β and IL-4 signaling.[99,100] Th9-polarized cells were capable of eliciting EAE in adoptive transfer recipients characterized by atypical meningeal and peripheral nervous system lesions, and acquisition of IFN-γ production by transferred Th9 cells.[101] IL-9 levels in plasma were increased in patients with chronic heart failure, in a manner that was inversely associated with ejection fraction among patients with an ischemic etiology.[102] Similar elevation of circulating IL-9 was detected in the heart failure of sarco-endoplasmic reticulum Ca^{2+} ATPase (SERCA2)–deficient mice.[103]

Effectors of CD4⁺ T cell–derived cytokines

If the very definition of a cytokine is to transduce signaling between cells, it stands to reason that identifying signaling targets may yield both mechanistic insights and potential therapeutic targets. Use of the first generation of anticytokine therapeutics in the clinic have indicated that cytokine-targeting strategies may be inherently rife with potential off-target or adverse effects, due to the pleiotropic nature of many cytokines.[104] We may treat heterogeneity among target cells as an added dimension of network complexity in understanding immunopathologic processes. Put another way, many cells, particularly within the immune system, exert specialized responses to cytokine signaling. The selective induction of nitric oxide production in macrophages by IFN-γ is a classic example of this principle. This section will discuss the responses of various cell populations, both hematopoietic and cardiac-resident, as signaling targets and subsequent effectors of cytokines produced by CD4⁺ T cells.

Monocytes and macrophages

High-resolution multicolor cytometric analysis of heart-infiltrating leukocytes in EAM has demonstrated that monocytes and macrophages are the most numerous population, implicating these cells as key effectors of the autoaggressive immunopathology of EAM.[105,106] Extensive heterogeneity among cells of the mononuclear phagocyte system (MPS), such as monocytes and macrophages, has been increasingly appreciated in recent years. Of the several frameworks within which to address this heterogeneity, one of the most used frameworks revolves around the responses of macrophages

to T cell–derived cytokines (Fig. 3). Classically activated—or M1 macrophages—undertake an antimicrobial program that is characterized by nitric oxide production, lysosomal uptake and killing, and enhanced antigen processing and presentation—in response to signaling by IFN-γ. In contrast, alternatively activated—or M2a macrophages—are directed by IL-4 and IL-13 signaling to a transcriptional profile associated with scavenging, wound healing, and fibrotic remodeling.[107] Our laboratory has reported on a unique profile of cytokine production elicited in primary macrophages by IL-17 signaling.[108]

It bears notice that this model of macrophage differentiation seemingly resembles Th1/Th2 models of CD4⁺ T cell lineage commitment; that is, for each Th subset there is a corresponding macrophage subset. This reductionist paradigm is probably less true of MPS-lineage cells than it is for T cells, as monocytes and macrophages are not thought to commit to lineage subsets in the same manner (although issues of T cell commitment and plasticity are ongoing, as discussed below). In addition, MPS-lineage cells integrate a great variety of activating, suppressive, and modulatory stimuli beyond cytokines derived from T cells.[109] It may be more useful to consider these model macrophage subpopulations as polar representatives on a continuous spectrum of possible differentiation states.[110]

Even with these qualifiers, it is clear that MPS-lineage cells are responsive to T cell cytokines in ways that bear on cardiac inflammation and remodeling. By examining the time course of expression of markers associated with the M1/M2 model, we have reported that heart-infiltrating macrophages acquire expression of ICAM1, a canonical IFN-γ–driven

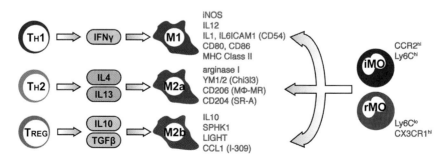

Figure 3. Schematic representation of putative relationships between CD4⁺ Th subsets and the heterogeneity of macrophages and monocytes. It should be noted that associations between monocytic precursors and specific macrophage activation phenotypes are not entirely clear.

target, and lose expression of the macrophage mannose receptor (CD206), a marker of M2 alternative-activation, over the course of EAM.[108] These data are consistent with reports from ischemic cardiac injury models in which monocytes most rapidly recruited to the myocardium are associated with inflammation, whereas monocytes associated with wound healing and fibrosis are recruited later during the recovery process.[111]

As discussed above, the protective effect of IL-13 in EAM was associated with enhanced lymphocytic activation in $Il13^{-/-}$ mice, in spite of the fact that mouse lymphocytes do not express receptors for IL-13. To address this, innate effector compartments were investigated, and we found fewer macrophages expressing markers of alternative activation, potentially pointing to a protective role for MPS-lineage cells responsive to IL-13. Alternatively, these data may also indicate that classically activated M1 macrophages mediate pathogenic functions.[50]

Suppressing nitric oxide production *in vivo* reduces cardiac inflammation, pointing to a net pathologic role for nitric oxide in myocarditis.[42,112,113] In spite of this, nitric oxide–dependent suppression of autoreactive lymphocytes has been implicated as a key mechanism of the protective effect of IFN-γ described above.[35,114] A recent study posited a fascinating mechanism by which expression of the macrophage inducible nitric oxide synthase (*Nos2*) is necessary for disease-protective differentiation of M-CSF–responsive macrophages.[115]

Neutrophils

Neutrophils are often considered to represent the major leukocytic effector of IL-17 responses, as IL-17 signaling potently elicits the production of growth factors associated with granulopoiesis, and chemokines that selectively recruit neutrophils.[116,117] Indeed, infiltration of the heart by neutrophils was significantly reduced in IL-17–deficient mice with EAM,[92] or animals with cardiac ischemia/reperfusion injury treated with anti-IL-17 antibodies.[118] Importantly, these diminutions of neutrophil recruitment were associated with improved cardiac function. Neutrophils also appeared to be Th1-responsive in CVB3 infection of IL-12p35–deficient mice.[119] In spite of this evidence, an understanding of the net pathogenic or protective functions of neutrophils has not been fully explored,

and may be dependent on model and experimental context. A pathogenic role for neutrophils has been described for a CD8+ T cell–dependent TCR transgenic model of myocarditis.[120] Blockade of the neutrophil chemotactic factor CXCL2/MIP2 limited cardiac inflammation following EMCV infection.[121] Similarly, CXCL1/KC-deficient animals were protected from myocarditis following infection with *Borrelia burgdorferi*.[122] Relative proportions of circulating neutrophils have been proposed as a predictor of poorer outcomes in patients with myocardial infarction.[123]

However, more generalized models of cardiac injury tend to point toward disease-protective functions of neutrophils, particularly regarding the neutrophil mobilization and differentiation factor G-CSF, although substantial controversy persists. Treating animals with G-CSF has been reported to improve cardiac function following infarct or ischemia,[124,125] although it is worthwhile to point out that the mechanism for this effect is thought to be via proangiogenic mobilization of stem cell precursors for cells that are not necessarily neutrophils. Clinical trials employing G-CSF treatment have reported improved cardiac outcomes in patients with myocardial infarction.[126,127] Treating animals with G-CSF has been reported to ameliorate cardiac inflammation in EAM.[128]

Eosinophils

Through IL-5 production, eosinophils are thought to participate in Th2 responses. Forms of myocarditis in humans resemble the canonical Th2 phenotype. Eosinophilic myocarditis possibly represents the most severe diagnostic category of myocarditis,[129] and etiologically, it may be associated with an atopic hypersensitivity response to drugs, or may often represent the most serious manifestation of hypereosinophilic syndrome.[130] Eosinophils are a feature of the Th2 disease of wild-type A/J mice,[49] as well as the severe EAM of IFN-γ–deficient animals.[35]

In infectious models, eosinophils are a clear participant in the cardiac inflammation of Chagas disease. Eosinophil-associated toxic granule products can be detected in the hearts of patients with Chagas cardiomyopathy.[131,132] Eosinophilic heart infiltrates are also associated with numerous other infectious agents, particularly parasites.[130,133] CVB3-infected animals treated with a novel Th2-promoting member of the IL-1 family, IL-33, developed eosinophilia and eosinophilic pericarditis. Surprisingly, rIL-33 treatment of naive mice by itself was sufficient to induce eosinophilic pericarditis.[134] The ability of IL-33 to induce eosinophilic pericarditis may interfere with targeting of IL-33 as a cardioprotective treatment, as IL-33 has been shown to be protective in myocardial infarction and hypertrophy models.[135,136]

Th subsets and cytokines in concert: interactions, deviation, and plasticity

Early work describing the differentiation of the CD4[+] T cell subsets generally considered the subsets to represent terminal phenotypes. It is now understood that *in vivo*, the various subsets retain substantial plasticity, that is, the ability to adopt alternate differentiation programs, according to specific rules and patterns.[137] Further complicating matters, developmental and effector pathways appear to be shared by at least some of the subsets in ways that are still under investigation.

In wild-type BALB/c mice, we have reported that heart-infiltrating CD4[+] T cells largely express either IFN-γ or IL-17A, indicating that Th1 and Th17 responses predominate the autoaggressive repertoire in this model. However, the diversity of disease subtypes seen in patients, as well as the ready deviations that can be elicited in mice deficient in, or depleted of, cytokines, indicate that myocarditis may be more etiologically diverse than has been previously appreciated.

Th1 and Th2 cells

Evidence of Th2 deviation can be found in mice with defects in Th1 programming with EAM, among other diseases. It has been reported that IL-4 production was increased by restimulated myosin-primed IL-12p40–deficient (*Il12b*[−/−]) splenocytes, as well as by increased class-switching to IgG1 serum autoantibodies.[31] Similar deviation to IL-4 production has been reported in T-bet knockout mice.[36] Conversely, treatment of mice with recombinant IL-12p70 suppressed the production of IL-4 and IL-10 in restimulated splenocytes.[30] Features of EAM in Th1-defective mice similarly show Th2 deviation, most notably the presence of eosinophilic infiltrates.[30,31,36]

Manipulations of Th2 cytokines did not appear to completely abrogate the skewed protection of p40-

deficient mice,[31] but simultaneous blockade of IL-4 and IFN-γ reversed the severe disease following the blockade of IFN-γ alone in A/J strain mice. As discussed above, the dependence of EAM on IL-4 depended on the strain background. IL-4 dependence of disease in A/J mice was associated with increased production of IFN-γ in IL-4–blocked animals.[49] Similar Th1 deviation was observed in *Il4*[−/−] A/J mice (unpublished data, D. Čiháková). In contrast, blockade or knockout of IL-4 on the BALB/c background had little effect on disease, and no impact on the production of IFN-γ.[50] Similar complex and confounding findings that did not conform to the dichomotous binary logic of the Th1/Th2 model had been reported in a variety of systems, in many ways presaging and foreshadowing the discovery of additional CD4[+] T cell subsets and associated cytokines.

Th1 and Th17 cells

The discovery of the Th17 lineage independently by several different laboratories in part involved the observation that the IL-12–related cytokine IL-23 exerted similar, but nonsynonymous, proinflammatory effects, particularly with regard to the programming of canonical Th1 IFN-γ production. By determining that IL-23, rather than IL-12, production was responsible for driving encephalitogenic CD4[+] T cells in EAE, the Kuchroo lab established that IL-23–responsive IL-17–producing cells were more central to the autoaggressive process than IL-12–responsive IFN-γ–producing Th1 cells.[138]

Expression of IFN-γ or IL-17 defines the bulk of infiltrating autoaggressive CD4[+] cells in the EAM of BALB/c mice.[92] In A/J mice, one study used tetramer technology to demonstrate myosin-specificity of Th1 and Th17 cells in EAM.[139] A recently developed TCR transgenic model responsive to cardiac myosin appears to depend on cooperation between both Th1 and Th17 responses for disease pathogenesis.[140] However, in the case of acute cardiotropic viral infection, cardiac expression of Th1- and CTL-associated signatures was recently reported, with little evidence for Th17 involvement.[62,141] Data from patients with unstable angina or acute infarct also provide evidence that Th1 and Th17 cells participate in the injury and healing responses to these acute coronary syndromes.[142]

In several of the original experiments characterizing the lineage identity of Th17 cells, IFN-γ signaling suppressed induction of IL-17 production by CD4[+] T cells,[81,82] consistent with the mutual counter-suppression premise of the original Th1/Th2 model.[20] There is evidence from a number of experimental systems clearly indicating heightened IL-17–associated responses in the absence of IFN-γ or T-bet.[143,144] It further stands to reason that amplified Th17 responses are responsible for the severe autoimmune disease elicited in animals with disrupted IFN-γ production or signaling, or other Th1 defects.[145]

The converse, that Th17 differentiation suppresses the Th1 program, remains less clear. In the EAM of *Il17a*[−/−] mice, cardiac expression of IFN-γ production was actually less than in wild-type controls.[92] Similarly, Th1-associated chemokines, such as CCL5/RANTES and CXCL10/IP10, were also diminished in IL-17–deficient animals, further supporting that autoaggressive Th1 responses were at least partly elicited by IL-17 signaling. Th17 cells have been shown to readily reprogram into Th1 cells *in vitro*, depending on the cytokine milieu.[146] Coexpression of IFN-γ and IL-17 has been widely reported in a subset of CD4[+] T cells, in a variety of experimental settings. Fating experiments in EAE using IL-17–reporter mice suggest that the Th17 program may, in part, represent an important transitional state in the induction of Th1 responses.[147] Evidence from psoriatic patients suggests that there are circumstances in which IFN-γ enables Th17 differentiation *in vivo*.[148]

T_{reg} versus T_{eff} cells

The premise of understanding the regulatory T cell is reflected in their name—that their purpose is to suppress inflammatory host immunity and defense. In specific pathophysiologic context, the diverse ontogeny and poorly understood mechanisms of suppression of these regulatory populations represents a major ongoing challenge in applying these cells to the rational design of therapeutics.

Transfer of T_{reg} cells into mice infected with CVB3 suppressed levels of IFN-γ and TNF-α in plasma, but also IL-10. These authors demonstrated that cardiac expression of TGF-β suppressed expression of the coxsackie-adenovirus receptor in T_{reg} cell recipients, providing a mechanism by which T_{reg} cell activity assisted in viral clearance.[64] Elimination of regulatory T cells by autoaggressive γδ T cells has been described in response to CVB3 in-

fection through a mechanism that seems to involve direct cytotoxic elimination.[149,150] Adenoviral gene therapy expression of IL-10 in EAM resulted in diminished expression of a broad variety of effector cytokines from restimulated splenocytes, including IFN-γ, IL-2, IL-4, IL-13, IL-17, and TNF-α.[151] In ischemic models, suppression of cardiac remodeling by the transfer of T_{reg} cells was associated with diminished IFN-γ expression,[152] as well as TNF-α and IL-1β.[153]

Clinical translation of T cell plasticity

Currently, giant cell myocarditis is treated with cyclosporine and corticosteroids. There has been some success with long-term immunosuppression in patients with chronic DCM.[154] Data from animal modeling suggest that myocarditis is driven by Th17 and Th1 cells, with Th17 cells being responsible for the cardiac remodeling and development of DCM. Patients with DCM have increased levels of IL-17A in sera and an increased frequency of Th17 cells in blood, supporting the clinical relevance of the animal mouse models.[92,155] Human data from heart biopsies of myocarditis patients to confirm the role of CD4[+] helper T cell-associated cytokines, and to appreciate the role of myeloid cells subtypes in the pathogenesis of the disease, are greatly needed. Increased risk of cardiovascular disease has been reported in several autoimmune and autoinflammatory diseases, including psoriasis and rheumatoid arthritis, consistent with the model that Th17 cells are pathogenic for the human heart.[156–158] In addition, 3–15% of systemic lupus erythematous (SLE) patients are diagnosed with myocarditis.[159,160] The coincidence of myocarditis with SLE is even greater in autopsy studies, indicating a clear association between systemic autoimmune disease and myocarditis, and further underscoring an autoimmune etiology for myocarditis.[161]

Due to the recent introduction of the first generation of biologic immunotherapeutics targeting Th1 and Th17 cells, it may be possible to examine the effect of these treatments on cardiovascular sequelae to understand how they may impact heart disease. Monoclonal antibodies targeting the shared p40 subunit of IL-12 and IL-23, ustekinumab and briakinumab, have been approved or investigated for plaque psoriasis, inflammatory bowel disorders, multiple sclerosis, and rheumatoid arthritis. Targeted blockade of IL-17A by

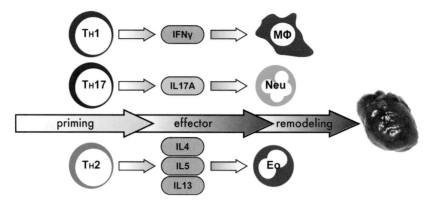

Figure 4. Schematic representation of the effector mechanisms driven by CD4⁺ T cell subsets in inflammatory heart disease.

secukinumab and ixekizumab remains under investigation for psoriasis, ankylosing spondylitis, noninfectious uveitis, and psoriatic arthritis. Surprisingly, usage of ustekinumab (anti-IL-12/23p40) in autoimmune disorders may be associated with altered risk of cardiovascular sequelae of psoriasis and arthritis.[162] Clinical investigation of briakinumab reported increased risk of cardiovascular events.[163,164] Some studies proposed that the IL-17 pathway might play a stabilizing role in atheromatous plaque,[165] while others suggest that both Th1 and Th17 induce plaque development through their proinflammatory effects.[166] As with many investigational drugs, substantial disagreement exists among cohorts and findings.[167–169]

On the Th2 side, asthma remains a key investigational target for clinical trials targeting IL-13 with lebrikizumab or IL-5 by mepolizumab and reslizumab. As autoimmune and autoinflammatory disorders are generally not thought to be Th2 dependent, limited data are available for examining the effectiveness of targeting these pathways. IL-13 blockade has been proposed for the treatment of childhood nephrotic syndrome, which may have autoimmune etiologies.[170] Logically, IL-5–blockading antibodies are being investigated for controlling several eosinophilic inflammatory disorders, including hypereosinophilic syndrome,[171–173] Churg-Strauss syndrome,[174,175] and eosinophilic gastroenteritis.[176,177] Additional targets of eosinophil recruitment may prove to be attractive therapies for eosinophilic myocarditities, among other eosinophilic inflammatory diseases.[178]

Conclusion

As the family of helper T cells expands, so does our understanding of the complexity in programming the differentiation, commitment, and effector programs of CD4⁺ T cells. Traditionally, autoimmune diseases have been considered to be driven by Th1. Following the discovery of Th17 cells, autoimmune inflammation was presented as Th17 dependent. We have discussed here that all CD4⁺ T cell subsets can drive autoimmune heart inflammation, depending on experimental or environmental context. We believe this to parallel human myocarditis, wherein necrotizing eosinophilic myocarditis represents Th2-driven disease, and giant cell myocarditis is most likely driven by a mixed Th1/Th17 response. It is notable that both of these disease classifications are regarded with poorer prognoses than lymphocytic myocarditis, suggesting that redundancy and competition among CD4⁺ T cell subsets possesses a homeostatic component and that a deviated response in any direction is less favorable. The association of these deviated diseases with specific effector cell types (Fig. 4) emphasizes the heterogeneity of autoimmune disease and underscores the need for tailored diagnostic procedures and targeted therapeutic strategies.

Acknowledgments

J.G.B. has been the Mary Renner Fellow in Autoimmune Disease Research, and the O'Leary-Wilson Fellow at the Johns Hopkins Autoimmune Disease Research Center, from the American Autoimmune-Related Disease Association. D.C. was supported by The Michel Mirowski MD Foundation; the W.W. Smith Charitable Trust, heart research grant H1103; and The Children's Cardiomyopathy Foundation.

Conflicts of interest

The authors declare no conflicts of interest.

References

1. Andreoletti, L. et al. 2009. Viral causes of human myocarditis. Arch. Cardiovasc. Dis. **102:** 559–568.
2. Frustaci, A. et al. 2003. Immunosuppressive therapy for active lymphocytic myocarditis: virological and immunologic profile of responders versus nonresponders. Circulation **107:** 857–863.
3. Frustaci, A., M.A. Russo & C. Chimenti. 2009. Randomized study on the efficacy of immunosuppressive therapy in patients with virus-negative inflammatory cardiomyopathy: the TIMIC study. Eur. Heart J.
4. Aretz, H.T. et al. 1987. Myocarditis. A histopathologic definition and classification. Am. J. Cardiovasc. Pathol. **1:** 3–14.
5. Basso, C. et al. 2012. Classification and histological, immunohistochemical, and molecular diagnosis of inflammatory myocardial disease. Heart Fail. Rev.
6. Elliott, P. et al. 2008. Classification of the cardiomyopathies: a position statement from the European Society Of Cardiology Working Group on Myocardial and Pericardial Diseases. Eur. Heart J. **29:** 270–276.
7. Maron, B. J. et al. 2006. Contemporary definitions and classification of the cardiomyopathies: an American Heart Association Scientific Statement from the Council on Clinical Cardiology, Heart Failure and Transplantation Committee; Quality of Care and Outcomes Research and Functional Genomics and Translational Biology Interdisciplinary Working Groups; and Council on Epidemiology and Prevention. Circulation **113:** 1807–1816.
8. Cooper, L.T. Jr. et al. 2008. Usefulness of immunosuppression for giant cell myocarditis. Am. J. Cardiol. **102:** 1535–1539.
9. Magnani, J.W. & G.W. Dec. 2006. Myocarditis: current trends in diagnosis and treatment. Circulation **113:** 876–890.
10. Felker, G.M. et al. 2000. Underlying causes and long-term survival in patients with initially unexplained cardiomyopathy. N. Engl. J. Med. **342:** 1077–1084.
11. Herskowitz, A. et al. 1993. Demographic features and prevalence of idiopathic myocarditis in patients undergoing endomyocardial biopsy. Am. J. Cardiol. **71:** 982–986.
12. Magnani, J.W. et al. 2006. Survival in biopsy-proven myocarditis: a long-term retrospective analysis of the histopathologic, clinical, and hemodynamic predictors. Am. Heart J. **151:** 463–470.
13. Rose, N.R. 2012. Infection and autoimmunity: theme and variations. Curr. Opin. Rheumatol. **24:** 380–382.
14. Neu, N. et al. 1987. Cardiac myosin induces myocarditis in genetically predisposed mice. J. Immunol. **139:** 3630–3636.
15. Cihakova, D. et al. 2004. Animal models for autoimmune myocarditis and autoimmune thyroiditis. Methods Mol. Med. **102:** 175–193.
16. Smith, S.C. & P.M. Allen. 1991. Myosin-induced acute myocarditis is a T cell-mediated disease. J. Immunol. **147:** 2141–2147.
17. Smith, S.C. & P.M. Allen. 1993. The role of T cells in myosin-induced autoimmune myocarditis. Clin. Immunol. Immunopathol. **68:** 100–106.
18. Gangaplara, A. et al. 2012. Coxsackievirus B3 infection leads to the generation of cardiac myosin heavy chain-alpha-reactive CD4 T cells in A/J mice. Clin. Immunol. **144:** 237–249.
19. Malkiel, S., S. Factor & B. Diamond. 1999. Autoimmune myocarditis does not require B cells for antigen presentation. J. Immunol. **163:** 5265–5268.
20. Mosmann, T.R. & R.L. Coffman. 1989. TH1 and TH2 cells: different patterns of lymphokine secretion lead to different functional properties. Annu. Rev. Immunol. **7:** 145–173.
21. Shioi, T., A. Matsumori & S. Sasayama. 1996. Persistent expression of cytokine in the chronic stage of viral myocarditis in mice. Circulation **94:** 2930–2937.
22. Schmidtke, M. et al. 2000. Cytokine profiles in heart, spleen, and thymus during the acute stage of experimental coxsackievirus B3-induced chronic myocarditis. J. Med. Virol. **61:** 518–526.
23. Luppi, P. et al. 2001. Analysis of TCR Vbeta repertoire and cytokine gene expression in patients with idiopathic dilated cardiomyopathy. J. Autoimmun. **16:** 3–13.
24. Luppi, P. et al. 2003. Expansion of specific alphabeta+ T-cell subsets in the myocardium of patients with myocarditis and idiopathic dilated cardiomyopathy associated with Coxsackievirus B infection. Hum. Immunol. **64:** 194–210.
25. Yamamoto, N. et al. 1998. Effects of intranasal administration of recombinant murine interferon-gamma on murine acute myocarditis caused by encephalomyocarditis virus. Circulation **97:** 1017–1023.
26. Taneja, V. & C.S. David. 2009. Spontaneous autoimmune myocarditis and cardiomyopathy in HLA-DQ8.NODAbo transgenic mice. J. Autoimmun. **33:** 260–269.
27. Taneja, V. et al. 2007. Spontaneous myocarditis mimicking human disease occurs in the presence of an appropriate MHC and non-MHC background in transgenic mice. J. Mol. Cell. Cardiol. **42:** 1054–1064.
28. Reifenberg, K. et al. 2007. Interferon-{gamma}induces chronic active myocarditis and cardiomyopathy in transgenic mice. Am. J. Pathol. **171:** 463–472.
29. Torzewski, M. et al. 2012. Chronic inflammatory cardiomyopathy of interferon gamma-overexpressing transgenic mice is mediated by tumor necrosis factor-alpha. Am. J. Pathol. **180:** 73–81.
30. Afanasyeva, M. et al. 2001. Interleukin-12 receptor/STAT4 signaling is required for the development of autoimmune myocarditis in mice by an interferon-gamma-independent pathway. Circulation **104:** 3145–3151.
31. Eriksson, U. et al. 2001. Dual role of the IL-12/IFN-gamma axis in the development of autoimmune myocarditis: induction by IL-12 and protection by IFN-gamma. J. Immunol. **167:** 5464–5469.

32. Okura, Y. *et al.* 1998. Recombinant murine interleukin-12 facilitates induction of cardiac myosin-specific type 1 helper T cells in rats. *Circ. Res.* **82:** 1035–1042.

33. Matthys, P. *et al.* 1999. Enhanced autoimmune arthritis in IFN-gamma receptor-deficient mice is conditioned by mycobacteria in Freund's adjuvant and by increased expansion of Mac-1$^+$ myeloid cells. *J. Immunol.* **163:** 3503–3510.

34. Caspi, R.R. *et al.* 1994. Endogenous systemic IFN-gamma has a protective role against ocular autoimmunity in mice. *J. Immunol.* **152:** 890–899.

35. Eriksson, U. *et al.* 2001. Lethal autoimmune myocarditis in interferon-gamma receptor-deficient mice: enhanced disease severity by impaired inducible nitric oxide synthase induction. *Circulation* **103:** 18–21.

36. Rangachari, M. *et al.* 2006. T-bet negatively regulates autoimmune myocarditis by suppressing local production of interleukin 17. *J. Exp. Med.* **203:** 2009–2019.

37. Fairweather, D. *et al.* 2004. Interferon-gamma protects against chronic viral myocarditis by reducing mast cell degranulation, fibrosis, and the profibrotic cytokines transforming growth factor-beta 1, interleukin-1 beta, and interleukin-4 in the heart. *Am. J. Pathol.* **165:** 1883–1894.

38. Afanasyeva, M. *et al.* 2005. Impaired up-regulation of CD25 on CD4$^+$ T cells in IFN-gamma knockout mice is associated with progression of myocarditis to heart failure. *Proc. Natl. Acad. Sci. USA* **102:** 180–185.

39. Afanasyeva, M. *et al.* 2004. Novel model of constrictive pericarditis associated with autoimmune heart disease in interferon-gamma-knockout mice. *Circulation* **110:** 2910–2917.

40. Tarrant, T.K. *et al.* 1999. Interleukin 12 protects from a T helper type 1-mediated autoimmune disease, experimental autoimmune uveitis, through a mechanism involving interferon gamma, nitric oxide, and apoptosis. *J. Exp. Med.* **189:** 219–230.

41. Dalton, D. K. *et al.* 2000. Interferon gamma eliminates responding CD4 T cells during mycobacterial infection by inducing apoptosis of activated CD4 T cells. *J. Exp. Med.* **192:** 117–122.

42. Barin, J.G. *et al.* 2010. Mechanisms of IFNgamma regulation of autoimmune myocarditis. *Exp. Mol. Pathol.* **89:** 83–91.

43. Dalton, D.K. *et al.* 1993. Multiple defects of immune cell function in mice with disrupted interferon-gamma genes. *Science* **259:** 1739–1742.

44. Chu, C.Q., S. Wittmer & D. K. Dalton. 2000. Failure to suppress the expansion of the activated CD4 T cell population in interferon gamma-deficient mice leads to exacerbation of experimental autoimmune encephalomyelitis. *J. Exp. Med.* **192:** 123–128.

45. Matthys, P., K. Vermeire & A. Billiau. 2001. Mac-1(+) myelopoiesis induced by CFA: a clue to the paradoxical effects of IFN-gamma in autoimmune disease models. *Trends Immunol.* **22:** 367–371.

46. Barin, J.G. *et al.* 2003. Thyroid-specific expression of IFN-gamma limits experimental autoimmune thyroiditis by suppressing lymphocyte activation in cervical lymph nodes. *J. Immunol.* **170:** 5523–5529.

47. Seko, Y. *et al.* 1997. Expression of cytokine mRNAs in murine hearts with acute myocarditis caused by coxsackievirus b3. *J. Pathol.* **183:** 105–108.

48. Han, R.O. *et al.* 1991. Detection of interleukin and interleukin-receptor mRNA in human heart by polymerase chain reaction. *Biochem. Biophys. Res. Commun.* **181:** 520–523.

49. Afanasyeva, M. *et al.* 2001. Experimental autoimmune myocarditis in A/J mice is an interleukin-4-dependent disease with a Th2 phenotype. *Am. J. Pathol.* **159:** 193–203.

50. Cihakova, D. *et al.* 2008. Interleukin-13 protects against experimental autoimmune myocarditis by regulating macrophage differentiation. *Am. J. Pathol.* **172:** 1195–1208.

51. Li, J. *et al.* 2007. Immunomodulation by interleukin-4 suppresses matrix metalloproteinases and improves cardiac function in murine myocarditis. *Eur. J. Pharmacol.* **554:** 60–68.

52. Satoskar, A.R. *et al.* 2000. Interleukin-4-deficient BALB/c mice develop an enhanced Th1-like response but control cardiac inflammation following Borrelia burgdorferi infection. *FEMS Microbiol. Lett.* **183:** 319–325.

53. Soares, M. B. *et al.* 2001. Modulation of chagasic cardiomyopathy by interleukin-4: dissociation between inflammation and tissue parasitism. *Am. J. Pathol.* **159:** 703–709.

54. Takemoto, N. *et al.* 1998. Th2-specific DNase I-hypersensitive sites in the murine IL-13 and IL-4 intergenic region. *Int. Immunol.* **10:** 1981–1985.

55. Loots, G.G. *et al.* 2000. Identification of a coordinate regulator of interleukins 4, 13, and 5 by cross-species sequence comparisons. *Science* **288:** 136–140.

56. Wills-Karp, M. 2004. Interleukin-13 in asthma pathogenesis. *Immunol. Rev.* **202:** 175–190.

57. Gor, D. O., N. R. Rose & N.S. Greenspan. 2003. TH1-TH2: a procrustean paradigm. *Nat. Immunol.* **4:** 503–505.

58. Shevach, E.M. 2000. Regulatory T cells in autoimmunity*. *Annu. Rev. Immunol.* **18:** 423–449.

59. Hori, S., T. Nomura & S. Sakaguchi. 2003. Control of regulatory T cell development by the transcription factor Foxp3. *Science* **299:** 1057–1061.

60. Fontenot, J.D., M.A. Gavin & A. Y. Rudensky. 2003. Foxp3 programs the development and function of CD4$^+$CD25$^+$ regulatory T cells. *Nat. Immunol.* **4:** 330–336.

61. Josefowicz, S.Z., L.F. Lu & A. Y. Rudensky. 2012. Regulatory T cells: mechanisms of differentiation and function. *Annu. Rev. Immunol.* **30:** 531–564.

62. Noutsias, M. *et al.* 2011. Expression of functional T-cell markers and T-cell receptor Vbeta repertoire in endomyocardial biopsies from patients presenting with acute myocarditis and dilated cardiomyopathy. *Eur. J. Heart Fail.* **13:** 611–618.

63. Ono, M. *et al.* 2006. Control of autoimmune myocarditis and multiorgan inflammation by glucocorticoid-induced TNF receptor family-related protein(high), Foxp3-expressing CD25$^+$ and CD25$^-$ regulatory T cells. *J. Immunol.* **176:** 4748–4756.

64. Shi, Y. *et al.* 2010. Regulatory T cells protect mice against coxsackievirus-induced myocarditis through the transforming growth factor beta-coxsackie-adenovirus receptor pathway. *Circulation* **121:** 2624–2634.

65. Mariano, F.S. *et al.* 2008. The involvement of CD4$^+$CD25$^+$ T cells in the acute phase of *Trypanosoma cruzi* infection. *Microbes Infect.* **10:** 825–833.

66. Fousteri, G. *et al.* 2011. Nasal cardiac myosin peptide treatment and OX40 blockade protect mice from acute and chronic virally-induced myocarditis. *J. Autoimmun.* **36:** 210–220.

67. Kaya, Z. *et al.* 2002. Cutting edge: a critical role for IL-10 in induction of nasal tolerance in experimental autoimmune myocarditis. *J. Immunol.* **168:** 1552–1556.

68. Horwitz, M.S. *et al.* 2006. Transforming growth factor-beta inhibits coxsackievirus-mediated autoimmune myocarditis. *Viral. Immunol.* **19:** 722–733.

69. Frisancho-Kiss, S. *et al.* 2009. Gonadectomy of male BALB/c mice increases Tim-3(+) alternatively activated M2 macrophages, Tim-3(+) T cells, Th2 cells and Treg in the heart during acute coxsackievirus-induced myocarditis. *Brain Behav. Immun.* **23:** 649–657.

70. Sardella, G. *et al.* 2007. Frequency of naturally-occurring regulatory T cells is reduced in patients with ST-segment elevation myocardial infarction. *Thromb. Res.* **120:** 631–634.

71. Ammirati, E. *et al.* 2010. Circulating CD4$^+$CD25^{hi}CD127^{lo} regulatory T-cell levels do not reflect the extent or severity of carotid and coronary atherosclerosis. *Arterios. Thromb. Vasc. Biol.* **30:** 1832–1841.

72. Carvalheiro, T. *et al.* 2012. Phenotypic and functional alterations on inflammatory peripheral blood cells after acute myocardial infarction. *J. Cardiovasc. Trans. Res.* **5:** 309–320.

73. Lv, H. *et al.* 2011. Impaired thymic tolerance to alpha-myosin directs autoimmunity to the heart in mice and humans. *J. Clin. Invest.* **121:** 1561–1573.

74. Tivol, E.A. *et al.* 1995. Loss of CTLA-4 leads to massive lymphoproliferation and fatal multiorgan tissue destruction, revealing a critical negative regulatory role of CTLA-4. *Immunity* **3:** 541–547.

75. Okazaki, T. *et al.* 2003. Autoantibodies against cardiac troponin I are responsible for dilated cardiomyopathy in PD-1-deficient mice. *Nat. Med.* **9:** 1477–1483.

76. Lucas, J.A. *et al.* 2008. Programmed death ligand 1 regulates a critical checkpoint for autoimmune myocarditis and pneumonitis in MRL mice. *J. Immunol.* **181:** 2513–2521.

77. Wang, J. *et al.* 2010. PD-1 deficiency results in the development of fatal myocarditis in MRL mice. *Int. Immunol.* **22:** 443–452.

78. Okazaki, T. *et al.* 2011. PD-1 and LAG-3 inhibitory co-receptors act synergistically to prevent autoimmunity in mice. *J. Exp. Med.* **208:** 395–407.

79. Wildin, R.S., S. Smyk-Pearson & A.H. Filipovich. 2002. Clinical and molecular features of the immunodysregulation, polyendocrinopathy, enteropathy, X linked (IPEX) syndrome. *J. Med. Genet.* **39:** 537–545.

80. Barzaghi, F., L. Passerini & R. Bacchetta. 2012. Immune dysregulation, polyendocrinopathy, enteropathy, X-linked syndrome: a paradigm of immunodeficiency with autoimmunity. *Front. Immunol.* **3:** 211.

81. Harrington, L.E. *et al.* 2005. Interleukin 17-producing CD4$^+$ effector T cells develop via a lineage distinct from the T helper type 1 and 2 lineages. *Nat. Immunol.* **6:** 1123–1132.

82. Park, H. *et al.* 2005. A distinct lineage of CD4 T cells regulates tissue inflammation by producing interleukin 17. *Nat. Immunol.* **6:** 1133–1141.

83. Veldhoen, M. *et al.* 2006. TGFbeta in the context of an inflammatory cytokine milieu supports de novo differentiation of IL-17-producing T cells. *Immunity* **24:** 179–189.

84. McGeachy, M.J. *et al.* 2009. The interleukin 23 receptor is essential for the terminal differentiation of interleukin 17-producing effector T helper cells in vivo. *Nat. Immunol.* **10:** 314–324.

85. Ivanov, II *et al.* 2006. The orphan nuclear receptor RORgammat directs the differentiation program of proinflammatory IL-17$^+$ T helper cells. *Cell* **126:** 1121–1133.

86. Langrish, C.L. *et al.* 2005. IL-23 drives a pathogenic T cell population that induces autoimmune inflammation. *J. Exp. Med.* **201:** 233–240.

87. Hu, Y. *et al.* 2011. The IL-17 pathway as a major therapeutic target in autoimmune diseases. *Ann. N.Y. Acad. Sci.* **1217:** 60–76.

88. Maddur, M.S. *et al.* 2012. Th17 cells: biology, pathogenesis of autoimmune and inflammatory diseases, and therapeutic strategies. *Am. J. Pathol.* **181:** 8–18.

89. Sonderegger, I. *et al.* 2008. GM-CSF mediates autoimmunity by enhancing IL-6-dependent Th17 cell development and survival. *J. Exp. Med.* **205:** 2281–2294.

90. Yamashita, T. *et al.* 2011. IL-6-mediated Th17 differentiation through RORgammat is essential for the initiation of experimental autoimmune myocarditis. *Cardiovasc. Res.* **91:** 640–648.

91. Chen, P. *et al.* 2012. Susceptibility to autoimmune myocarditis is associated with intrinsic differences in CD4(+) T cells. *Clin. Exp. Immunol.* **169:** 79–88.

92. Baldeviano, G.C. *et al.* 2010. Interleukin-17A is dispensable for myocarditis but essential for the progression to dilated cardiomyopathy. *Circ. Res.* **106:** 1646–1655.

93. Wilson, M.S. *et al.* 2010. Bleomycin and IL-1beta-mediated pulmonary fibrosis is IL-17A dependent. *J. Exp. Med.* **207:** 535–552.

94. Yuan, J. *et al.* 2010. Th17 cells contribute to viral replication in coxsackievirus B3-induced acute viral myocarditis. *J. Immunol.* **185:** 4004–4010.

95. da Matta Guedes, P.M. *et al.* 2010. IL-17 produced during *Trypanosoma cruzi* infection plays a central role in regulating parasite-induced myocarditis. *PLoS Neglect. Trop. Dis.* **4:** e604.

96. Yuan, J. *et al.* 2010. Th17 cells facilitate the humoral immune response in patients with acute viral myocarditis. *J. Clin. Immunol.* **30:** 226–234.

97. Ding, L. *et al.* 2010. Lipocalin-2/neutrophil gelatinase-B associated lipocalin is strongly induced in hearts of rats with autoimmune myocarditis and in human myocarditis. *Circ. J.* **74:** 523–530.

98. Palmer, M.T. & C.T. Weaver. 2010. Autoimmunity: increasing suspects in the CD4$^+$ T cell lineup. *Nat. Immunol.* **11:** 36–40.

99. Dardalhon, V. *et al.* 2008. IL-4 inhibits TGF-beta-induced Foxp3$^+$ T cells and, together with TGF-beta, generates IL-9$^+$ IL-10$^+$ Foxp3(-) effector T cells. *Nat. Immunol.* **9:** 1347–1355.

100. Veldhoen, M. *et al.* 2008. Transforming growth factor-beta 'reprograms' the differentiation of T helper 2 cells and promotes an interleukin 9-producing subset. *Nat. Immunol.* **9:** 1341–1346.

101. Elyaman, W. *et al.* 2009. IL-9 induces differentiation of TH17 cells and enhances function of FoxP3+ natural regulatory T cells. *Proc. Natl. Acad. Sci. USA* **106:** 12885–12890.

102. Cappuzzello, C. *et al.* 2011. Increase of plasma IL-9 and decrease of plasma IL-5, IL-7, and IFN-gamma in patients with chronic heart failure. *J. Transl. Med.* **9:** 28.

103. Vistnes, M. *et al.* 2010. Circulating cytokine levels in mice with heart failure are etiology dependent. *J. Appl. Physiol.* **108:** 1357–1364.

104. Aaltonen, K.J. *et al.* 2012. Systematic review and meta-analysis of the efficacy and safety of existing TNF blocking agents in treatment of rheumatoid arthritis. *PLoS One* **7:** e30275.

105. Afanasyeva, M. *et al.* 2004. Quantitative analysis of myocardial inflammation by flow cytometry in murine autoimmune myocarditis: correlation with cardiac function. *Am. J. Pathol.* **164:** 807–815.

106. Barin, J.G. *et al.* 2012. Macrophages participate in IL-17-mediated inflammation. *Eur. J. Immunol.* **42:** 726–736.

107. Gordon, S. 2003. Alternative activation of macrophages. *Nat. Rev. Immunol.* **3:** 23–35.

108. Barin, J.G., N. R. Rose & D. Cihakova. 2012. Macrophage diversity in cardiac inflammation: a review. *Immunobiology* **217:** 468–475.

109. Mantovani, A., A. Sica & M. Locati. 2005. Macrophage polarization comes of age. *Immunity* **23:** 344–346.

110. Mosser, D.M. & J.P. Edwards. 2008. Exploring the full spectrum of macrophage activation. *Nat. Rev. Immunol.* **8:** 958–969.

111. Nahrendorf, M. *et al.* 2007. The healing myocardium sequentially mobilizes two monocyte subsets with divergent and complementary functions. *J. Exp. Med.* **204:** 3037–3047.

112. Ishiyama, S. *et al.* 1997. Nitric oxide contributes to the progression of myocardial damage in experimental autoimmune myocarditis in rats. *Circulation* **95:** 489–496.

113. Shin, T. *et al.* 1998. An inhibitor of inducible nitric oxide synthase ameliorates experimental autoimmune myocarditis in Lewis rats. *J. Neuroimmunol.* **92:** 133–138.

114. Valaperti, A. *et al.* 2008. CD11b$^+$ monocytes abrogate Th17 CD4$^+$ T cell-mediated experimental autoimmune myocarditis. *J. Immunol.* **180:** 2686–2695.

115. Blyszczuk, P. *et al.* 2012. Nitric oxide synthase 2 is required for conversion of pro-fibrogenic inflammatory CD133$^+$ progenitors into F4/80$^+$ macrophages in experimental autoimmune myocarditis. *Cardiovasc. Res.*

116. Khader, S.A., S.L. Gaffen & J.K. Kolls. 2009. Th17 cells at the crossroads of innate and adaptive immunity against infectious diseases at the mucosa. *Mucosal. Immunol.* **2:** 403–411.

117. Kolls, J.K. & A. Linden. 2004. Interleukin-17 family members and inflammation. *Immunity* **21:** 467–476.

118. Liao, Y.H. *et al.* 2012. Interleukin-17A contributes to myocardial ischemia/reperfusion injury by regulating cardiomyocyte apoptosis and neutrophil infiltration. *J. Am. Coll. Cardiol.* **59:** 420–429.

119. Fairweather, D. *et al.* 2005. IL-12 protects against coxsackievirus B3-induced myocarditis by increasing IFN-gamma and macrophage and neutrophil populations in the heart. *J. Immunol.* **174:** 261–269.

120. Grabie, N. *et al.* 2003. Neutrophils sustain pathogenic CD8$^+$ T cell responses in the heart. *Am. J. Pathol.* **163:** 2413–2420.

121. Kishimoto, C. *et al.* 2001. Enhanced production of macrophage inflammatory protein 2 (MIP-2) by in vitro and in vivo infections with encephalomyocarditis virus and modulation of myocarditis with an antibody against MIP-2. *J. Virol.* **75:** 1294–1300.

122. Ritzman, A.M. *et al.* 2010. The chemokine receptor CXCR2 ligand KC (CXCL1) mediates neutrophil recruitment and is critical for development of experimental Lyme arthritis and carditis. *Infect. Immun.* **78:** 4593–4600.

123. Arruda-Olson, A.M. *et al.* 2009. Neutrophilia predicts death and heart failure after myocardial infarction: a community-based study. *Circ. Cardiovasc. Qual. Outcom.* **2:** 656–662.

124. Minatoguchi, S. *et al.* 2004. Acceleration of the healing process and myocardial regeneration may be important as a mechanism of improvement of cardiac function and remodeling by postinfarction granulocyte colony-stimulating factor treatment. *Circulation* **109:** 2572–2580.

125. Orlic, D. *et al.* 2001. Mobilized bone marrow cells repair the infarcted heart, improving function and survival. *Proc. Natl. Acad. Sci. USA* **98:** 10344–10349.

126. Kang, H.J. *et al.* 2012. Five-year results of intracoronary infusion of the mobilized peripheral blood stem cells by granulocyte colony-stimulating factor in patients with myocardial infarction. *Eur. Heart J.*

127. Honold, J. *et al.* 2012. G-CSF-stimulation and coronary reinfusion of mobilized circulating mononuclear proangiogenic cells in patients with chronic ischemic heart disease: five year results of the TOPCARE- G-CSF Trial. *Cell Transplant.*

128. Shimada, K. *et al.* 2010. Therapy with granulocyte colony-stimulating factor in the chronic stage, but not in the acute stage, improves experimental autoimmune myocarditis in rats via nitric oxide. *J. Mol. Cell. Cardiol.* **49:** 469–481.

129. Parrillo, J.E. 1990. Heart disease and the eosinophil. *N. Engl. J. Med.* **323:** 1560–1561.

130. Ginsberg, F. & J.E. Parrillo. 2005. Eosinophilic myocarditis. *Heart Fail. Clin.* **1:** 419–429.

131. Molina, H.A. & F. Kierszenbaum. 1989. Eosinophil activation in acute and chronic chagasic myocardial lesions and deposition of toxic eosinophil granule proteins on heart myofibers. *J. Parasitol.* **75:** 129–133.

132. Molina, H.A. & F. Kierszenbaum. 1988. Immunohistochemical detection of deposits of eosinophil-derived neurotoxin and eosinophil peroxidase in the myocardium of patients with Chagas' disease. *Immunology* **64:** 725–731.

133. Spry, C.J., M. Take & P.C. Tai. 1985. Eosinophilic disorders affecting the myocardium and endocardium: a review. *Heart Vess. Suppl.* **1:** 240–242.

134. Abston, E.D. *et al.* 2012. IL-33 independently induces eosinophilic pericarditis and cardiac dilation: ST2 improves cardiac function. *Circ. Heart Fail.* **5:** 366–375.

135. Sanada, S. *et al.* 2007. IL-33 and ST2 comprise a critical biomechanically induced and cardioprotective signaling system. *J. Clin. Invest.* **117:** 1538–1549.

136. Seki, K. *et al.* 2009. Interleukin-33 prevents apoptosis and improves survival after experimental myocardial infarction through ST2 signaling. *Circ. Heart Fail.* **2:** 684–691.

137. Lee, Y.K. *et al.* 2009. Developmental plasticity of Th17 and Treg cells. *Curr. Opin. Immunol.*

138. Bettelli, E. *et al.* 2006. Reciprocal developmental pathways for the generation of pathogenic effector TH17 and regulatory T cells. *Nature* **441:** 235–238.

139. Massilamany, C. *et al.* 2011. Identification of novel mimicry epitopes for cardiac myosin heavy chain-alpha that induce autoimmune myocarditis in A/J mice. *Cell Immunol.* **271:** 438–449.

140. Nindl, V. *et al.* 2012. Cooperation of Th1 and Th17 cells determines transition from autoimmune myocarditis to dilated cardiomyopathy. *Eur. J. Immunol.* **42:** 2311–2321.

141. Noutsias, M., V.J. Patil & B. Maisch. 2012. Cellular immune mechanisms in myocarditis. *Herz*

142. Zhao, Z. *et al.* 2011. Activation of Th17/Th1 and Th1, but not Th17, is associated with the acute cardiac event in patients with acute coronary syndrome. *Atherosclerosis* **217:** 518–524.

143. Berghmans, N. *et al.* 2011. Interferon-gamma orchestrates the number and function of Th17 cells in experimental autoimmune encephalomyelitis. *J. Interferon Cytokine Res.* **31:** 575–587.

144. Nakae, S. *et al.* 2007. Phenotypic differences between Th1 and Th17 cells and negative regulation of Th1 cell differentiation by IL-17. *J. Leukoc. Biol.* **81:** 1258–1268.

145. Kelchtermans, H. *et al.* 2009. Effector mechanisms of interleukin-17 in collagen-induced arthritis in the absence of interferon-gamma and counteraction by interferon-gamma. *Arthr. Res. Ther.* **11:** R122.

146. Lee, Y.K. *et al.* 2009. Late developmental plasticity in the T helper 17 lineage. *Immunity* **30:** 92–107.

147. Hirota, K. *et al.* 2011. Fate mapping of IL-17-producing T cells in inflammatory responses. *Nat. Immunol.* **12:** 255–263.

148. Kryczek, I. *et al.* 2008. Induction of IL-17+ T cell trafficking and development by IFN-gamma: mechanism and pathological relevance in psoriasis. *J. Immunol.* **181:** 4733–4741.

149. Huber, S.A. 2010. gammadelta T lymphocytes kill T regulatory cells through CD1d. *Immunology* **131:** 202–209.

150. Huber, S.A. 2009. Depletion of gammadelta+ T cells increases CD4+ FoxP3 (T regulatory) cell response in coxsackievirus B3-induced myocarditis. *Immunology* **127:** 567–576.

151. Kaya, Z. *et al.* 2011. Comparison of IL-10 and MCP-1–7ND gene transfer with AAV9 vectors for protection from murine autoimmune myocarditis. *Cardiovasc. Res.* **91:** 116–123.

152. Matsumoto, K. *et al.* 2011. Regulatory T lymphocytes attenuate myocardial infarction-induced ventricular remodeling in mice. *Int. Heart J.* **52:** 382–387.

153. Tang, T.T. *et al.* 2012. Regulatory T cells ameliorate cardiac remodeling after myocardial infarction. *Basic Res. Cardiol.* **107:** 232.

154. Cooper, L.T., Jr., G.J. Berry & R. Shabetai. 1997. Idiopathic giant-cell myocarditis–natural history and treatment. Multicenter Giant Cell Myocarditis Study Group Investigators. *N. Engl. J. Med.* **336:** 1860–1866.

155. Yi, A. *et al.* 2009. The prevalence of Th17 cells in patients with dilated cardiomyopathy. Clinical and investigative medicine.*Medecine Clinique Et Experimentale.* **32:** E144–E150.

156. Ong, K.L. *et al.* 2013. Arthritis: its prevalence, risk factors, and association with cardiovascular diseases in the United States, 1999 to 2008. *Ann. Epidemiol.* **23:** 80–86.

157. Gisondi, P. *et al.* 2010. Usefulness of the framingham risk score in patients with chronic psoriasis. *Am. J. Cardiol.* **106:** 1754–1757.

158. Mehta, N.N. *et al.* 2011. Attributable risk estimate of severe psoriasis on major cardiovascular events. *Am. J. Med.* **124:** 775 e771–776.

159. Tincani, A. *et al.* 2006. Heart involvement in systemic lupus erythematosus, anti-phospholipid syndrome and neonatal lupus. *Rheumatology.* **45** (Suppl. 4): iv8–13.

160. Abdel-Aty, H. *et al.* 2008. Myocardial tissue characterization in systemic lupus erythematosus: value of a comprehensive cardiovascular magnetic resonance approach. *Lupus* **17:** 561–567.

161. Panchal, L. *et al.* 2006. Cardiovascular involvement in systemic lupus erythematosus: an autopsy study of 27 patients in India. *J. Postgrad. Med.* **52:** 5–10; discussion 10.

162. Puig, L. 2012. Cardiovascular risk and psoriasis: the role of biologic therapy. *Actas Dermo-Sifiliograficas.* **103:** 853–862.

163. Langley, R.G. *et al.* 2012. Safety results from a pooled analysis of randomized, controlled phase II and III clinical trials and interim data from an open-label extension trial of the interleukin-12/23 monoclonal antibody, briakinumab, in moderate to severe psoriasis. *J. Eur. Acad. Dermatol. Venereol.*

164. Gordon, K.B. *et al.* 2012. A phase III, randomized, controlled trial of the fully human IL-12/23 mAb briakinumab in moderate-to-severe psoriasis. *J. Invest. Dermatol.* **132:** 304–314.

165. Taleb, S. *et al.* 2009. Loss of SOCS3 expression in T cells reveals a regulatory role for interleukin-17 in atherosclerosis. *J. Exp. Med.* **206:** 2067–2077.

166. Armstrong, A.W. *et al.* 2011. A tale of two plaques: convergent mechanisms of T-cell-mediated inflammation in psoriasis and atherosclerosis. *Exp. Dermatol.* **20:** 544–549.

167. Tzellos, T., A. Kyrgidis & C.C. Zouboulis. 2012. Re-evaluation of the risk for major adverse cardiovascular events in patients treated with anti-IL-12/23 biological agents for chronic plaque psoriasis: a meta-analysis of randomized controlled trials. *J. Eur. Acad. Dermatol. Venereol.*

168. Ryan, C. *et al.* 2011. Association between biologic therapies for chronic plaque psoriasis and cardiovascular events: a

meta-analysis of randomized controlled trials. *JAMA* **306:** 864–871.

169. Reich, K. *et al.* 2011. Cardiovascular safety of ustekinumab in patients with moderate to severe psoriasis: results of integrated analyses of data from phase II and III clinical studies. *Br. J. Dermatol.* **164:** 862–872.

170. Greenbaum, L.A., R. Benndorf & W.E. Smoyer. 2012. Childhood nephrotic syndrome—current and future therapies. *Nat. Rev. Nephrol.* **8:** 445–458.

171. Garrett, J.K. *et al.* 2004. Anti-interleukin-5 (mepolizumab) therapy for hypereosinophilic syndromes. *J. Allergy Clin. Immunol.* **113:** 115–119.

172. Plotz, S.G. *et al.* 2003. Use of an anti-interleukin-5 antibody in the hypereosinophilic syndrome with eosinophilic dermatitis. *N. Engl. J. Med.* **349:** 2334–2339.

173. Rothenberg, M.E. *et al.* 2008. Treatment of patients with the hypereosinophilic syndrome with mepolizumab. *N. Engl. J. Med.* **358:** 1215–1228.

174. Moosig, F. *et al.* 2011. Targeting interleukin-5 in refractory and relapsing Churg-Strauss syndrome. *Ann. Intern. Med.* **155:** 341–343.

175. Kim, S. *et al.* 2010. Mepolizumab as a steroid-sparing treatment option in patients with Churg-Strauss syndrome. *J. Allergy Clin. Immunol.* **125:** 1336–1343.

176. Kim, Y.J. *et al.* 2004. Rebound eosinophilia after treatment of hypereosinophilic syndrome and eosinophilic gastroenteritis with monoclonal anti-IL-5 antibody SCH55700. *J. Allergy Clin. Immunol.* **114:** 1449–1455.

177. Klion, A.D. *et al.* 2004. Safety and efficacy of the monoclonal anti-interleukin-5 antibody SCH55700 in the treatment of patients with hypereosinophilic syndrome. *Blood* **103:** 2939–2941.

178. Wechsler, M.E. *et al.* 2012. Novel targeted therapies for eosinophilic disorders. *J. Allergy Clin. Immunol.* **130:** 563–571.

179. Pummerer, C.L. *et al.* 1996. Identification of cardiac myosin peptides capable of inducing autoimmune myocarditis in BALB/c mice. *J. Clin. Invest.* **97:** 2057–2062.

180. Donermeyer, D.L. *et al.* 1995. Myocarditis-inducing epitope of myosin binds constitutively and stably to I-Ak on antigen-presenting cells in the heart. *J. Exp. Med.* **182:** 1291–1300.

181. Kaya, Z. *et al.* 2008. Identification of cardiac troponin I sequence motifs leading to heart failure by induction of myocardial inflammation and fibrosis. *Circulation* **118:** 2063–2072.

182. Jane-wit, D. *et al.* 2002. A novel class II-binding motif selects peptides that mediate organ-specific autoimmune disease in SWXJ, SJL/J, and SWR/J mice. *J. Immunol.* **169:** 6507–6514.

Ann. N.Y. Acad. Sci. ISSN 0077-8923

ANNALS OF THE NEW YORK ACADEMY OF SCIENCES
Issue: *The Year in immunology*

Human B-1 cells take the stage

Thomas L. Rothstein,[1,2] Daniel O. Griffin,[1] Nichol E. Holodick,[1] Tam D. Quach,[1] and Hiroaki Kaku[1]

[1]Center for Oncology and Cell Biology, The Feinstein Institute for Medical Research, and [2]Departments of Medicine and Molecular Medicine, Hofstra North Shore-LIJ School of Medicine, Manhasset, New York

Address for correspondence: Thomas L. Rothstein, The Feinstein Institute for Medical Research, 350 Community Drive, Room 3354, Manhasset, NY. tr@nshs.edu

B-1 cells play critical roles in defending against microbial invasion and in housekeeping removal of cellular debris. B-1 cells secrete natural antibody and manifest functions that influence T cell expansion and differentiation and in these and other ways differ from conventional B-2 cells. B-1 cells were originally studied in mice where they are easily distinguished from B-2 cells, but their identity in the human system remained poorly defined for many years. Recently, functional criteria for human B-1 cells were established on the basis of murine findings, and reverse engineering resulted in identification of the phenotypic profile, $CD20^+CD27^+CD43^+CD70^-$, for B-1 cells found in both umbilical cord blood and adult peripheral blood. Human B-1 cells may contribute to multiple disease states through production of autoantibody and stimulation/modulation of T cell activity. Human B-1 cells could be a rich source of antibodies useful in treating diseases present in elderly populations where natural antibody protection may have eroded. Manipulation of human B-1 cell numbers and/or activity may be a new avenue for altering T cell function and treating immune dyscrasias.

Keywords: B-1; B cells; lymphocytes; antibody

Introduction

The immune system is an intricate and multifaceted device. It comprises numerous cell types and structures that respond in a measured way to microbial assaults with actions that arise appropriately, end promptly, and, for the most part, do not damage normal tissue, all the while maintaining tolerance for self structures and symbiotic microorganisms. B cells are the key effectors of serological immunity, responsible for generation of life-saving antibody in response to microbial invasion (and intentional vaccination), and possibly malignant transformation. In the past, B cells have often been envisioned as simple antibody production facilities responding to antigen binding and signals derived from other cell types, although they are clearly capable of presenting antigen and influencing T cells, among other activities.[1] In recent years the marked clinical success of B cell depletion therapy with anti-CD20 antibody in several autoimmune diseases[2–8] has sug-

gested that B cells may be prime movers in some and possibly many immune dyscrasias. This has evoked considerable renewed interest in the physiological and pathological functions and roles of B cells.

B cells are divided into separate populations, each recognized by a particular phenotypic array of surface markers. These include transitional, follicular, germinal center, and memory (isotype switched and unswitched) B cells. Together these populations constitute conventional B cells that react adaptively to new antigenic challenges with antibody responses produced by differentiated plasmablasts and plasma cells that are generally characterized by affinity maturation.[9] Separate and apart from these conventional populations of B cells stand B cells that can be classified as elements of the innate immune system: marginal zone (MZ) B cells that specialize in responses to blood-borne pathogens and may represent a type of memory B cell,[10,11] and B-1 cells, that constitutively and spontaneously secrete "natural"

doi: 10.1111/nyas.12137

Table 1. Phenotypic properties of mouse and human B cell subsets

	Mouse					Human			
	B-1	FO	MZ	Memory		B-1	Naive	IgM memory	Switched memory
CD5	+	−	−	−	CD5	+/−*	+/−**	+/−**	−
CD9	++/−*	−	++	ND					
CD11b	++/−[a]	−	−	−	CD11b	++/−**	−	−	−
CD19	+++	++	++	++	CD19	++	++	++	++
CD21	+	++	+++	+/−*	CD20	++	++	++	++
CD23	+/−**	+++	+	+/−**					
CD25	+/−**	−	−	ND	CD27	++	−	++	++
CD38	+++	++	++	++					
CD43	++	−	−	−	CD43	++	+/−**	−	−
CD44	++	−	++	++					
CD45[b]	+	++	++	++	CD45[b]	++	++	++	++
CD80	+++	−	+	+/−**					
CD86	+/−**	−	+	+	CD86	++/−**	−	++/−**	++/−**
CD273[c]	+/−*	−	−	+/−**					
IL-5R	+	−	ND	ND					
IgM	+++	+	+++	+/−**	IgM	++/−*	++	+++	+/−**
IgD	+	+++	+	+/−**	IgD	++/−*	+++	++	−

NOTE : Phenotypic properties are shown for peritoneal B-1a (B-1), splenic follicular (FO), splenic marginal zone (MZ), and memory B (memory) cells from BALB/c mice. Phenotypic properties are shown for human peripheral B cell subsets, wherein B-1 cells are $CD27^+CD43^+$, mature naive B cells are $CD27^-IgD^+$, IgM memory B cells are $CD27^+IgM^+IgD^+$, and switched memory B cells are $CD27^+IgD^-$. Phenotypic markers for all cells are described for cells taken *ex vivo* and unstimulated. + = low expression; ++ = moderate expression; +++ = high expression; − = no expression; ND = not determined. *50% or more of the population express the indicated marker. **50% or more of the population lack expression of indicated marker.
[a]CD11b characterizes most B-1 cells in the peritoneum; absence of CD11b defines a distinct subset of $CD5^+$ B-1 cells.
[b]B220.
[c]PD-L2.

antibody and influence other elements of immune activity.[12]

Identification of B-1 cells, a relatively small but unique B cell population, emerged from the initial finding over three decades ago that malignant cells of human and mouse B cell leukemias and lymphomas incongruously express the T cell antigen, CD5.[13,14] It was subsequently determined that CD5 expression is a characteristic feature of a small population of normal B cells[15,16] that may be the cell of origin for, or transform into, B cell malignancy. CD5 expression on $CD5^+$ B cells is dim, much less than that of T cells, for which reason $CD5^+$ B cells can be identified by flow cytometry with its use of photomultiplier detectors but for all practical purposes cannot be detected by fluorescence microscopy. In the mouse system B-1 cell expression of CD5 correlates with expression of several other distinctive markers ($IgM^{hi}IgD^{lo}CD45^{lo}CD23^{lo/-}CD43^+$; also mostly $CD11b^+$ in the peritoneal cavity and $CD9^+$ shared with MZ B cells) such that B-1 cells are readily identifiable and cleanly separable from conventional B (B-2) cells and can thus be individually examined (Table 1). Of note, two kinds of B-1 cells have been described in mice: B-1a cells, with the phenotype noted above; and, B-1b cells, that bear all B-1a cell surface markers except CD5. B-1b cells are regulated separately from B-1a cells, fulfill distinct immune functions, and appear to develop in concert with B-2 cells.[17–22] Intensive study in the murine system has demonstrated that B-1a cells (denoted B-1 cells in the foregoing except where specified) are quite different from conventional B-2 cells in many ways, as discussed in the next five sections, after which the nature of human B-1 cells is addressed in the remaining sections.

B-1 cells secrete protective natural antibody

Mouse B-1 cells are predominantly located in the peritoneal cavity, but are also found in the pleural cavity, the spleen, and the bone marrow, with little representation in lymph nodes or blood.[23,24] The principal function unique to B-1 cells is spontaneous, constitutive secretion of antibody. This antibody accumulates as baseline or resting immunoglobulin, termed *natural antibody* that appears in the absence of infection or immunization. It is predominantly IgM, and it is estimated that 80–90% of resting serum IgM, and perhaps 50% of resting serum IgA (the major isotype of switched B-1 cell immunoglobulin) is derived from B-1 cells.[25–27] More specifically, serum IgM is preferentially produced by B-1 cells in the spleen that secrete much more antibody than peritoneal B-1 cells, and by B-1 cells in the bone marrow.[28,29] There is evidence that peritoneal B-1 cells migrate to the spleen under certain activation conditions and upregulate antibody secretion there,[30–33] although it is possible that splenic B-1 cells represent a separate, high-secreting subpopulation. It has also been suggested that the splenic environment is critical to B-1 cell generation.[34,35] Recent results suggest that for at least one antigen, and maybe more, B-1 cells in the spleen are activated by immunization in a T-independent fashion to become memory B cells that reside in the peritoneal cavity and, upon rechallenge, return to the spleen where they differentiate to antigen-specific, high-secreting plasma cells.[36,37] These findings raise the possibility that many B-1 cells located in the peritoneum may represent memory cells, a status that had not been thought to exist among B-1 cells.

Mouse B-1 cell natural antibody is distinctive and differs from conventional B-2 cell adaptive antibody in many ways, including repertoire, structure, and development. Natural antibody tends to be polyreactive, autoreactive, and antimicrobial at relatively modest affinity.[38–41] B-1 cell natural antibody is highly effective, such that animal recovery from a number of experimental infections depends on the joint action of B-1 and B-2 cell-derived antibod-

ies as mice with only B-1 cells or only B-2 cells do poorly.[22,42–45] The success of B-1 cell natural antibody may depend, in part, on polyreactivity, which provides the means for a single antibody to heteroligate different, each possibly widely spaced, surface antigens, thereby increasing effective avidity.[46] Alternatively, or in addition, B-1 cell natural antibody may succeed as a result of the specific nature of putative conformational changes in the Fc region following antigen binding, in that effector function typically depends on engagement of other cell types and immune elements. Because B-1 cell natural antibody is secreted spontaneously and constitutively, it forms a pre-existing shield against infection that provides protection during the lag period required for germinal center formation and adaptive antibody production (Fig 1). A major component of natural antibody recognizes phosphorylcholine (PC), a key and invariant constituent of Gram positive microbial pathogen membranes, including the *Streptococcus pneumoniae* bacterial cell wall, and is often encoded by $V_H S107.1$.[45,47]

Anti-PC antibodies do not just recognize PC on pneumococci, as PC is also present on a number of other bacterial pathogens, apoptotic cell membranes, and oxidized lipids.[48] Another important component of natural antibody recognizes phosphatidylcholine (PtC), a key constituent of senescent red blood cell membranes, that is encoded primarily by $V_H 11$ and $V_H 12$.[49,50] These and other examples of autoreactivity have given rise to the concept that a second, parallel function of B-1 cell natural antibody lies in housekeeping or homeostatic activity that speeds elimination of dead and dying cells and cellular debris. In so doing, potentially inflammatory and/or toxic molecules are removed before damage in the form of immune cell priming or direct tissue injury can occur. This anti-inflammatory effect can involve deposition of complement and suppression of accessory cell function.[51] Thus, mice lacking natural IgM antibody are prone to accelerated development of autoantibodies and more severe autoimmune disease,[52] presumably because antigens and inflammation associated with apoptotic cell debris stimulate B-2 cell responses when not properly cleared in a timely fashion. Further, B-1 cell-derived natural IgM has been shown to be protective against atherosclerosis in a mouse model of cardiovascular disease, presumably as a result of efficient disposal of oxidized low

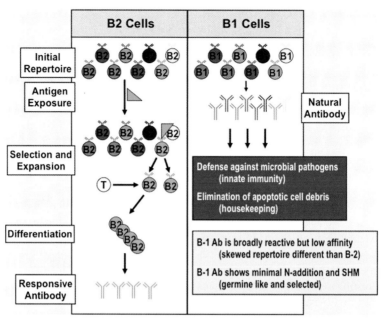

Figure 1. B-1 cells secrete protective natural antibody. B-1 and B-2 cells fulfill different functions in generating serological immunity as shown in the right and left panels. B-2 cells express immunoglobulin molecules that are junctionally diverse as a result of N-region addition. Following antigen/microbial/vaccination activation, B-2 cells undergo multiple steps to produce antibody secreting cells that require substantial periods of time to develop after initial exposure. Specific B-2 cells that bind antigen are selected to develop germinal centers during which marked B cell expansion is accompanied by somatic hypermutation (and isotype switching), resulting in further repertoire diversity and selection on the basis of antigen-binding affinity. Differentiation to antibody secreting plasma cells (and memory B cells) completes the process. In contrast, B-1 cells express immunoglobulin molecules that are less diverse as a result of minimal N-region addition and minimal somatic hypermutation. Although many B-1 cell antibodies manifest modest affinity, they are often polyreactive, and the latter feature may assist in functional efficacy. B-1 cells constitutively and spontaneously secrete the range of antibodies (mostly IgM) they express, without the need for stimulation or activation (although immunoglobulin secretion may be increased by certain TLR agonists). This "natural" antibody constitutes the bulk of normal baseline or resting IgM. The B-1 cell repertoire represents a pre-existing antimicrobial shield and functions to dispose of cellular debris and toxic molecules. Because B-1 cell antibodies closely mirror germline sequences, the B-1 cell repertoire is considered to have been optimized for survival over evolutionary time. Thus B-1 cell antibodies are selected for function whereas B-2 cell antibodies are selected for affinity. Erosion of the natural antibody repertoire with increasing age may underlie susceptibility of older individuals to certain infectious and degenerative diseases. Because B-1 cell antibodies are often autoreactive, imposition of somatic hypermutation and isotype switching could result in production of typical pathogenic autoantibodies.

density lipoprotein (LDL) and similar pathogenic lipids.[53–55] Thus natural antibody produced by B-1 cells is considered to fulfill two important functions: immediate defense against microbial pathogens and housekeeping removal of cellular debris.

The structure of B-1 cell natural antibody differs markedly from B-2 cell adaptive antibody in being more germline-like. In comparison to B-2 cell antibody, B-1 cell antibody contains little or no somatic hypermutation and much reduced, or nonexistent, N-region addition.[49,56–58] This means B-1 cell antibodies more or less exactly reflect germline $V_H D_H J_H / V_L J_L$ sequences. A good example of this is the prototypic, pneumococcal-protective anti-PC

antibody, T15, that is completely germline and contains no somatic mutation or N-addition.[47] Somatic mutation and N-addition would be expected to increase repertoire diversity by altering antibody structure, but at the same time could change the original binding specificity of the germline sequence. In fact, enforced N-addition in transgenic mice results in loss of T15 antibody and loss of protection against pneumococcal infection.[59] Notably N-region addition is determined during V_H-D_H-J_H and V_L-J_L joining early in B cell development and requires the enzyme terminal deoxynucleotidyl transferase (TdT), which adds nontemplated nucleotides;[60] somatic mutation occurs in the course of antigen-triggered expansion of mature B-2 cells during residence in transient, specialized germinal center structures.[61] Because B-1 cell antibodies tend to reflect sequences delineated in the genome largely without alteration, and because B-1 cell antibodies play a critical role in antimicrobial defense, it has been suggested that the B-1 cell repertoire is "tuned" over evolutionary time, obeying Darwinian precepts such that sequences functioning to promote survival are retained.[47] This then differs from the situation with B-2 cell antibodies in which the principal criterion for retention is affinity. In this view, B-1 cell antibodies may represent the very best antibodies for functional protection against some infectious pathogens and, by extension, the very best antibodies for disposing of apoptotic cellular constituents.

B-1 cells constitute a separate B cell lineage

The origin of B-1 cells has been the subject of much debate over many years' time, involving two distinct hypotheses of lineage versus differentiation. Early adoptive transfer experiments indicated that adult bone marrow does not reconstitute the B-1 cell population; instead, reconstitution only occurs if/when B-1 cells (e.g., peritoneal B-1 cells) are transferred along with bone marrow cells.[62] However, both B-1 and B-2 cells are generated after adoptive transfer of fetal liver cells. Moreover, cells from omental tissue give rise predominantly to B-1 cells.[63] These results suggest that B-1 cells only arise early in ontogeny and cannot be generated later in life. The early appearance of B-1 cells is the reason this population is designated "B-1" and conventional B cells that arise later are termed "B-2".[64] Consistent with an early, restricted origin for B-1 cells is the special property of self-renewal, in which mature, surface immunoglobulin-bearing B-1 cells give rise to their own progeny, unlike B-2 cells that derive from immature, immunoglobulin-negative progenitors.[65,66] All together these findings suggest that B-1 cells emerge early in the life of the animal as a separate and distinct lineage that maintains itself through self-renewal without further input from other sources. The sequential timing of B-1 and B-2 cell development suggests an ontological "switch" in development from production of B-1 cells to production of B-2 cells.[67] Similar changes in T cell development (from $\gamma\delta$ to $\alpha\beta$ antigen receptors) and red blood cell development (from fetal to adult hemoglobin) support the hypothesis that a generalized ontological switch involving multiple hematopoietic lineages occurs around the time of birth.[68] Lin28b may dictate that switch, and results with enforced expression of Lin28b support the notion that ontological switching occurs.[69]

An alternative to this paradigm was advanced by the finding that CD5 expression is induced on conventional B-2 cells after stimulation by BCR crosslinking.[70] This suggests that CD5[+] B-1 cells are generated by stimulation of B cells at a relatively mature stage.[71] Strong support for this idea comes from the construction of immunoglobulin transgenic mice in which the BCR is fixed as a typical antiphosphatidylcholine specificity; B cells in these mice ($V_H12V_\kappa4$ and $V_H11V_\kappa9$) are overwhelmingly phenotypic B-1 cells,[72,73] implying that the events responsible for producing B-1 cells occur subsequent to immunoglobulin rearrangement. The failure of B-1 cell development in animals with dysfunctional mediators of BCR signaling, such as *xid* animals with mutant Btk,[23,24,74] lends further support to the idea that BCR signaling is necessary for B-1 cell development, which occurs after the BCR is expressed. Along the same lines, mutation of SHP tyrosine phosphatase involved in modulating BCR signaling cascades leads to increased numbers of B-1 cells.[27,75,76] Because the B-1 cell repertoire is selected for certain specificities like PtC and PC, taken together these results infer that B-1 cells arise not from a separate lineage but from a differentiative process triggered by ligand interactions with B cell receptors capable of recognizing certain self-antigens.[77]

This controversy regarding lineage and differentiation was resolved by the discovery of a specific progenitor that gives rise to B-1 cells, but not B-2 cells, and phenotypes as lineage-negative (lin[−]) CD45[lo/−]CD19[+], in contradistinction to the conventional B-2 cell developmental pathway in which CD45 expression precedes expression of CD19.[78,79] This lin[−]CD45[lo/−]CD19[+] B-1 cell progenitor arises from yolk sac and para-aortic splanchnopleura tissues and is abundantly present in mouse fetal liver;[80] although a small number of B-1 cell progenitors are found in adult bone marrow, these do not appear to function as efficiently as phenotypically similar progenitors present earlier in life.[81] B-1 cell progenitors are also present, albeit quiescent, in adult spleen but can respond to inflammation.[80,82] Although it cannot be said with certainty that every B-1 cell derives from the identified progenitor, these findings clearly indicate that at least some, and likely most if not all, B-1 cells constitute a separate lymphocyte lineage derived from a distinct, surface immunoglobulin negative progenitor. Commitment to the B-1 cell lineage appears to occur prior to the acknowledged $CD45^{lo/-}CD19^+$ B-1 cell progenitor, at least as early as the common lymphocyte precursor (CLP) stage.[18,81]

These results also support the notion that B cell development occurs in waves, with B-1 cells generated initially and B-2 cells after that. However, B-1 cells can be divided based on relative expression or lack thereof for CD11b, CD25, PD-L2, and PC-1, among other surface antigens,[17,83–85b] and thus it remains possible that a particular subpopulation could be generated through a distinct pathway separate from the identified B-1 cell progenitor. Of note, earlier work had indicated that developing B-1 cells are affected differently than developing B-2 cells by strong BCR binding of self-antigens;[86–89] whereas B-2 cells are deleted, B-1 cell development is promoted.[88,90,91] Along the same lines, strong signaling for B-1 cell development may be produced by the BCR autonomously in the absence of antigen.[92] This positive response specifically in B-1 cells may explain the necessity for intact BCR signaling during B-1 cell development and, along with other functional differences between B-1 and B-2 cells, can now be ascribed to the distinct lineages of which these cells are the mature, differentiated end products.

B-1 cell natural antibody changes with advancing age

Although reduced in number and function, bone marrow B-1 cell progenitors do, in fact, generate B-1 cells after adoptive transfer.[93–96] However, the B-1 cells produced by adult bone marrow, though authentic in phenotype and function, differ in one important respect from the native B-1 cells that populate young animals: bone marrow-derived B-1 cells express antibodies that contain abundant N-region additions, in contrast to native B-1 cells from young animals.[94,95] In fact, the number of bone marrow-derived B-1 cells that lack N-addition at both the D_H–J_H and V_H–D_H junctions approximates the very low level present in native B-2 cells from young animals.[94] At the same time, among wild-type mice,

B-1 cells in older animals express antibodies that contain much more N-addition compared to B-1 cells in younger animals;[56,94] in other words, as mice age, the level of N-addition in B-1 cell antibody increases. Taken together, these results infer that bone marrow progenitors give rise to mature B-1 cells that over time become part of the native B-1 cell pool. In other words, the early B-1 cell population is not completely perpetuated (via self-renewal) without change, but rather appears to accumulate bone marrow immigrants that, with increasing age, alter the overall composition of the native B-1 cell pool. Such changing composition may actually amount to erosion of beneficial germline-determined specificities because the abundance of N-addition in bone marrow-derived B-1 cell antibodies can alter CDR3 combining site structures. If germline-like natural antibody is evolutionarily tuned for efficacy, then with increasing age B-1 cell natural antibody may become less and less effective in carrying out its key functions of microbial defense and debris disposition. This process could play a role in the increased susceptibility of older individuals to a variety of diseases whose incidence is age-related, such as the aforementioned pneumococcal pneumonia and cardiovascular disease. Going further, the existence of human natural antibodies against pathogenic amyloid peptides and tumor-associated gangliosides and other antigens[97–100] raises the possibility that erosion of the B-1 cell repertoire could degrade defense against neurodegenerative and neoplastic diseases.

Chronically signaling B-1 cells stimulate and regulate T cell responses

Beyond natural antibody secretion and its key role in infection remediation and apoptotic housekeeping, B-1 cell activities affect other elements of the immune system in both stimulatory and suppressive ways. B-1 cells strongly induce activation and proliferation of naive T cells across an allogeneic barrier, indicating that B-1 cells are efficient antigen presenting cells, as effective as dendritic cells.[101–103] Among mouse B-1 cells, the PD-L2$^+$ subpopulation is particularly adept at stimulating T cell expansion and particularly engaged in producing autoantibodies.[104] T cell stimulation by B-1 cells is evident directly *ex vivo* without any activation or further manipulation of B-1 cells, and can be attributed at least in part to constitutively elevated expression of the costimulatory molecule, CD86 and, to a lesser extent, CD80.[101,102] Upregulated expression of CD86 joins several other characteristics of "resting" B-1 cells that are similar to features of activated B-2 cells, including upregulated expression of phosphorylated ERK, phosphorylated STAT3, NF-AT, and CD44.[105–109] Constitutively phosphorylated ERK would seem incongruous because ERK phosphorylation occurs downstream of BCR signaling, yet it has long been known that BCR signaling is impaired in B-1 cells; in B-1 cells, unlike B-2 cells, BCR triggering fails to induce cellular proliferation or NF-κB activation.[110–112] Further, signaling mediators between BCR and ERK are not constitutively phosphorylated in B-1 cells, further clouding the origin of pERK. However, BCR signaling intermediates are indeed responsible for constitutive ERK phosphorylation in B-1 cells, as evidenced by recent work showing that various signalosome inhibitors quickly eliminate phospho-ERK, and that phosphatase inhibitors result in accumulation of phosphorylated forms of BCR signaling intermediates.[113] It is speculated, then, that B-1 cells are chronically signaling as a result of self-recognizing BCR specificities or autonomous BCR activity, but that signaling for phosphorylation of most intermediates is exactly matched by upregulated phosphatase activity, except in the case of ERK, and so becomes apparent only in the presence of phosphatase inhibition. This more active physiology and enhanced signal modulation may explain, as a form of tachyphylaxis, why acute BCR triggering has little effect on NF-κB activation. Because BCR signaling induces CD86 expression,[114] these studies suggest a mechanism for baseline upregulated expression of CD86 by B-1 cells, and indeed inhibition of the signalosome element, PI-3K, produces a rapid decline in B-1 cell CD86 that is reversed upon removal of the inhibitor.[113] Thus, in this case, lineage and BCR structure/specificity appear to encode destiny, producing chronic signaling that leads to increased CD86 expression that contributes to strong antigen presentation and efficient T cell stimulation.

Beyond stimulating T cell expansion, B-1 cells can influence T cell function. B-1 cells induce differentiation of naive, CD4$^+$ T cells to IL-17-expressing pro-inflammatory Th17 cells, whereas B-2 cells induce T cell differentiation to regulatory T (T_{reg}) cells.[102,104,115] Although no direct mechanism for B-1 cell-induced Th17 cell differentiation is known,

costimulatory molecules CD80 and CD86 play a role (albeit a smaller role than in stimulation for T cell expansion), as does CD44 through binding of osteopontin.[115] It is also possible that cytokine secretion by B-1 cell-stimulated T cells, or by B-1 cells themselves, could play a role.[102,104] Induction of Th17 cell differentiation is not unique to B-1 cells, as B-2 cells can do the same, but only after activation, which upregulates CD80, CD86 and CD44, among other molecules.[115]

These stimulatory effects contrast with B cell–mediated suppression, identified early on as a key element in recovery from experimental autoimmune encephalomyelitis (EAE).[116] The beneficial effects of B cells in modulating EAE result from IL-10.[117] Inasmuch as B-1 cells have long been known to secrete IL-10,[118] the property of T cell regulation by B cells would appear to be another unique characteristic of B-1 cells, not shared with unstimulated B-2 cells. However, it is not clear that regulatory B cells secreting IL-10 and B-1 cells are synonymous groupings. IL-10 secreting B cells have been reported to express CD5 and high level CD1d, and to consist mostly of B-1 cells but to also overlap phenotypically with some MZ B cells.[119] Alternatively, IL-10 secreting B cells have been reported to express CD23 and CD21 and high level CD1d, and to consist primarily of T2-MZ precursor B cells.[120] Adding to confusion regarding identity is the possibility of other mechanisms for B cell–mediated suppression, including secretion of TGF-β; expression of FasL, TRAIL and PD-L2; and production of adenosine.[84,121–126] Although it is clear that B cells can exert suppression, and it seems likely that B-1 cells are responsible through IL-10 secretion, the role of other actors and other mechanisms remains uncertain, including the role of B-2 cells following activation.

Considering that B-1 cells are capable of presenting antigen to T cells and stimulating T cell expansion, inducing Th17 cell differentiation, and suppressing T cell activity, they would appear to be in a position to heavily influence the nature and direction of T cell responses, depending on whether stimulatory or suppressive activities dominate (Fig. 2). It may be speculated, then, that excessive or inappropriate B-1 cell activity may be involved in the pathophysiology of autoimmune dyscrasias by presenting autoantigen or stimulating effector T cell expansion, inducing Th17 cell differentiation, and/or failing to suppress T cell function at the

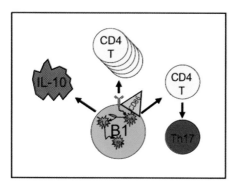

Figure 2. Chronically signaling B-1 cells stimulate and regulate T cell responses. B-1 cells affect immune system function in several ways beyond antibody production. B-1 cells strongly present antigen and stimulate T cell proliferation, which depends on baseline enhanced expression of CD86, absent any stimulation or activation. Upregulated CD86 in turn depends on chronic signaling that is presumably generated by B cell receptor binding to self-antigen, but could represent antigen independent activity. Further, B-1 cells promote CD4 T cell differentiation to pro-inflammatory IL-17-containing Th17 cells, a process that also depends on CD86. Whereas these activities promote inflammation, B-1 cells also produce and secrete immunosuppressive IL-10. Thus, B-1 cells manifest a full suite of immune system modulatory activities that include T cell expansion, inflammation, and immunosuppression. As such, B-1 cells express countervailing activities, the balance of which may regulate the direction of normal T cell immune responses and, under pathologic conditions, may contribute to autoimmunity.

proper time and place. The role of B-1 cells could even include production of pathological autoantibodies, if the infrequent events of isotype switching and somatic mutation are determinative for the infrequent occurrence of autoimmune dyscrasias. Evidence implicating B-1 cells in some autoimmune animal models supports this connection.[101,103, 104,127]

B-1 cells are distinguished from B-2 cells in other ways

B-1 cells differ from resting B-2 cells in a number of characteristics beyond surface antigen expression, natural antibody secretion, chronic intracellular signaling, and, T cell stimulation, differentiation and suppression. Some additional features that have been reported to distinguish B-1 cells in comparison to B-2 cells include larger overall size; enhanced survival *ex vivo*; resistance to Fas-mediated apoptosis; unique expression of gene transcripts and proteins; distinct signaling characteristics, including responsiveness to phorbol ester and increased intracellular Ca^{2+}; and, developmental indepen-

dence from BAFF/BLys and IL-7 (Table 2).[108,109, 111,128–142] These findings have resulted for the most part from comparisons between peritoneal B-1 cells and splenic B-2 cells, and it should be noted that splenic B-1 cells are not in every respect the same as peritoneal B-1 cells.[73,106] However, the range and extent of B-1 cell characteristics that differ from B-2 cells are consistent with the current view that B-1 cells represent a separate lineage borne of a distinct progenitor.

Human CD5+ B cells are not synonymous with human B-1 cells

Following the initial finding that human chronic lymphocytic leukemia (CLL) malignant B cells express CD5, the presumed normal counterpart, a CD5-expressing B cell, was identified in healthy individuals.[143] Human CD5+ B cells were reported to produce polyreactive autoantibodies much like mouse B-1 cells, to be expanded in autoimmune rheumatoid arthritis, and to represent 15–30% of circulating B cells and up to 75% of umbilical cord blood B cells.[144–149] However, it is now clear that CD5 is not an exclusive marker of B-1 cells in many species, especially in *Homo sapiens*, where CD5 is expressed on prenaive, transitional, and activated B-2 cell populations.[150–154] This somewhat promiscuous expression of CD5 on various B cell populations may explain the relatively large numbers of circulating CD5+ B cells identified in early human studies.

The uncertainty regarding markers for B-1 cells in non-*Mus* species raised the possibility that this population is a limited idiosyncrasy and possibly a feature not found in the wild but restricted to inbred strains of mice,[155] and therefore of little clinical significance. This minimalist view was counterbalanced by the implied role of CD5+ B cells in human disease and the important physiological functions extrapolated for human B-1 cells on the basis of murine studies.

Human B-1 cells are identified through a functional reverse-engineering strategy

To identify human B-1 cells, the typical discovery vector from recognizing phenotype to ascertaining function, which served to identify and characterize mouse B-1 cells, was reversed. In this approach, several distinctive functional features of mouse B-1 cells were collected as a set of index characteristics that any putative human B-1 cell population should fulfill to be validated as such. These key features are (1) spontaneous IgM secretion; (2) efficient T cell stimulation; and (3) chronic intracellular signaling. Spontaneous IgM secretion, assessed by ELISPOT

Table 2. Functional properties of mouse and human B cell subsets*

Functional properties	Mouse		Human	
	B-1	FO	B-1	Naive
Natural antibody	Yes	No	Yes	No
Few N additions	Yes	No	ND	No
Skewed repertoire	Yes	No	ND	No
Anti-PtC[a] antibody	Yes	No	ND	ND
Anti-PC[b] antibody	Yes	No	Yes	No
Signaling				
Chronic signaling[c]	Yes	No	Yes	No
Constitutive pERK	Yes	No	ND	ND
Constitutive pSTAT3	Yes	No	ND	ND
Constitutive NFAT	Yes	No	ND	ND
Allogeneic T cell stimulation	Yes	No	Yes	No
Induction of Th17 differentiation	Yes	No	ND	ND
Spontaneous IL-10 secretion	Yes	No	Yes	No
Sensitivity to Fas induced apoptosis[d]	No[e]	Yes	ND	Yes
Response to phorbol ester	Yes	No	ND	Yes
Unique gene/protein expression of				
Elfin	Yes	No	ND	ND
Annexin II	Yes	No	ND	ND
S100A6	Yes	No	ND	ND
Transgelin 2	Yes	No	ND	ND
Development				
Specific progenitor	Yes	Yes	ND	Yes
BAFF dependent	No	Yes	ND	Yes
IL-7 dependent	No	Yes	ND	No
TSLP responsive	Yes	No	ND	Yes
Btk dependent	Yes	No[f]	ND[g]	Yes
CD19 dependent	Yes	No[f]	ND	ND
Proliferation in response to				
LPS	Yes	Yes	ND	No
Anti-IgM	No	Yes	ND	No
CD40L	Yes	Yes	ND	No

assay, was used for initial screening and CD20 was used to mark B cells because it is lost during mature B cell differentiation,[156] unlike CD19, and thus insures that immunoglobulin-secreting plasmablasts and plasma cells are excluded. Various populations of sort-purified CD20[+] B cells expressing different combinations of surface markers were isolated and tested for function *in vitro*, beginning with umbilical cord blood, because in mice B-1 cells predominate early in ontogeny. A particularly interesting, albeit small, population of CD27[+] B cells was identified that had previously been noted as infrequently present in cord blood.[157] Cord blood CD27[+] B cells are not memory B cells, because immunoglobulin sequencing shows a dearth of somatic mutation, unlike adult peripheral blood CD27[+] B cells.[158] Instead, cord blood CD27[+] B cells spontaneously secrete IgM and fulfill the other criteria for B-1 cell status.[159,160] They also express CD43, a surface antigen that is expressed on mouse B-1 cells.[161] Thus, umbilical cord blood B cells that coexpress CD20, CD27, and CD43 fulfill the three-fold criteria for B-1 status and hence by that functional definition can be said to represent human B-1 cells.

The same phenotype, CD20[+]CD27[+]CD43[+], recognizes a small number of B cells in adult peripheral blood samples. However, unlike cord blood, expression of CD27 and CD43 in adult blood do not coincide; rather, CD43 identifies a small subset within the overall CD27[+] B cell population, heretofore presumed to consist entirely of memory

Table 2. *Continued*

NOTE: Functional properties are shown for mouse peritoneal B-1a (B-1) and splenic follicular (FO) B cells. Functional properties are shown for human circulating B-1 and mature naive B cells as noted in the footnote to Table 1. Functional properties are described for cells taken *ex vivo* and unstimulated, except as noted. ND = not determined.
[a]Phosphatidylcholine.
[b]Phosphorylcholine.
[c]All B cells require a degree of tonic signaling for continued viability, separate from chronic signaling.
[d]Assessed after stimulation and upregulation of CD95 (Fas) expression.
[e]Sensitive but reduced in comparison to FO B cell.
[f]Present in deficient animals but reduced in number.
[g]Most likely yes, because Btk mutant XLA patients have little resting serum immunoglobulin and few if any circulating B cells.

B cells. This previously unrecognized population of CD20[+]CD27[+] B cells that coexpress CD43 spontaneously secretes IgM, efficiently stimulates T cells, and evidences chronic intracellular signaling, and thus parallels its cord blood counterpart in fulfilling the criteria for B-1 cell status (Table 1).[159,160] These CD20[+]CD27[+]CD43[+] B cells preferentially bind PC, as well as the DWEYS peptide mimetope of DNA,[162] two typical mouse B-1 cell specificities, unlike CD20[+]CD27[+]CD43[−] memory B cells and CD20[+]CD27[−]CD43[−] naive B cells, which fail to do so, lending further support to their designation as B-1 cells. Of note, CD43 is inducible on conventional B-2 cells following some forms of stimulation, but this is not the mechanism for CD43 expression on B-1 cells because stimulated, CD43[+] B-2 cells always express typical activation markers CD69 and CD70, whereas CD43[+] B-1 cells express neither.[159,160] Unlike the B-1 cell marker CD43, CD5 is found on the majority of, but not all, human B-1 cells, whereas most CD5[+] B cells are other than B-1 cells, in keeping with the different human B cell types known to express CD5.[159,160]

As noted above, CD27 has been considered to constitute a marker for memory B cells in the human system.[158,163] The finding that a portion of CD27[+] B cells are B-1 cells raises questions regarding the validity of conclusions reached during studies of what is now shown to be a heterogeneous population. The observation that CD27[+]CD43[+] B-1 cells secrete antibody that recognizes PC, a major antigenic determinant of pneumococci, suggests the possibility that previous work indicating that IgM[+]CD27[+] memory B cells are responsible for controlling pneumococcal infection[164,165] may actually represent the activity of B-1 cells coexisting with memory B cells in the CD27[+] B cell pool. Thus, it may be necessary to re-evaluate the features of memory B cells, particularly IgM memory B cells, after removal of CD27[+] B cells that also express CD43.

Determination of human B-1 cell frequencies can be difficult

Although confocal microscopy has verified the existence of B cells that coexpress CD20, CD27 and CD43,[160] enumeration of B-1 cells by flow cytometry can be difficult, depending as it does on multiple parameters, a partial listing of which includes efficiency of antibody binding; brightness of fluorescence signals; sensitivity of fluorescence detection; nature and hierarchy of gating strategy, and competency of computerized algorithms for data analysis.[166] For these reasons, results from different laboratories using different staining panels, different gates, different instruments, and different software may well differ, above and beyond differences in donor characteristics. A particularly difficult issue is posed by expression of CD27 and CD43 on most normal T cells, as well as other non-B cell types.[167,168] Because peripheral blood contains many more T cells than B cells, any stochastic tendency of (non-B-1) B cells to form doublets with another lymphocyte is likely to produce B:T doublets rather than B:B doublets. B:T doublets would express CD20, contributed by the B cell constituent, and CD27/CD43, contributed by the T cell constituent. In other words, a B:T doublet would express CD20, CD27 and CD43, and could easily be confused with an authentic CD20[+]CD27[+]CD43[+] B-1 cell.[169] In fact, B:T doublets can form under certain conditions. The most effective counter measure is taken before cytometry to avoid doublets in the first place, by briefly agitating samples just prior to analysis, by including EDTA in cell suspensions, and by examining samples at low concentrations.[160,166] If present, B:T doublets can be removed from consideration by area/height or pulse-width doublet discrimination, keeping in mind that doublet discrimination is geared around small, spherical cells so that excessively tight gating may exclude large normal cells such as B-1 cells.[160,166] B:T doublets can also be removed from consideration by staining for, and excluding, all CD3[+] cells.[160,166] However, the presence of substantial fractions of CD3[+]CD20[+] doubly positive events, and/or the presence of substantial fractions of doublet excluded cells, suggests suboptimal initial cell preparation and the likelihood that results obtained will not be truly representative of the sample at hand.

There is much individual and age-related variability among healthy donors in the fraction of circulating CD20[+] B cells that are B-1 cells,[166] and so large numbers of determinations are required to arrive at normal values for any given population. At present the frequency of B-1 cells among B cells in peripheral blood samples from normal individuals is estimated to vary from 1% to 9% and to decline with advancing age.[159,160,170] Although 1–9% covers a wide range (and some values are still higher and some lower than these limits), it is important to keep in mind that thus far no tissue reservoir for human B-1 cells has been identified, unlike the situation in mice where B-1 cells are concentrated in coelomic cavities. And with or without a reservoir, the endogenous and/or environmental factors that regulate the free circulation of B-1 cells on a day to day, week to week, or longer basis are at present unknown.

Since the first publication delineating the phenotype of human B-1 cells, several studies have appeared in which $CD20^+CD27^+CD43^+$ cells were examined. These investigations report the frequency of $CD20^+CD27^+CD43^+$ cells among B cells obtained from adult peripheral blood as 2.2% ($n = 8$), approximately 1–2.5% ($n = 5$), and 4.1% ($n = 33$).[169,171,172] The latter two studies included assay of CD5 expression, finding markedly contrasting results, with 65.6% of B-1 cells, and 11.5% of B-1 cells, positive for CD5.[171,172] Despite variable results regarding CD5 staining, these studies are consistent in supporting the new phenotypic identity of human B-1 cells. Further support derives from study of the response to *Borrelia* infection in immunodeficient NSG mice engrafted by human hematopoietic stem cells (human immune system, or HIS, mice). B-1b cells are responsible for resolving *Borrelia* infection in normal, wild-type (WT) mice.[173] HIS mice counteract *Borrelia* infection, unlike unengrafted NSG mice, and contain $CD20^+CD27^+CD43^+$ B cells, suggesting that stem cell derived human B-1 cells in HIS mice fulfill a function carried out by murine B-1b cells in WT mice.[174]

Human B-1 cell antibodies may have therapeutic benefit

As noted earlier, natural antibodies are pivotal in defending against microbial pathogens and in disposing of cellular debris and molecular toxins. And because natural antibodies tend to reflect sequences found in the genome, it is likely that they are subject to evolutionary selection. In other words, natural antibodies produced by B-1 cells are likely to be optimized for effectiveness in doing what they do (which is likely to be different than being optimized for binding affinity). However, in mouse studies B-1 cell antibodies change with advancing age in a way that erodes germline configuration.[94,95] Moreover, in humans B-1 cell numbers decline with advancing age.[159] Taken together these results suggest that protection afforded by B-1 cell-derived natu-

ral antibody declines with age; this in turn may increase susceptibility to several diseases that are more common in the elderly. In both human and mouse studies, natural antibodies have been implicated in protection against illnesses ranging from microbial infection to atherosclerosis to neurodegenerative diseases to cancer, and intravenous immunoglobulin has been used therapeutically in some of these dyscrasias.[22,55,98,175–177] One could speculate then that passive immunization with specific natural antibodies, against PC, oxidized LDL, tau, amyloid, or NeuGcGanglioside, by supplying repertoire elements that are missing or deficient, might prevent or treat one or more diseases of aging. Methods for generating human monoclonal antibodies from individual cells by single cell PCR/expression cloning have been described[178] and can be used to obtain antibodies from members of small cell populations, such as B-1 cells. Generation of completely human antibodies from B-1 cells or other infrequent B cell populations with the goal of passive immunization may well constitute the next phase of monoclonal antibody therapy and bypass the need for, and issues associated with, "humanizing" antibodies obtained from other species. Alternatively, as more is learned about human B-1 cell development, and the potential role and behavior of a putative lineage-specific human B-1 cell progenitor, it may be possible to upregulate B-1 cell numbers and/or function as individuals age and thereby maintain a "young" natural antibody protective/homeostatic shield.

Human B-1 cells may regulate immune responses

Regulatory B cells can modulate immune responses.[126,179,180] Several candidates for putative human B_{reg} cells that express IL-10 have been suggested, including in particular B cells that are $CD24^{hi}CD38^{hi}$ and B cells that are $CD24^{hi}CD27^+$.[181–183] The recognition early on that B-1 cells are a key source of IL-10 in the mouse system suggested the possibility that human B-1 cells might similarly express and secrete IL-10.

Two subpopulations of human B-1 cells have been defined on the basis of CD11b expression: $CD11b^-$ B-1 cells are the predominant population whereas $CD11b^+$ B-1 cells are the minor population.[184] $CD11b^-$ B-1 cells secrete IgM robustly (and constitutively) in comparison to the much smaller amounts constitutively secreted by $CD11b^+$ B-1 cells; CD11b$^+$ B-1 cells stimulate T cell expansion strongly in comparison to the much weaker stimulation produced by CD11b$^-$ B-1 cells. This dichotomy is similar to the functional differences between PC-1^{hi} and PC-1^{lo} murine B-1 cells.[85b] Although the possibility that CD11b$^+$ B-1 cells represent B cell:monocyte doublets has been raised,[185] confocal microscopy, light microscopy and flow cytometry results support the existence of human B-1 cells expressing CD11b.[184,186] The impression that CD11b$^+$ B-1 cells could be monocytes/macrophages may derive at least in part from the many similarities between B-1 cells and myeloid cells delineated in the mouse system that include phagocytosis (and antigen presentation) and have led to the idea that the two derive from the same developmental pathway and share elements of lineage.[187–189]

Both CD11b$^-$ and CD11b$^+$ B-1 cells, along with naive mature and true memory B cells, have been examined for IL-10 expression and secretion.[190] Among these four B cell populations, the very small pool of CD11b$^+$ B-1 cells expresses and secretes IL-10 at baseline, in the absence of any stimulation, in contrast to all other B cells. Moreover, CD11b$^+$ B-1 cells suppress naive CD4$^+$ T cell activation as judged by expression of TNF-α, and do so in an IL-10-dependent manner, unlike CD11b$^-$ B-1 cells or naive or memory B cells, which do not suppress. Thus, human B-1 cells, like their murine counterparts, are capable of suppressing immune responses via production of IL-10.

These results on B-1 cell-generated IL-10 and immunosuppression, combined with B-1 cell-induced T cell stimulation, indicate that human B-1 cells, like mouse B-1 cells, manifest potentially countervailing tendencies toward immune regulation with respect to B:T interaction. In view of the therapeutic efficacy of B cell depletion therapy in a variety of autoimmune diseases, it may be speculated that human B-1 cells play a role in pathogenesis or pathopersistence through dysfunctional or skewed immunoregulation, beyond the potential production of autoantibodies. Excessive B-1 cell activity in terms of driving T cell expansion (and, extrapolating from mouse B-1 cell function, also in terms of inducing proinflammatory Th17 cell differentiation), or diminished B-1 cell activity in terms of IL-10 secretion and immunosuppression, could contribute to inflammation and disease. In fact, in a small survey of lupus patients, CD11b$^+$ B-1 cells were found to be increased.[184] In other words, deletion or immunoregulation of B-1 cells, rather than total B cell depletion, may constitute a means to influence the course of autoimmune and other dyscrasias in which the immune system plays a role.

Concluding remarks

Building on the remarkable foundation provided by decades of research on mouse B-1 cells by many investigators, the anonymity with which human B-1 cells eluded serious scrutiny over the last 30 years has now been lifted by elucidation of the human B-1 cell phenotypic profile. Human B-1 cells share functional characteristics with mouse B-1 cells by definition; in addition, human and mouse B-1 cells share expression of CD43 and for most, CD5, although other surface antigens differ. There are many questions about human B-1 cells yet to be resolved, from simple (e.g., what is the normal level of B-1 cells in healthy individuals) to complex (e.g., how does the B-1 cell antibody repertoire compare to that of B-2 cells). However, previous work with mouse B-1 cells and early work with human B-1 cells suggests that a fuller understanding of B-1 cells in ill patients and healthy donors may favorably impact prevention and treatment of disease. Human B-1 cells are likely to be a rich source of fully humanized antibodies obtained for prevention and/or treatment of microbial pathogens and degenerative diseases associated with the accumulation of toxic molecules. Moreover, through production of autoantibody and through countervailing effects on T cells, human B-1 cells may instigate, perpetuate or exacerbate autoimmune and inflammatory diseases. Thus, a full and complete understanding of B-1 cell physiology and pathology is likely to contribute to new insights into human illness and to open new avenues for treatment of autoimmune dyscrasias and other diseases of humankind.

Acknowledgments

The authors thank Dr. Franak Batliwalla for critical review of the manuscript, Dr. Ana Maria Hernandez for sharing unpublished data, and Teresa Vizconde for assistance with figures. The authors are very grateful for continuing support provided by the National Institutes of Health over many years time for studies of B-1 cells.

Conflicts of interest

The authors declare no conflicts of interest.

References

1. Tony, H.P. & D.C. Parker. 1985. Major histocompatibility complex-restricted, polyclonal B cell responses resulting from helper T cell recognition of antiimmunoglobulin presented by small B lymphocytes. *J. Exp. Med.* **161:** 223–241.

2. Emery, P., R. Fleischmann, A. Filipowicz-Sosnowska, *et al.* 2006. The efficacy and safety of rituximab in patients with active rheumatoid arthritis despite methotrexate treatment: results of a phase IIB randomized, double-blind, placebo-controlled, dose-ranging trial. *Arthr. Rheum* **54:** 1390–1400.

3. Edwards, J.C., L. Szczepanski, J. Szechinski, *et al.* 2004. Efficacy of B-cell-targeted therapy with rituximab in patients with rheumatoid arthritis. *N. Engl., J. Med.* **350:** 2572–2581.

4. Cohen, S.B., P. Emery, M.W. Greenwald, *et al.* 2006. Rituximab for rheumatoid arthritis refractory to anti-tumor necrosis factor therapy: results of a multicenter, randomized, double-blind, placebo-controlled, phase III trial evaluating primary efficacy and safety at twenty-four weeks. *Arthr. Rheum* **54:** 2793–2806.

5. Lu, T.Y., K.P. Ng, G. Cambridge, *et al.* 2009. A retrospective seven-year analysis of the use of B cell depletion therapy in systemic lupus erythematosus at University College London Hospital: the first fifty patients. *Arthr. Rheum* **61:** 482–487.

6. Looney, R.J., J.H. Anolik, D. Campbell, *et al.* 2004. B cell depletion as a novel treatment for systemic lupus erythematosus: a phase I/II dose-escalation trial of rituximab. *Arthr. Rheum* **50:** 2580–2589.

7. Merrill, J.T., C.M. Neuwelt, D.J. Wallace, *et al.* 2010. Efficacy and safety of rituximab in moderately-to-severely active systemic lupus erythematosus: the randomized, double-blind, phase II/III systemic lupus erythematosus evaluation of rituximab trial. *Arthr. Rheum* **62:** 222–233.

8. Coca, A. & I. Sanz. 2009. B cell depletion in lupus and Sjogren's syndrome: an update. *Curr. Opin. Rheumatol.* **21:** 483–488.

9. Steiner, L.A. & H.N. Eisen. 1967. Sequential changes in the relative affinity of antibodies synthesized during the immune response. *J. Exp. Med.* **126:** 1161–1183.

10. Martin, F., A.M. Oliver & J.F. Kearney. 2001. Marginal zone and B1 B cells unite in the early response against T-independent blood-borne particulate antigens. *Immunity* **14:** 617–629.

11. Dunn-Walters, D.K., P.G. Isaacson & J. Spencer. 1995. Analysis of mutations in immunoglobulin heavy chain variable region genes of microdissected marginal zone (MGZ) B cells suggests that the MGZ of human spleen is a reservoir of memory B cells. *J. Exp. Med.* **182:** 559–566.

12. Baumgarth, N. 2011. The double life of a B-1 cell: self-reactivity selects for protective effector functions. *Nat. Rev. Immunol.* **11:** 34–46.

13. Wang, C.Y., R.A. Good, P. Ammirati, *et al.* 1980. Identification of a p69,71 complex expressed on human T cells sharing determinants with B-type chronic lymphatic leukemic cells. *J. Exp. Med.* **151:** 1539–1544.

14. Lanier, L.L., N.L. Warner, J.A. Ledbetter & L.A. Herzenberg. 1981. Expression of Lyt-1 antigen on certain murine B cell lymphomas. *J. Exp. Med.* **153:** 998–1003.

15. Manohar, V., E. Brown, W.M. Leiserson & T.M. Chused. 1982. Expression of Lyt-1 by a subset of B lymphocytes. *J. Immunol.* **129:** 532–538.

16. Hardy, R.R., K. Hayakawa, J. Haaijman & L.A. Herzenberg. 1982. B-cell subpopulations identifiable by two-color fluorescence analysis using a dual-laser FACS. *Ann. N.Y. Acad. Sci.* **399:** 112–121.

17. Kantor, A.B., A.M. Stall, S. Adams & L.A. Herzenberg. 1992. Differential development of progenitor activity for three B-cell lineages. *Proc. Natl. Acad. Sci. USA* **89:** 3320–3324.

18. Ghosn, E.E., R. Yamamoto, S. Hamanaka, *et al.* 2012. Distinct B-cell lineage commitment distinguishes adult bone marrow hematopoietic stem cells. *Proc. Natl. Acad. Sci. USA* **109:** 5394–5398.

19. Tornberg, U.C. & D. Holmberg. 1995. B-1a, B-1b and B-2 B cells display unique VHDJH repertoires formed at different stages of ontogeny and under different selection pressures. *Embo J.* **14:** 1680–1689.

20. Vink, A., G. Warnier, F. Brombacher & J.C. Renauld. 1999. Interleukin 9-induced in vivo expansion of the B-1 lymphocyte population. *J. Exp. Med.* **189:** 1413–1423.

21. Alugupalli, K.R., J.M. Leong, R.T. Woodland, *et al.* 2004. B1b lymphocytes confer T cell-independent long-lasting immunity. *Immunity* **21:** 379–390.

22. Haas, K.M., J.C. Poe, D.A. Steeber & T.F. Tedder. 2005. B-1a and B-1b cells exhibit distinct developmental requirements and have unique functional roles in innate and adaptive immunity to S. pneumoniae. *Immunity* **23:** 7–18.

23. Hayakawa, K., R.R. Hardy, D.R. Parks & L.A. Herzenberg. 1983. The "Ly-1 B" cell subpopulation in normal immunodefective, and autoimmune mice. *J. Exp. Med.* **157:** 202–218.

24. Hayakawa, K., R.R. Hardy & L.A. Herzenberg. 1986. Peritoneal Ly-1 B cells: genetic control, autoantibody production, increased lambda light chain expression. *Eur. J. Immunol.* **16:** 450–456.

25. Ishida, H., R. Hastings, J. Kearney & M. Howard. 1992. Continuous anti-interleukin 10 antibody administration depletes mice of Ly-1 B cells but not conventional B cells. *J. Exp. Med.* **175:** 1213–1220.

26. Kroese, F.G., W.A. Ammerlaan & A.B. Kantor. 1993. Evidence that intestinal IgA plasma cells in mu, kappa transgenic mice are derived from B-1 (Ly-1 B) cells. *Int. Immunol.* **5:** 1317–1327.

27. Sidman, C.L., L.D. Shultz, R.R. Hardy, *et al.* 1986. Production of immunoglobulin isotypes by Ly-1$^+$ B cells in viable motheaten and normal mice. *Science* **232:** 1423–1425.

28. Holodick, N.E., J.R. Tumang & T.L. Rothstein. 2010. B1 cells constitutively secrete IgM independently of IRF4. *Eur. J. Immunol.* **40:** 3007–3016.

29. Choi, Y.S., J.A. Dieter, K. Rothaeusler, *et al.* B-1 cells in the bone marrow are a significant source of natural IgM. *Eur. J. Immunol.* **42:** 120–129.

30. Kawahara, T., H. Ohdan, G. Zhao, *et al.* 2003. Peritoneal cavity B cells are precursors of splenic IgM natural antibody-producing cells. *J. Immunol.* **171:** 5406–5414.

31. Itakura, A., M. Szczepanik, R.A. Campos, *et al.* 2005. An hour after immunization peritoneal B-1 cells are activated to migrate to lymphoid organs where within 1 day they produce IgM antibodies that initiate elicitation of contact sensitivity. *J. Immunol.* **175:** 7170–7178.

32. Ha, S.A., M. Tsuji, K. Suzuki, *et al.* 2006. Regulation of B1 cell migration by signals through Toll-like receptors. *J. Exp. Med.* **203:** 2541–2550.

33. Yang, Y., J.W. Tung, E.E. Ghosn, *et al.* 2007. Division and differentiation of natural antibody-producing cells in mouse spleen. *Proc. Natl. Acad. Sci. USA* **104:** 4542–4546.

34. Wardemann, H., T. Boehm, N. Dear & R. Carsetti. 2002. B-1a B cells that link the innate and adaptive immune responses are lacking in the absence of the spleen. *J. Exp. Med.* **195:** 771–780.

35. Kretschmer, K., J. Stopkowicz, S. Scheffer, *et al.* 2004. Maintenance of peritoneal B-1a lymphocytes in the absence of the spleen. *J. Immunol.* **173:** 197–204.

36. Yang, Y., E.E. Ghosn, L.E. Cole, *et al.* 2012. Antigen-specific memory in B-1a and its relationship to natural immunity. *Proc. Natl. Acad. Sci. USA* **109:** 5388–5393.

37. Yang, Y., E.E. Ghosn, L.E. Cole, *et al.* 2012. Antigen-specific antibody responses in B-1a and their relationship to natural immunity. *Proc. Natl. Acad. Sci. USA* **109:** 5382–5387.

38. Baccala, R., T.V. Quang, M. Gilbert, *et al.* 1989. Two murine natural polyreactive autoantibodies are encoded by non-mutated germ-line genes. *Proc. Natl. Acad. Sci. USA* **86:** 4624–4628.

39. Hartman, A.B., C.P. Mallett, J. Srinivasappa, *et al.* 1989. Organ reactive autoantibodies from non-immunized adult BALB/c mice are polyreactive and express non-biased VH gene usage. *Mol. Immunol.* **26:** 359–370.

40. Lalor, P.A. & G. Morahan. 1990. The peritoneal Ly-1 (CD5) B cell repertoire is unique among murine B cell repertoires. *Eur. J. Immunol.* **20:** 485–492.

41. Klinman, D.M. & K.L. Holmes. 1990. Differences in the repertoire expressed by peritoneal and splenic Ly-1 (CD5)$^+$ B cells. *J. Immunol.* **144:** 4520–4525.

42. Ochsenbein, A.F., T. Fehr, C. Lutz, *et al.* 1999. Control of early viral and bacterial distribution and disease by natural antibodies. *Science* **286:** 2156–2159.

43. Baumgarth, N., O.C. Herman, G.C. Jager, *et al.* 2000. B-1 and B-2 cell-derived immunoglobulin M antibodies are nonredundant components of the protective response to influenza virus infection. *J. Exp. Med.* **192:** 271–280.

44. Boes, M., A.P. Prodeus, T. Schmidt, *et al.* 1998. A critical role of natural immunoglobulin M in immediate defense against systemic bacterial infection. *J. Exp. Med.* **188:** 2381–2386.

45. Briles, D.E., M. Nahm, K. Schroer, *et al.* 1981. Antiphosphocholine antibodies found in normal mouse serum are protective against intravenous infection with type 3 streptococcus pneumoniae. *J. Exp. Med.* **153:** 694–705.

46. Mouquet, H., J.F. Scheid, M.J. Zoller, *et al.* 2010. Polyreactivity increases the apparent affinity of anti-HIV antibodies by heteroligation. *Nature* **467:** 591–595.

47. Briles, D.E., C. Forman, S. Hudak & J.L. Claflin. 1982. Anti-phosphorylcholine antibodies of the T15 idiotype are optimally protective against Streptococcus pneumoniae. *J. Exp. Med.* **156:** 1177–1185.

48. Shaw, P.X., C.S. Goodyear, M.K. Chang, *et al.* 2003. The autoreactivity of anti-phosphorylcholine antibodies for atherosclerosis-associated neo-antigens and apoptotic cells. *J. Immunol.* **170:** 6151–6157.

49. Hardy, R.R., C.E. Carmack, S.A. Shinton, *et al.* 1989. A single VH gene is utilized predominantly in anti-BrMRBC hybridomas derived from purified Ly-1 B cells. Definition of the VH11 family. *J. Immunol.* **142:** 3643–3651.

50. Pennell, C.A., K.M. Sheehan, P.H. Brodeur & S.H. Clarke. 1989. Organization and expression of VH gene families preferentially expressed by Ly-1$^+$ (CD5) B cells. *Eur. J. Immunol.* **19:** 2115–2121.

51. Chen, Y., S. Khanna, C.S. Goodyear, *et al.* 2009. Regulation of dendritic cells and macrophages by an anti-apoptotic cell natural antibody that suppresses TLR responses and inhibits inflammatory arthritis. *J. Immunol.* **183:** 1346–1359.

52. Boes, M., T. Schmidt, K. Linkemann, *et al.* 2000. Accelerated development of IgG autoantibodies and autoimmune disease in the absence of secreted IgM. *Proc. Natl. Acad. Sci. USA* **97:** 1184–1189.

53. Tsimikas, S., E.S. Brilakis, R.J. Lennon, *et al.* 2007. Relationship of IgG and IgM autoantibodies to oxidized low density lipoprotein with coronary artery disease and cardiovascular events. *J. Lipid Res.* **48:** 425–433.

54. Soto, Y., H. Conde, R. Aroche, *et al.* 2009. Autoantibodies to oxidized low density lipoprotein in relation with coronary artery disease. *Hum. Antibodies* **18:** 109–117.

55. Kyaw, T., C. Tay, S. Krishnamurthi, *et al.* 2011. B1a B lymphocytes are atheroprotective by secreting natural IgM that increases IgM deposits and reduces necrotic cores in atherosclerotic lesions. *Circ. Res.* **109:** 830–840.

56. Gu, H., I. Forster & K. Rajewsky. 1990. Sequence homologies, N sequence insertion and JH gene utilization in VHDJH joining: implications for the joining mechanism and the ontogenetic timing of Ly1 B cell and B-CLL progenitor generation. *Embo J.* **9:** 2133–2140.

57. Forster, I., H. Gu & K. Rajewsky. 1988. Germline antibody V regions as determinants of clonal persistence and malignant growth in the B cell compartment. *Embo J.* **7:** 3693–3703.

58. Pennell, C.A., T.J. Mercolino, T.A. Grdina, *et al.* 1989. Biased immunoglobulin variable region gene expression by Ly-1 B cells due to clonal selection. *Eur. J. Immunol.* **19:** 1289–1295.

59. Benedict, C.L. & J.F. Kearney. 1999. Increased junctional diversity in fetal B cells results in a loss of protective anti-phosphorylcholine antibodies in adult mice. *Immunity* **10:** 607–617.

60. Desiderio, S.V., G.D. Yancopoulos, M. Paskind, *et al.* 1984. Insertion of N regions into heavy-chain genes is correlated with expression of terminal deoxytransferase in B cells. *Nature* **311:** 752–755.

61. Jacob, J., G. Kelsoe, K. Rajewsky & U. Weiss. 1991. Intraclonal generation of antibody mutants in germinal centres. *Nature* **354:** 389–392.

62. Hayakawa, K., R.R. Hardy & L.A. Herzenberg. 1985. Progenitors for Ly-1 B cells are distinct from progenitors for other B cells. *J. Exp. Med.* **161:** 1554–1568.

63. Solvason, N., A. Lehuen & J.F. Kearney. 1991. An embryonic source of Ly1 but not conventional B cells. *Int. Immunol.* **3:** 543–550.

64. Kantor, A. 1991. A new nomenclature for B cells. *Immunol. Today* **12:** 388.

65. Hayakawa, K., R.R. Hardy, A.M. Stall & L.A. Herzenberg. 1986. Immunoglobulin-bearing B cells reconstitute and maintain the murine Ly-1 B cell lineage. *Eur. J. Immunol.* **16:** 1313–1316.

66. Forster, I. & K. Rajewsky. 1987. Expansion and functional activity of Ly-1$^+$ B cells upon transfer of peritoneal cells into allotype-congenic, newborn mice. *Eur. J. Immunol.* **17:** 521–528.

67. Hardy, R.R. & K. Hayakawa. 1991. A developmental switch in B lymphopoiesis. *Proc. Natl. Acad. Sci. USA* **88:** 11550–11554.

68. Kantor, A.B. & L.A. Herzenberg. 1993. Origin of murine B cell lineages. *Annu. Rev. Immunol.* **11:** 501–538.

69. Yuan, J., C.K. Nguyen, X. Liu, *et al.* Lin28b reprograms adult bone marrow hematopoietic progenitors to mediate fetal-like lymphopoiesis. *Science* **335:** 1195–1200.

70. Cong, Y.Z., E. Rabin & H.H. Wortis. 1991. Treatment of murine CD5$^-$ B cells with anti-Ig, but not LPS, induces surface CD5: two B-cell activation pathways. *Int. Immunol.* **3:** 467–476.

71. Clarke, S.H. & L.W. Arnold. 1998. B-1 cell development: evidence for an uncommitted immunoglobulin (Ig)M$^+$ B cell precursor in B-1 cell differentiation. *J. Exp. Med.* **187:** 1325–1334.

72. Arnold, L.W., C.A. Pennell, S.K. McCray & S.H. Clarke. 1994. Development of B-1 cells: segregation of phosphatidyl choline-specific B cells to the B-1 population occurs after immunoglobulin gene expression. *J. Exp. Med.* **179:** 1585–1595.

73. Chumley, M.J., J.M. Dal Porto, S. Kawaguchi, *et al.* 2000. A VH11V kappa 9 B cell antigen receptor drives generation of CD5$^+$ B cells both in vivo and in vitro. *J. Immunol.* **164:** 4586–4593.

74. Fruman, D.A., A.B. Satterthwaite & O.N. Witte. 2000. Xid-like phenotypes: a B cell signalosome takes shape. *Immunity* **13:** 1–3.

75. Kozlowski, M., I. Mlinaric-Rascan, G.S. Feng, *et al.* 1993. Expression and catalytic activity of the tyrosine phosphatase PTP1C is severely impaired in motheaten and viable motheaten mice. *J. Exp. Med.* **178:** 2157–2163.

76. Shultz, L.D., P.A. Schweitzer, T.V. Rajan, *et al.* 1993. Mutations at the murine motheaten locus are within the hematopoietic cell protein-tyrosine phosphatase (Hcph) gene. *Cell* **73:** 1445–1454.

77. Wortis, H.H. & R. Berland. 2001. Cutting edge commentary: origins of B-1 cells. *J. Immunol.* **166:** 2163–2166.

78. Montecino-Rodriguez, E., H. Leathers & K. Dorshkind. 2006. Identification of a B-1 B cell-specified progenitor. *Nat. Immunol.* **7:** 293–301.

79. Herzenberg, L.A. & J.W. Tung. 2006. B cell lineages: documented at last! *Nat. Immunol.* **7:** 225–226.

80. Yoshimoto, M., E. Montecino-Rodriguez, M.J. Ferkowicz, *et al.* 2011. Embryonic day 9 yolk sac and intra-embryonic hemogenic endothelium independently generate a B-1 and marginal zone progenitor lacking B-2 potential. *Proc. Natl. Acad. Sci. USA* **108:** 1468–1473.

81. Barber, C.L., E. Montecino-Rodriguez & K. Dorshkind. 2011. Reduced production of B-1-specified common lymphoid progenitors results in diminished potential of adult marrow to generate B-1 cells. *Proc. Natl. Acad. Sci. USA* **108:** 13700–13704.

82. Ghosn, E.E., P. Sadate-Ngatchou, Y. Yang & L.A. Herzenberg. 2011. Distinct progenitors for B-1 and B-2 cells are present in adult mouse spleen. *Proc. Natl. Acad. Sci. USA* **108:** 2879–2884.

83. Hastings, W.D., S.M. Gurdak, J.R. Tumang & T.L. Rothstein. 2006. CD5$^+$/Mac-1$^-$ peritoneal B cells: a novel B cell subset that exhibits characteristics of B-1 cells. *Immunol. Lett.* **105:** 90–96.

84. Zhong, X., J.R. Tumang, W. Gao, *et al.* 2007. PD-L2 expression extends beyond dendritic cells/macrophages to B1 cells enriched for V(H)11/V(H)12 and phosphatidylcholine binding. *Eur. J. Immunol.* **37:** 2405–2410.

85a. Tumang, J.R., N.E. Holodick, T.C. Vizconde, *et al.* 2011. A CD25-positive population of activated B1 cells expresses LIFR and responds to LIF. *Front. Immunol.* **2:** 1–8.

85b. Wang, H., D.-M. Shin, S. Abbasi, *et al.* 2012. Expression of plasma cell alloantigen 1 defines layered development of B-1a B-cell subsets with distinct innate-like functions. *Proc. Natl. Acad. Sci. USA* **109:** 20077–20082.

86. Haury, M., A. Sundblad, A. Grandien, *et al.* 1997. The repertoire of serum IgM in normal mice is largely independent of external antigenic contact. *Eur. J. Immunol.* **27:** 1557–1563.

87. Wasserman, R., Y.S. Li, S.A. Shinton, *et al.* 1998. A novel mechanism for B cell repertoire maturation based on response by B cell precursors to pre-B receptor assembly. *J. Exp. Med.* **187:** 259–264.

88. Qian, Y., C. Santiago, M. Borrero, *et al.* 2001. Lupus-specific antiribonucleoprotein B cell tolerance in nonautoimmune mice is maintained by differentiation to B-1 and governed by B cell receptor signaling thresholds. *J. Immunol.* **166:** 2412–2419.

89. Lam, K.P. & K. Rajewsky. 1999. B cell antigen receptor specificity and surface density together determine B-1 versus B-2 cell development. *J. Exp. Med.* **190:** 471–477.

90. Hayakawa, K., M. Asano, S.A. Shinton, *et al.* 1999. Positive selection of natural autoreactive B cells. *Science* **285:** 113–116.

91. Hayakawa, K., M. Asano, S.A. Shinton, *et al.* 2003. Positive selection of anti-thy-1 autoreactive B-1 cells and natural serum autoantibody production independent from bone marrow B cell development. *J. Exp. Med.* **197:** 87–99.

92. Duhren-von Minden, M., R. Ubelhart, D. Schneider, *et al.* 2012. Chronic lymphocytic leukaemia is driven by antigen-independent cell-autonomous signalling. *Nature* **489:** 309–312.

93. Huang, C.A., C. Henry, J. Iacomini, *et al.* 1996. Adult bone marrow contains precursors for CD5$^+$ B cells. *Eur. J. Immunol.* **26:** 2537–2540.

94. Holodick, N.E., K. Repetny, X. Zhong & T.L. Rothstein. 2009. Adult BM generates CD5⁺ B1 cells containing abundant N-region additions. *Eur. J. Immunol.* **39:** 2383–2394.

95. Duber, S., M. Hafner, M. Krey, *et al.* 2009. Induction of B-cell development in adult mice reveals the ability of bone marrow to produce B-1a cells. *Blood* **114:** 4960–4967.

96. Esplin, B.L., R.S. Welner, Q. Zhang, *et al.* 2009. A differentiation pathway for B1 cells in adult bone marrow. *Proc. Natl. Acad. Sci. USA* **106:** 5773–5778.

97. Szabo, P., N. Relkin & M.E. Weksler. 2008. Natural human antibodies to amyloid beta peptide. *Autoimmun. Rev.* **7:** 415–420.

98. Britschgi, M., C.E. Olin, H.T. Johns, *et al.* 2009. Neuroprotective natural antibodies to assemblies of amyloidogenic peptides decrease with normal aging and advancing Alzheimer's disease. *Proc. Natl. Acad. Sci. USA* **106:** 12145–12150.

99. Chapman, C.J., A. Murray, J.E. McElveen, *et al.* 2008. Autoantibodies in lung cancer: possibilities for early detection and subsequent cure. *Thorax* **63:** 228–233.

100. Mizutamari, R.K., H. Wiegandt & G.A. Nores. 1994. Characterization of anti-ganglioside antibodies present in normal human plasma. *J. Neuroimmunol.* **50:** 215–220.

101. Sato, T., S. Ishikawa, K. Akadegawa, *et al.* 2004. Aberrant B1 cell migration into the thymus results in activation of CD4 T cells through its potent antigen-presenting activity in the development of murine lupus. *Eur. J. Immunol.* **34:** 3346–3358.

102. Zhong, X., W. Gao, N. Degauque, *et al.* 2007. Reciprocal generation of Th1/Th17 and T(reg) cells by B1 and B2 B cells. *Eur. J. Immunol.* **37:** 2400–2404.

103. Mohan, C., L. Morel, P. Yang & E. K. Wakeland. 1998. Accumulation of splenic B1a cells with potent antigen-presenting capability in NZM2410 lupus-prone mice. *Arthr. Rheum* **41:** 1652–1662.

104. Zhong, X., S. Lau, C. Bai, *et al.* 2009. A novel subpopulation of B1 B cells is enriched with autoreactivity in normal and lupus-prone mice. *Arthr. Rheum* **60:** 3734–3743.

105. Murphy, T.P., D.L. Kolber & T.L. Rothstein. 1990. Elevated expression of Pgp-1 (Ly-24) by murine peritoneal B lymphocytes. *Eur. J. Immunol.* **20:** 1137–1142.

106. Tumang, J.R., W.D. Hastings, C. Bai & T.L. Rothstein. 2004. Peritoneal and splenic B-1 cells are separable by phenotypic, functional, and transcriptomic characteristics. *Eur. J. Immunol.* **34:** 2158–2167.

107. Karras, J.G., Z. Wang, L. Huo, *et al.* 1997. Signal transducer and activator of transcription-3 (STAT3) is constitutively activated in normal, self-renewing B-1 cells but only inducibly expressed in conventional B lymphocytes [see comments]. *J. Exp. Med.* **185:** 1035–1042.

108. Wong, S.C., W.K. Chew, J.E. Tan, *et al.* 2002. Peritoneal CD5⁺ B-1 cells have signaling properties similar to tolerant B cells. *J. Biol. Chem.* **277:** 30707–30715.

109. Berland, R. & H.H. Wortis. 2003. Normal B-1a cell development requires B cell-intrinsic NFATc1 activity. *Proc. Natl. Acad. Sci. USA* **100:** 13459–13464.

110. Rothstein, T.L. & D.L. Kolber. 1988. Anti-Ig antibody inhibits the phorbol ester-induced stimulation of peritoneal B cells. *J. Immunol.* **141:** 4089–4093.

111. Morris, D.L. & T.L. Rothstein. 1994. Decreased surface IgM receptor-mediated activation of phospholipase C gamma 2 in B-1 lymphocytes. *Int. Immunol.* **6:** 1011–1016.

112. Morris, D.L. & T.L. Rothstein. 1993. Abnormal transcription factor induction through the surface immunoglobulin M receptor of B-1 lymphocytes. *J. Exp. Med.* **177:** 857–861.

113. Holodick, N.E., J.R. Tumang & T.L. Rothstein. 2009. Continual signaling is responsible for constitutive ERK phosphorylation in B-1a cells. *Mol. Immunol.* **46:** 329–30360.

114. Hathcock, K.S., G. Laszlo, C. Pucillo, *et al.* 1994. Comparative analysis of B7–1 and B7–2 costimulatory ligands: expression and function. *J. Exp. Med.* **180:** 631–640.

115. Wang, Y. & T.L. Rothstein. 2012. Induction of Th17 cell differentiation by B-1 cells. *Front. Immunol.* **3:** 281.

116. Wolf, S.D., B.N. Dittel, F. Hardardottir & C.A. Janeway, Jr. 1996. Experimental autoimmune encephalomyelitis induction in genetically B cell-deficient mice. *J. Exp. Med.* **184:** 2271–2278.

117. Fillatreau, S., C.H. Sweenie, M.J. McGeachy, *et al.* 2002. B cells regulate autoimmunity by provision of IL-10. *Nat. Immunol.* **3:** 944–950.

118. O'Garra, A., R. Chang, N. Go, *et al.* 1992. Ly-1 B (B-1) cells are the main source of B cell-derived interleukin 10. *Eur. J. Immunol.* **22:** 711–717.

119. Yanaba, K., J.D. Bouaziz, K.M. Haas, *et al.* 2008. A regulatory B cell subset with a unique CD1dʰⁱCD5⁺ phenotype controls T cell-dependent inflammatory responses. *Immunity* **28:** 639–650.

120. Evans, J.G., K.A. Chavez-Rueda, A. Eddaoudi, *et al.* 2007. Novel suppressive function of transitional 2 B cells in experimental arthritis. *J. Immunol.* **178:** 7868–7878.

121. Tian, J., D. Zekzer, L. Hanssen, *et al.* 2001. Lipopolysaccharide-activated B cells down-regulate Th1 immunity and prevent autoimmune diabetes in nonobese diabetic mice. *J. Immunol.* **167:** 1081–1089.

122. Hahne, M., T. Renno, M. Schroeter, *et al.* 1996. Activated B cells express functional Fas ligand. *Eur. J. Immunol.* **26:** 721–724.

123. Mariani, S.M. & P.H. Krammer. 1998. Surface expression of TRAIL/Apo-2 ligand in activated mouse T and B cells. *Eur. J. Immunol.* **28:** 1492–1498.

124. Strater, J., S.M. Mariani, H. Walczak, *et al.* 1999. CD95 ligand (CD95L) in normal human lymphoid tissues: a subset of plasma cells are prominent producers of CD95L. *Am. J. Pathol.* **154:** 193–201.

125. Lundy, S.K. & D.L. Boros. 2002. Fas ligand-expressing B-1a lymphocytes mediate CD4(+)-T-cell apoptosis during schistosomal infection: induction by interleukin 4 (IL-4) and IL-10. *Infect. Immun.* **70:** 812–819.

126. Ring, S., A.H. Enk & K. Mahnke. 2011. Regulatory T cells from IL-10-deficient mice fail to suppress contact hypersensitivity reactions due to lack of adenosine production. *J. Invest. Dermatol.* **131:** 1494–1502.

127. Murakami, M., H. Yoshioka, T. Shirai, *et al.* 1995. Prevention of autoimmune symptoms in autoimmune-prone mice by elimination of B-1 cells. *Int. Immunol.* **7:** 877–882.

128. Rothstein, T.L. & D.L. Kolber. 1988. Peritoneal B cells respond to phorbol esters in the absence of co-mitogen. *J. Immunol.* **140:** 2880–2885.

129. Miller, D.J. & C.E. Hayes. 1991. Phenotypic and genetic characterization of a unique B lymphocyte deficiency in strain A/WySnJ mice. *Eur. J. Immunol.* **21:** 1123–1130.

130. Masuda, K., J. Wang & T. Watanabe. 1997. Reduced susceptibility to Fas-mediated apoptosis in B-1 cells. *Eur. J. Immunol.* **27:** 449–455.

131. Chumley, M.J., J.M. Dal Porto & J.C. Cambier. 2002. The unique antigen receptor signaling phenotype of B-1 cells is influenced by locale but induced by antigen. *J. Immunol.* **169:** 1735–1743.

132. Sen, G., H.J. Wu, G. Bikah, *et al.* 2002. Defective CD19-dependent signaling in B-1a and B-1b B lymphocyte subpopulations. *Mol. Immunol.* **39:** 57–68.

133. Morris, D.L. & T.L. Rothstein. 1994. "CD5$^+$ B (B-1) cells and immunity." In *Handbook of B and T Lymphocytes.* E. C. Snow, Eds.: 421–445 Academic Press, Inc. San Diego.

134. Bikah, G., J. Carey, J.R. Ciallella, *et al.* 1996. CD5-mediated negative regulation of antigen receptor-induced growth signals in B-1 B cells. *Science* **274:** 1906–1909.

135. Frances, R., J.R. Tumang & T.L. Rothstein. 2007. Extreme skewing of annexin II and S100A6 expression identified by proteomic analysis of peritoneal B-1 cells. *Int. Immunol.* **19:** 59–65.

136. Frances, R., J.R. Tumang, H. Kaku, *et al.* 2006. B-1 cells express transgelin 2: Unexpected lymphocyte expression of a smooth muscle protein identified by proteomic analysis of peritoneal B-1 cells. *Mol. Immunol.* **43:** 2124–2129.

137. Fischer, G.M., L.A. Solt, W.D. Hastings, *et al.* 2001. Splenic and peritoneal B-1 cells differ in terms of transcriptional and proliferative features that separate peritoneal B-1 from splenic B-2 cells. *Cell Immunol.* **213:** 62–71.

138. Tanguay, D.A., T.P. Colarusso, S. Pavlovic, *et al.* 1999. Early induction of cyclin D2 expression in phorbol ester-responsive B-1 lymphocytes. *J. Exp. Med.* **189:** 1685–1690.

139. Tanguay, D.A., T.P. Colarusso, C. Doughty, *et al.* 2001. Cutting edge: differential signaling requirements for activation of assembled cyclin D3-cdk4 complexes in B-1 and B-2 lymphocyte subsets. *J. Immunol.* **166:** 4273–4277.

140. Mataraza, J.M., J.R. Tumang, M.R. Gumina, *et al.* 2006. Disruption of cyclin D3 blocks proliferation of normal B-1a cells but loss of cyclin D3 is compensated by cyclin D2 in cyclin D3-deficient mice. *J. Immunol.* **177:** 787–795.

141. Dasu, T., V. Sindhava, S.H. Clarke & S. Bondada. 2009. CD19 signaling is impaired in murine peritoneal and splenic B-1 B lymphocytes. *Mol. Immunol.* **46:** 2655–2665.

142. Carvalho, T.L., T. Mota-Santos, A. Cumano, *et al.* 2001. Arrested B lymphopoiesis and persistence of activated B cells in adult interleukin 7$^{-/-}$ mice. *J. Exp. Med.* **194:** 1141–1150.

143. Caligaris-Cappio, F., M. Gobbi, M. Bofill & G. Janossy. 1982. Infrequent normal B lymphocytes express features of B-chronic lymphocytic leukemia. *J. Exp. Med.* **155:** 623–628.

144. Casali, P., S.E. Burastero, M. Nakamura, *et al.* 1987. Human lymphocytes making rheumatoid factor and antibody to ssDNA belong to Leu-1$^+$ B-cell subset. *Science* **236:** 77–81.

145. Hardy, R.R., K. Hayakawa, M. Shimizu, *et al.* 1987. Rheumatoid factor secretion from human Leu-1$^+$ B cells. *Science* **236:** 81–83.

146. Plater-Zyberk, C., R.N. Maini, K. Lam, *et al.* 1985. A rheumatoid arthritis B cell subset expresses a phenotype similar to that in chronic lymphocytic leukemia. *Arthr. Rheum* **28:** 971–976.

147. Taniguchi, O., H. Miyajima, T. Hirano, *et al.* 1987. The Leu-1 B-cell subpopulation in patients with rheumatoid arthritis. *J. Clin. Immunol.* **7:** 441–448.

148. Burastero, S.E., P. Casali, R.L. Wilder & A.L. Notkins. 1988. Monoreactive high affinity and polyreactive low affinity rheumatoid factors are produced by CD5$^+$ B cells from patients with rheumatoid arthritis. *J. Exp. Med.* **168:** 1979–1992.

149. Nakamura, M., S.E. Burastero, A.L. Notkins & P. Casal. 1988. Human monoclonal rheumatoid factor-like antibodies from CD5 (Leu-1)$^+$ B cells are polyreactive. *J. Immunol.* **140:** 4180–4186.

150. Sims, G.P., R. Ettinger, Y. Shirota, *et al.* 2005. Identification and characterization of circulating human transitional B cells. *Blood* **105:** 4390–4398.

151. Lee, J., S. Kuchen, R. Fischer, *et al.* 2009. Identification and characterization of a human CD5$^+$ pre-naive B cell population. *J. Immunol.* **182:** 4116–4126.

152. Freedman, A.S., G. Freeman, J. Whitman, *et al.* 1989. Studies of in vitro activated CD5$^+$ B cells. *Blood* **73:** 202–208.

153. Raman, C. & K.L. Knight. 1992. CD5$^+$ B cells predominate in peripheral tissues of rabbit. *J. Immunol.* **149:** 3858–3864.

154. Wilson, S.M. & B.N. Wilkie. 2007. B-1 and B-2 B-cells in the pig cannot be differentiated by expression of CD5. *Vet. Immunol. Immunopathol.* **115:** 10–16.

155. Thiriot, A., A.M. Drapier, P. Vieira, *et al.* 2007. The Bw cells, a novel B cell population conserved in the whole genus Mus. *J. Immunol.* **179:** 6568–6578.

156. Jego, G., R. Bataille & C. Pellat-Deceunynck. 2001. Interleukin-6 is a growth factor for nonmalignant human plasmablasts. *Blood* **97:** 1817–1822.

157. Scheeren, F.A., M. Nagasawa, K. Weijer, *et al.* 2008. T cell-independent development and induction of somatic hypermutation in human IgM$^+$ IgD$^+$ CD27$^+$ B cells. *J. Exp. Med.* **205:** 2033–2042.

158. Klein, U., K. Rajewsky & R. Kuppers. 1998. Human immunoglobulin (Ig)M$^+$IgD$^+$ peripheral blood B cells expressing the CD27 cell surface antigen carry somatically mutated variable region genes: CD27 as a general marker for somatically mutated (memory) B cells. *J. Exp. Med.* **188:** 1679–1689.

159. Griffin, D.O., N.E. Holodick & T.L. Rothstein. 2011. Human B1 cells in umbilical cord and adult peripheral blood express the novel phenotype CD20$^+$CD27$^+$CD43$^+$CD70. *J. Exp. Med.* **208:** 67–80.

160. Griffin, D.O., N.E. Holodick & T.L. Rothstein. 2011. Human B1 cells are CD3$^-$: a reply to "A human equivalent of mouse B-1 cells?" and "The nature of circulating CD27$^+$CD43$^+$ B cells." *J. Exp. Med.* **208:** 2566–2569.

161. Wells, S.M., A.B. Kantor & A.M. Stall. 1994. CD43 (S7) expression identifies peripheral B cell subsets. *J. Immunol.* **153:** 5503–5515.

162. Jacobi, A.M., J. Zhang, M. Mackay, *et al.* 2009. Phenotypic characterization of autoreactive B cells—checkpoints of B

cell tolerance in patients with systemic lupus erythematosus. *PLoS One* **4**: e5776.

163. Agematsu, K., H. Nagumo, F.C. Yang, *et al.* 1997. B cell subpopulations separated by CD27 and crucial collaboration of CD27$^+$ B cells and helper T cells in immunoglobulin production. *Eur. J. Immunol.* **27**: 2073–2079.

164. Kruetzmann, S., M.M. Rosado, H. Weber, *et al.* 2003. Human immunoglobulin M memory B cells controlling Streptococcus pneumoniae infections are generated in the spleen. *J. Exp. Med.* **197**: 939–945.

165. Shi, Y., T. Yamazaki, Y. Okubo, *et al.* 2005. Regulation of aged humoral immune defense against pneumococcal bacteria by IgM memory B cell. *J. Immunol.* **175**: 3262–3267.

166. Griffin, D.O. & T.L. Rothstein. 2012. Human B1 cell frequency: isolation and analysis of human B1 cells. *Front. Immunol.* **3**: 122.

167. Carlsson, S.R. & M. Fukuda. 1986. Isolation and characterization of leukosialin, a major sialoglycoprotein on human leukocytes. *J. Biol. Chem.* **261**: 12779–12786.

168. van Lier, R.A., J. Borst, T. M. Vroom, *et al.* 1987. Tissue distribution and biochemical and functional properties of Tp55 (CD27), a novel T cell differentiation antigen. *J. Immunol.* **139**: 1589–1596.

169. Descatoire, M., J.C. Weill, C.A. Reynaud & S. Weller. 2011. A human equivalent of mouse B-1 cells? *J. Exp. Med.* **208**: 2563–2564.

170. Perez-Andres, M., C. Grosserichter-Wagener, C. Teodosio, *et al.* 2011. The nature of circulating CD27$^+$CD43$^+$ B cells. *J. Exp. Med.* **208**: 2565–2566; author reply 2566–2569.

171. Verbinnen, B., K. Covens, L. Moens, *et al.* 2012. Human CD20$^+$CD43$^+$CD27$^+$CD5$^-$ B cells generate antibodies to capsular polysaccharides of Streptococcus pneumoniae. *J. Allergy Clin. Immunol.* **130**: 272–275.

172. Suchanek, O., R. Sadler, E.A. Bateman, *et al.* 2012. Immunophenotyping of putative human B1 B cells in healthy controls and common variable immunodeficiency (CVID) patients. *Clin. Exp. Immunol.* **170**: 333–341.

173. Alugupalli, K.R., R.M. Gerstein, J. Chen, *et al.* 2003. The resolution of relapsing fever borreliosis requires IgM and is concurrent with expansion of B1b lymphocytes. *J. Immunol.* **170**: 3819–3827.

174. Vuyyuru, R., H. Liu, T. Manser & K.R. Alugupalli. 2011. Characteristics of Borrelia hermsii infection in human hematopoietic stem cell-engrafted mice mirror those of human relapsing fever. *Proc. Natl. Acad. Sci. USA* **108**: 20707–20712.

175. Istrin, G., E. Bosis & B. Solomon. 2006. Intravenous immunoglobulin enhances the clearance of fibrillar amyloid-beta peptide. *J. Neurosci. Res.* **84**: 434–443.

176. Sapir, T. & Y. Shoenfeld. 2005. Uncovering the hidden potential of intravenous immunoglobulin as an anticancer therapy. *Clin. Rev. Allergy Immunol.* **29**: 307–310.

177. Rodriguez-Zhurbenko, N., D. Martinez, R. Blanco, *et al.* 2013. Human antibodies reactive to NeuGcGM3 ganglioside have cytotoxic anti-tumor properties. *Eur. J. Immunol.* **43**: 826–837.

178. Tiller, T., E. Meffre, S. Yurasov, *et al.* 2008. Efficient generation of monoclonal antibodies from single human B cells by single cell RT-PCR and expression vector cloning. *J. Immunol. Methods* **329**: 112–124.

179. Mauri, C. & A. Bosma. 2012. Immune regulatory function of B cells. *Annu. Rev. Immunol.*

180. Bouaziz, J.D., K. Yanaba & T.F. Tedder. 2008. Regulatory B cells as inhibitors of immune responses and inflammation. *Immunol. Rev.* **224**: 201–214.

181. Blair, P.A., L.Y. Norena, F. Flores-Borja, *et al.* 2010. CD19(+)CD24(hi)CD38(hi) B cells exhibit regulatory capacity in healthy individuals but are functionally impaired in systemic Lupus Erythematosus patients. *Immunity* **32**: 129–140.

182. Iwata, Y., T. Matsushita, M. Horikawa, *et al.* 2010. Characterization of a rare IL-10-competent B-cell subset in man that parallels mouse regulatory B10 cells. *Blood* **117**: 530–541.

183. Bouaziz, J.D., S. Calbo, M. Maho-Vaillant, *et al.* 2010. IL-10 produced by activated human B cells regulates CD4(+) T-cell activation in vitro. *Eur. J. Immunol.* **40**: 2686–2691.

184. Griffin, D.O. & T.L. Rothstein. 2011. A small CD11b$^+$ human B1 cell subpopulation stimulates T cells and is expanded in lupus. *J. Exp. Med.* **208**: 2591–2598.

185. Reynaud, C.A. & J.C. Weill. 2012. Gene profiling of CD11b(+) and CD11b(-) B1 cell subsets reveals potential cell sorting artifacts. *J. Exp. Med.* **209**: 433–434; author reply 434–436.

186. Griffin, D.O., T. Quach, F. Batliwalla, *et al.* 2012. Human CD11b$^+$ B1 cells are not monocytes: a reply to "Gene profiling of CD11b$^+$ and CD11b$^-$ B1 cell subsets reveals potential cell sorting artifacts." *J. Exp. Med.* **209**: 434–436.

187. Parra, D., A.M. Rieger, J. Li, *et al.* 2012. Pivotal advance: peritoneal cavity B-1 B cells have phagocytic and microbicidal capacities and present phagocytosed antigen to CD4$^+$ T cells. *J. Leukoc. Biol.* **91**: 525–536.

188. Cumano, A., C.J. Paige, N.N. Iscove & G. Brady. 1992. Bipotential precursors of B cells and macrophages in murine fetal liver. *Nature* **356**: 612–615.

189. Montecino-Rodriguez, E., H. Leathers & K. Dorshkind. 2001. Bipotential B-macrophage progenitors are present in adult bone marrow. *Nat. Immunol.* **2**: 83–88.

190. Griffin, D.O. & T.L. Rothstein. 2012. Human CD11b$^+$ B1 cells spontaneously secrete IL-10 and regulate T cell activity. *Mol. Med.* **18**: 1003–1008.

Ann. N.Y. Acad. Sci. ISSN 0077-8923

ANNALS OF THE NEW YORK ACADEMY OF SCIENCES
Issue: *The Year in Immunology*

Reverse vaccinology in the 21st century: improvements over the original design

Claudio Donati and Rino Rappuoli

Novartis Vaccines and Diagnostics, Siena, Italy

Address for correspondence: Rino Rappuoli, Novartis Vaccines and Diagnostics, Via Fiorentina 1, 53100 Siena, Italy. rino.rappuoli@novartis.com

Reverse vaccinology (RV), the first application of genomic technologies in vaccine research, represented a major revolution in the process of discovering novel vaccines. By determining their entire antigenic repertoire, researchers could identify protective targets and design efficacious vaccines for pathogens where conventional approaches had failed. Bexsero, the first vaccine developed using RV, has recently received positive opinion from the European Medicines Agency. The use of RV initiated a cascade of changes that affected the entire vaccine development process, shifting the focus from the identification of a list of vaccine candidates to the definition of a set of high throughput screens to reduce the need for costly and labor intensive tests in animal models. It is now clear that a deep understanding of the epidemiology of vaccine candidates, and their regulation and role in host-pathogen interactions, must become an integral component of the screening workflow. Far from being outdated by technological advancements, RV still represents a paradigm of how high-throughput technologies and scientific insight can be integrated into biotechnology research.

Keywords: reverse vaccinology; vaccines; bacteria; genomics; proteomics

Introduction

In its original formulation, vaccination is the practice by which individuals injected with inactivated or attenuated forms of an infectious agent become immune to infection from the injected agent. The application of this practice has essentially remained unchanged for nearly two centuries. The first major revolution was the development of subunit vaccines, when it was realized that components of the microorganism could be sufficient to elicit immune response, decreasing the probability of unwanted side effects. Since then most efforts in vaccine research have been dedicated to identifying the component or mixture of components able to protect against the disease. The main characteristics of these molecules are their presence and conservation in the infectious agent, their visibility to the host immune system, and their ability to elicit a protective immune response. Given these assumptions, the preferred method for vaccine target identification has been the analysis of sera from infected individuals who are protected from reinfection. This procedure is usually able to identify a restricted set of candidates that dominate the host immune response; it fails to identify those components that are not highly immunogenic during infection, but are able to confer protective immunity. A typical example is tetanus toxin.

Since the late 1990s, the development of sequencing technologies has changed the landscape of the slowly evolving field of vaccinology. When the genome of the first living organism was sequenced in 1995,[1] it was realized that genomic technologies, by determining the whole proteomic potential of the infectious organism, could boost the chances of identifying the protein, or mixture of proteins, that could be used to develop an efficacious vaccine. The method, reverse vaccinology (RV), offered two main advantages. First, it allowed identification of a much broader spectrum of candidates, including proteins that had not been identified before because they were masked by other, immunodominant targets. Second, it allowed the identification of potential

doi: 10.1111/nyas.12046

vaccine targets in organisms that were difficult to cultivate in the laboratory.

The RV protocol was originally developed to overcome the hurdles that had hampered the development of an efficacious vaccine against serogroup B *Neisseria meningitidis* (MenB), a gram-negative bacterium responsible for about 50% of the bacterial meningitis worldwide.[2] *N. meningitidis* is a natural component of the commensal flora that colonizes the upper respiratory tract of healthy individuals. In a small proportion of cases, the bacterium can invade the host bloodstream and, after crossing the blood–brain barrier, cause meningitis. To escape reconnaissance by the host immune system and survive in blood, *N. meningitidis* is coated by a polysaccharide capsule that, based on its chemical properties, is classified into five major serogroups: A, B, C, Y, and W135. Given its exposure on the surface of the cell and role in pathogenicity, the capsular polysaccharide constitutes the antigen of choice for the meningococcus, and is an excellent target for bactericidal antibodies elicited by conjugate vaccines against serogroups A, C, Y, and W135. However, in the case of serogroup B, the conjugate vaccine was not feasible because the capsular polysaccharide is an $\alpha(2, 8)$ polysialic acid, identical to the polysialic acid present in human glycoproteins such as N-CAM. The capsule of MenB is thus a human self-antigen, and much effort has been directed toward the development of a protein-based vaccine specific for it. In the mid 1990s, all of these efforts were frustrated by the inconsistency of the protection data, in that there was extreme variability in the surface proteins tested as vaccine antigens.

The term *reverse vaccinology* originates from the change in perspective allowed by the advancements in sequencing technologies. The entire genome of the virulent MC58 strain was sequenced,[3] and from the genomic data, potential vaccine targets were selected.[2] The main idea behind the procedure was that all of the successful examples of protein-based vaccines include targets that are either exposed on the surface of the cell or secreted into the extracellular milieu. Starting from the 2,158 proteins encoded in the MC58 sequenced genome, bioinformatic analysis predicted that over 600 were either exposed on the surface or secreted. Of these, 350 were cloned in *Escherichia coli*, successfully expressed in soluble form, purified, and used to immunize mice. The sera of immunized animals were then screened in a serum bactericidal assay that is known to correlate with protection. At each of these steps, candidates not satisfying quality criteria were discarded; the process led to the identification of five previously unknown vaccine candidates[4] that subsequently have completed clinical trials in a vaccine combination known as 4CMenB, and received a positive opinion from the European Medicines Agency (and approved with the commercial name of Bexsero®). Since the pioneering MenB project, the RV approach has been applied to a variety of other important pathogens, including *Streptococcus pneumonia*,[5] *Porphyromonas gingivalis*,[6] *Chlamydia pneumoniae*,[7] *Streptococcus agalactiae*,[8] *E. coli*,[9] *Leishmania major*, and *L. infantum*,[10] and has earned a dedicated entry on Wikipedia (http://en.wikipedia.org/wiki/Reverse_vaccinology).

When first proposed, the idea behind the RV approach was for it to be the definitive solution to the problem of antigen discovery. Once all the genes encoded in the genome of a pathogenic species are known, the list of vaccine candidates is finite and, in principle, can be tested in animal models. Therefore, protective antigens would not be missed, although it might take time and effort to find them and to define the most effective vaccine formulation. However, in each of the vaccine projects based on RV, the original design had to be modified to adapt to the peculiarities of the target species. In turn, following the enormous research effort that was needed to overcome many unforeseen difficulties, there is a clearer understanding of many aspects of bacterial population biology and of the interactions between pathogens and the human host, as well as how they impact the development of a vaccine.

The experience accumulated in the last decade has demonstrated that the formulation of a vaccine able to guarantee broad coverage requires a deep understanding of the population structure of the pathogen. Theoretical and experimental work of sequence analysis has shown that a certain degree of strain-to-strain variability, both in sequence and expression level, is an unavoidable characteristic of the antigens identified using RV. Thanks to the advent of high-throughput sequencing technologies, it is now feasible to determine the complete genome sequences of hundreds of bacterial isolates and to use these, instead of a single genome, as a starting point for the vaccine target selection process.

In this way, epidemiological characterization of the pathogen has become an integral part of the RV approach.

The testing of vaccine candidates in animal models—a step at the end of which usually only a handful of the screened candidates proves to induce protective immunity—still produces the major bottleneck of the entire RV process. Therefore, a large effort has been devoted to defining a set of screening procedures that could integrate the original bioinformatic selection to significantly reduce the number of candidates that need to be tested in animal models. New technologies, including microarrays, RNA-Seq, and proteomics, are now providing data that, integrated into the RV process, can turn the original brute force approach into a much more efficient and streamlined process. In addition, there has been a general technological advancement in the software tools that are used throughout the selection process, and in many cases their predictions can now be tested using new experimental methods.

In the following pages we will review the major improvements of the original RV workflow that occurred in the last decade, with particular attention to those genome-wide experimental methods that constitute a valuable complement to bioinformatic screening. In doing so, we will also review the major discoveries that were made in the context of RV projects (Table 1).

Genomic variability

Fifteen years ago the sequencing of the entire genome of a single bacterial isolate was a significant achievement; thanks to improvements in sequencing technologies within the last decade, the sequencing of hundreds of bacterial genomes is now routinely done at a fraction of the cost of that of a single genome at the beginning of the RV era. Comparative analysis of multiple genomes of the same bacterial species has shown that genomic variability in bacteria is much more extensive than initially anticipated, and is a mechanism by which bacterial species are able to adapt to many different environments and escape reconnaissance by the host immune system. There are two main ways in which this affects the selection of a vaccine candidate: different strains can have different antigenic repertoires, and the sequence of shared antigens can vary from strain to strain. This highlights the importance of characterizing the epidemiology of selected candidates that

Table 1. Major milestones in the evolution of reverse vaccinology

1995	First complete genome sequence of a living organism.[1]
2000	First application of whole genome sequencing in vaccine research: formulation of the reverse vaccinology approach.[2]
2002	First application of DNA microarray technology to antigen discovery.[96,97]
2005	First comparative genomic study of multiple isolates of the same bacterial species and formulation of the pan-genome concept.[17]
2005	First rational design of a multi-component protein vaccine for GBS based on the analysis and screening of multiple bacterial genomes.[8]
2006	First formulation of a broadly protective vaccine against MenB based on reverse vaccinology.[4]
2006	First use of proteomics to identify surface exposed proteins in the screening of vaccine candidates.[83]
2011	First rational, structure-based design of an antigen inducing broad protective immunity against heterologous strains for MenB.[136]

might require the development of an entirely new typing system.

Variability of genome content: core and pan-genome

When RV was first proposed, several aspects of bacterial population genomics were not known in detail. Although it was clear that at the genomic level bacteria are more variable than species in other realms of life, the extent of this variability was not fully understood, and it was thought to be confined to a few structures, known as pathogenicity islands (PI), strictly involved in interaction with the host.[11] These regions, usually including more than 10 kb of sequences, are present in pathogenic strains and absent from non-pathogenic strains of a given species, are frequently associated with mobile elements, and can often be identified from a distinct GC content from the hosting genome that is a relic of their recent acquisition from a foreign origin. Well-studied examples include the PI in uropathogenic *E. coli*,[12] the SPI-1 and SPI-2 islands in *Salmonella*,[13] the Yop virulon in *Yersinia pestis*,[14] and the Cag island in *Helicobacter pylori*.[15]

This anthropocentric vision was put into a wider perspective when the availability of multiple genomes of the same bacterial species showed that a certain degree of variability in gene content is not an exceptional phenomenon limited to PI, but is instead an essential component of bacterial population biology with profound implications for the way bacteria adapt to changing environments. Comparing the genomic sequences of eight strains of *S. agalactiae* (group B *Streptococcus*, GBS), it was shown that each strain had genes that were missing from one or more of the other strains. Mathematical extrapolation of this concept led to the definition of the *core genome* of a species (i.e., the portion of the genome that is shared by all strains). In the case of GBS, the core genome is composed of 1806 genes, representing approximately 80% of the genome of any given strain.[16] The remaining 20% includes genes either shared only by a subset of the strains or that are strain-specific. The surprising result of this analysis was the prediction that even after a large number of strains have been sequenced, each new sequence will contribute an average of thirty-three new genes, suggesting that the size of the pan-genome (i.e., the total set of distinct genes that can be found in at least one strain of a named species) can continue to grow as more strains are sequenced.

This model can be applied to any bacterial species.[17] The size of the core genome reflects the evolutionary history and lifestyle of each species, and can be as little as 42% of the genome in species, such as *E. coli,* that are able to colonize very different environments. In addition, although the core genome mostly encodes metabolic functions that are essential for cell viability, the rest of the genome that was, perhaps inappropriately, defined as dispensable is comparatively rich in poorly characterized genes and genes associated with mobile and extrachromosomal elements, supporting the hypothesis that the majority of strain-specific traits depend on lateral gene transfer events.[16,18]

Later analysis has shown that the size of a species pan-genome can be related to fundamental parameters of the population genetics of a species,[19] supporting a vision in which bacterial cells have access to a large pool of genes (the species pan-genome) from which they occasionally derive traits that are not essential for survival.[20] In the case of *E. coli,* the pool of genes present at least once in a panel of 100 genomic sequences of randomly chosen isolates was estimated to include 17,838 genes, almost four times bigger than the average size of *E. coli* genomes with 4,721 genes;[18] in contrast, for the same number of strains, the pan-genome of *S. pneumonia* was predicted to include 3,221 genes, compared with the 2,104 genes encoded, on average, in each *S. pneumoniae* genome.[19]

The probability of exchange of genetic material among intracellular pathogens that have a low chance of sharing the same environment with unrelated strains is low.[17] However, it has recently been shown that even in a strictly intracellular pathogen such as *Chlamydia trachomatis* horizontal gene transfer is an important phenomenon essentially shaping the phylogeny of the species.[21] The frequency at which gene exchange occurs can be significantly increased by natural processes such as inflammation, or by selective pressure induced by clinical intervention. An example of the former is the boost of the efficiency of plasmid exchange between *Salmonella enteric* serovar Typhimurium and *E. coli* following pathogen-driven inflammatory responses in the gut.[22] Frequent capsular exchange between pneumococcal strains following the introduction of a capsular polysaccharide vaccine, and spread of antibiotic resistance loci identified in *S. pneumoniae*, are clear examples of the latter.[23]

Recently, advancements in sequencing technologies, allowing characterization of the genetic composition of entire microbial communities (the microbiome), have shown that even the pan-genome concept is probably too restrictive, and that a network of gene exchange connects the bacteria forming the normal commensal flora of the human body, where the main limitation is the ecology of the microbial species.[24] This is especially relevant in vaccine research for those bacterial pathogens, such as *N. meningitidis*, that are essentially harmless components of the human microbial flora of the upper respiratory tract and only cause life-threatening disease in a small minority of cases for reasons that are still poorly understood.

From a vaccine discovery perspective, the distinction between core and pan-genome can be seen as both a limitation and an opportunity. If it is required that a single antigen protects against all strains, the antigen needs to be part of the core genome, thus limiting the panel of potential candidates. On the

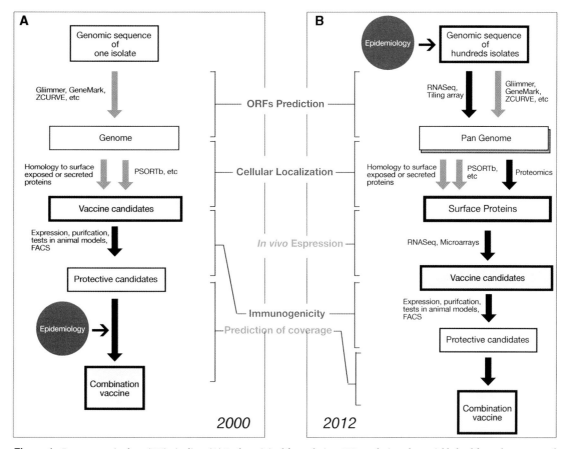

Figure 1. Reverse vaccinology (RV) pipeline. (A) In the original formulation, RV was designed to quickly lead from the genome of a single virulent isolate of a bacterial pathogen to the definition of a list of vaccine candidates through bioinformatics screening (grey arrows). The process involved the testing of a large panel of candidates in animal models, and only at the end, epidemiological data were generated for the protective antigens. (B) In the latest applications of RV, several steps have been modified and bioinformatic predictions have been complemented by experimental screenings (black arrows). The process starts with the sequencing of the genomes of a panel of representative isolates selected on the basis of epidemiological data. The complete set of genes encoded by these isolates (the pan-genome) is determined using bioinformatic predictions and transcriptome analysis. A list of surface-exposed proteins is extracted using bioinformatic predictions and refined using proteomic analysis, and additionally filtered using expression studies. This produces a focused list of high priority candidates to be tested in animal models. The ability of the selected antigens to protect against heterologous strains is tested, and a combination guaranteeing broad coverage is identified on the basis of epidemiology. Besides the introduction of several experimental steps to reduce the number of candidates to be tested in animal models, the main innovation is the use of next generation sequencing technologies to sequence large collections of isolates as a starting point for the selection pipeline. In this way, the conservation and epidemiology of a vaccine target is taken into account at the beginning of the process.

other hand, vaccine candidates able to guarantee partial protection can be derived from a gene pool that is larger than the genome of a single strain, and multicomponent vaccines including two or more of these antigens might guarantee broad protection. However, identification of the best combination requires a deep understanding of the epidemiology of the species, as an essential component of the initial screening of candidates (Fig. 1).

Variability of the antigens

The screening of large collections of isolates has shown that, even in the case of core genes, an aspect that must be taken into account is the sequence variability of the antigens and the effect that this has on their ability to elicit protection against heterologous strains. In an epidemiological study of a sample of 107 isolates, *fetA*, one of the major antigens in MenB, was found to have 56 distinct amino acid sequences.[25] Five major variant families were identified, and polyclonal mouse sera raised against four of the variants were shown to react poorly with other variants. Similarly, one of the antigens that was selected in the first RV project, the factor H binding protein (fHbp), was found in three major variants that are not cross protective.[26] Subsequent studies showed that distinct subvariants differ in their level of surface accessibility and intrinsic reactivity to serum from a vaccinated individual.[27] Given its importance as an antigen, the epidemiology of fHbp has been extensively characterized.[28–32] Presently, more than 570 distinct peptide sequences have been deposited in a public database (http://pubmlst.org/neisseria/fHbp/).

Theoretical considerations and studies based on sequence analysis have shown that the high variability of the molecules having antigenic properties is related to the pressure exerted by the host immune response. In the case of PorB, another major meningococcal antigen, the variable regions of the protein coincide with the loops that are exposed on the surface of the bacterial cell and display a higher than expected rate of nonsynonymous mutation,[33] a phenomenon that is known as positive selection. Similar results have been shown for other antigens in MenB[34] and in other species, such as internalin A (inlA) in *Listeria monocytogenes*,[33] the antigenic membrane protein (Amp) in the plant pathogen *Phytoplasmas*,[35] the Hrp pilin HrpE of the plant pathogen *Xanthomonas*,[36] the intimin protein in *E. coli*,[37] the outer surface protein OspC in *Borrelia burgdoferi*,[38] and the major structural components RrgA and RrgB of the pilus in *S. pneumoniae*.[39]

Such results in many different species and for many different surface-exposed proteins suggest that a certain degree of variability of those proteins that are able to elicit a protective immune response is an unavoidable consequence of the evolutionary pressures exerted by their interaction with the host immune system and that select for the maintenance of polymorphisms within pathogen populations. Therefore, vaccine projects based on RV should take into account the possibility of having vaccine candidates with a low degree of cross protection against heterologous strains. To overcome these difficulties, strategies should be devised based on extensive characterization of the epidemiology of the candidate, or candidates of interest, in order to individuate the main variants and formulate a combination that is broadly cross protective. These variants can be expressed independently, or fused into a single construct.[40] Alternatively, a promising approach is the use of structural information of the target protein to rationally design a chimera that merges the major antigenic regions of the main variants into a single molecule, as recently shown in pioneering work on meningococcal fHbp.[41]

Population genomics and epidemiology of the bacterial species

Given the sequence variability often found in vaccine candidates, it is essential that sequences are characterized from a panel of isolates representative of the target bacterial population. This procedure requires an adequate description of the population structure of the pathogen. Considerable effort has been devoted to the definition of typing schema, such as multilocus sequence typing (MLST), based on the sequencing of small numbers of carefully chosen genomic loci (typically seven, but extended schema have also been proposed[42]); online databases for many pathogens are available.[43–49] Once a panel of strains reproducing the relevant characteristics of the population of circulating strains has been selected (in terms of, for instance, MLST typing), the antigens are sequenced and alignment pipelines, based on software tools like BLAST,[50] FastA,[51] ClustalW,[52] or MUSCLE,[53] are used to determine their variability and the distribution of distinct allelic variants. Since the advent of next generation sequencing (NGS),[10] it is often more practical to sequence the entire genome of representative strains and then extract the sequences of the MLST loci and the potential vaccine candidates from the genome. Two computational procedures are possible. The short sequencing reads can be directly aligned against one or more reference genomes to identify structural genomic variants, such as substitutions or short indels, using dedicated software suites.[54,55] Alternatively, the genomes can first be assembled and then the sequences of the potential antigens can be extracted and aligned. Although the first approach is usually quicker, given the short reads generated by NGS it can be applied only in the case of highly similar sequences, whereas preliminary assembly is required in the case of variable sequences, as is the case for many candidate antigens.

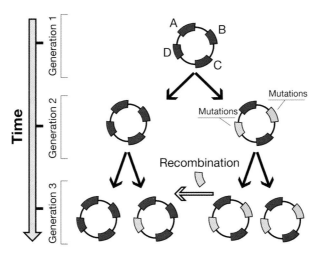

Figure 2. Clonal relationships and gene content. By transferring portions of the genome between unrelated strains, recombination events break the correlation between clonal relationships and gene content. Therefore, the presence, absence or allelic form of a given antigen cannot be predicted on the basis of the molecular typing of the strains. In the example sketched here, typing of isolates using loci A and B can predict the allelic state of locus D at generation 2, but not at generation 3, after an event of homologous recombination.

The work on MenB and GBS has shown that novel vaccine antigens do not necessarily follow the typing systems currently used and described in the textbooks, complicating the task of predicting which strains will be covered by the vaccine and, ultimately, the expected decrease in the number of disease cases following vaccination. Therefore, developing a vaccine based on RV may require developing a new typing system and educating the scientific community accordingly. A typical example is the 4CMenB vaccine against *N. meningitidis*. Pathogenic *N. meningitidis* is classified into serogroups A, B, C, Y, W-135, and X based on the chemical composition of the capsular polysaccharide, and on clonal complexes and sequence types based on the genetic make-up of the seven genes defined by the MLST schema.[43] It was found that neither of these typing systems was able to accurately describe the potential strain coverage of the 4CMenB vaccine. This lack of predictive value was attributed, on one hand, to the confounding effect of homologous recombination that breaks the linkage between the MLST loci and the antigens[28–32] and, on the other hand, to the lack of correlation between expression of the antigens and molecular typing (Fig. 2). As a generalization of MLST, sequencing of complete genomes is now increasingly used to gain a deeper understanding of the relation between bacterial strains,[21,23,56] and will soon become the tool of choice for the typing of bacterial species. The high resolution guaranteed by whole genome typing can readily be used to dissect finer relationships within known clades,[23,56] and these efforts are likely to result in improved phylogenetic characterization of bacterial species.[57] However, although in principle genomic data contain all of the information concerning the expression, surface exposure, and accessibility of each antigen, using them to predict coverage by a given vaccine formulation is still not feasible.

For this reason the meningococcal antigen typing system (MATS) was developed to predict the coverage of the 4CMenB vaccine (Fig. 3).[35] MATS combines a series of three antigen-specific sandwich ELISA assays for fHbp, NadA, and NHBA, with genotyping of the variable region of the PorA component. MATS ELISA simultaneously quantifies the amount of the antigens expressed by a given bacterial isolate and its immunological cross-reactivity with the antigens present in the 4CMenB vaccine. Given the correlation between MATS typing and susceptibility to killing in a serum bactericidal assay, MATS has the potential to predict vaccine coverage in large panels of strains, a result that even genome-based typing schema cannot presently guarantee.

Improvements to the antigen prediction pipeline

There has been a general evolution of the quality and accuracy of the bioinformatics tools that can be used to perform the selection of antigens, rivaling

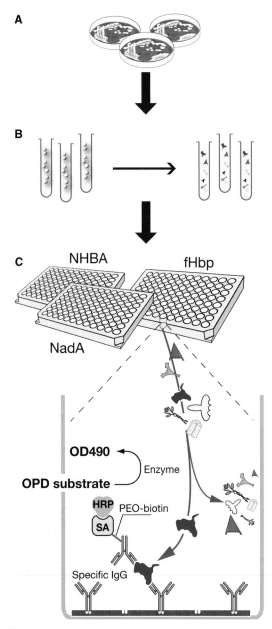

Figure 3. MATS typing system for the 4CMenB vaccine. (A) MenB bacteria are grown overnight on chocolate agar. (B) A suspension of bacteria taken from the plate is prepared to a specified OD600, and detergent is added to the suspension to extract the capsule and expose the antigens. (C) Serial dilutions of extract are tested in the MATS ELISA. A specific capture antibody binds one of the antigens from the extract, which is then detected with a specific biotin-labeled antibody and a streptavidin–enzyme conjugate. Plates are read in an ELISA reader.

in many cases the accuracy of experimental methods. The bioinformatics pipeline of RV involves several prediction steps, including (1) prediction of the protein open reading frames (ORFs), (2) annotation of the ORFs, and (3) prediction of the cellular localization of proteins. Because of the increasing popularity of the RV approach and the need for tools that allow its application, including by research groups that could not afford a large team of bioinformatics experts, dedicated software platforms were developed,[26–29] often using machine learning methods that leverage on accumulated knowledge from the experimental screens of large sets of potential vaccine candidates. Moreover, the increased availability of genome-scale experimental protocols, in many cases, now allows independent confirmation of bioinformatics predictions; in particular, it is now feasible to experimentally validate the gene prediction algorithms and the cellular localization algorithms at the genomic level. These experimental techniques are both able to correct errors and to identify new genes or surface-exposed proteins that were missed in the predictions.

Experimental validation of gene prediction algorithms

In the original RV efforts, identification of protein coding genes was based on gene prediction algorithms such a Glimmer,[58–61] GeneMark,[62] ZCURVE,[63] EasyGene,[64] or MED.[65] Despite continuous improvements, these algorithms suffer from systematic errors that are often not easy to quantify because of the relatively low prevalence of experimentally confirmed protein coding sequences in the genomic databases. Critical reannotation of 143 prokaryotic genomes has shown that the number of genes for which the wrong starting site has been predicted can be as high as 60%, especially for GC–rich genomes.[66] Given that, in many cases, the signal for cellular localization of the proteins is encoded near the start site, accuracy of the gene prediction is vital for the RV selection process of vaccine candidates.

Tiling arrays and RNA-Seq experiments can identify protein coding regions, transcriptional units, and regulatory elements independently from prediction algorithms.[67–69] Dedicated software suites for the assembly of RNA-Seq data are continuously improving our understanding of the structure of transcriptional units in both eukaryotes and prokaryotes.[70,71] Previously unpredicted coding sequences, alternative transcripts, and regulatory elements have been identified in *Mycoplasma pneumoniae*, one of the smallest self-replicating organisms.[72] Alternatively, proteomic approaches using high resolution mass spectra obtained by tandem mass spectrometry can experimentally validate gene predictions by directly identifying peptides from expressed proteins. A proteome-derived ORF model for *M. pneumoniae* was able to confirm 81% of the predicted ORFs, additionally discovering 16 previously unknown ORFs and extending 19 ORFs at their N-termini.[73] In a recent genome-wide study on *S. typhimurium*, MS-based proteomics confirmed more than 40% of the predicted ORFs, correcting 47 start sites and identifying 12 novel genes not predicted by current gene-finding algorithms.[74]

Improved bioinformatics algorithms

Experimental determination of the cellular localization of proteins is a time consuming task that is difficult to perform on a genomic scale. Therefore, RV projects usually rely on teams of experts that complement protein cellular localization predictions provided by computational tools with literature-based searches of experimental evidence.[2] In the last ten years, the accuracy of computational predictions has greatly improved, limiting the need for expert supervision.

In bacteria, proteins are synthesized in the cytoplasm and then directed to specific sites or cell compartment by signals that are encoded in their amino-acid sequences. Although the nature of these signals is not completely known, their existence allows one to approach the protein localization problem through bioinformatics tools. The computational pipelines leading to a reliable prediction can be roughly classified into two main categories: homology-based inferences in which databases of proteins whose cellular localization has been experimentally determined are scanned to identify possible homologies with the unknown protein, and tools based on the identification of sequence-encoded signals known to influence protein localization. The homology-based method relies on the assumption that a certain degree of sequence conservation will lead to conservation of localization,[75] and its high accuracy is supported by the surprisingly sharp transition found in the relation between sequence similarity and identity in subcellular localization.[76]

Other studies have shown that the level of homology needed for an accurate prediction of localization can be as low as 30%.[77]

In the last decade, many computational methods for predicting cellular localization based on machine learning algorithms have been introduced.[77–82] Because the first version was applicable only to Gram-negative bacteria, PSORTb[83] has been the most widely used localization prediction tool in RV projects. PSORTb has now been updated to include Gram-positive bacteria and to increase its coverage, while maintaining high precision.[84,85] Web-accessible databases of precompiled PSORTb predictions for most of the sequenced genomes also exist.[86] Other methods, combining more than one predictor, have been proposed.[87–89] Comprehensive databases that include the predictions of many computational tools for large samples of bacterial genomes are now freely available on the web.[90] Using these methods it is now possible to predict the cellular localization of large protein datasets with a precision that exceeds that of many experimental methods.[91] An approach that could substantially further improve the accuracy of computational methods is the integration of the available knowledge from the body of scientific literature using text mining and machine learning approaches,[92] supporting the role of human experts with modern tools of knowledge management. More generally, literature mining methods have been developed to identify proteins involved in host–pathogen interaction that could therefore constitute promising vaccine targets.[93]

Proteomics

The availability of bacterial genomes, together with the advancement of bioinformatic analysis tools, has greatly improved the ability of mass spectroscopy to identify bacterial proteins in uncharacterized samples. Using these technologies, known as *proteomics*, the large scale identification of proteins exposed on the surface of bacterial cells (the *surfome*) is now feasible.[94] In Gram-positive bacteria, the technology is based on "shaving" the surface of bacteria with proteases under conditions that preserve bacterial viability.[95] For Gram-negatives, the technology leverages on the fact that these organisms naturally release outer membrane vesicles (OMVs), organelles that bud out of the outer membranes without impairing cell viability. OMVs are then purified and their protein content, prevalently composed by membrane-associated proteins, is characterized.[96,97]

Surfome analysis has allowed confirmation of surface localization predictions obtained by computational tools in many bacteria, and to identify previously unknown antigens. Novel antigens were identified by 2D gel electrophoresis of membrane extracts followed by MALDI-TOF identification in *Clostridium difficile*[98] and *Bordetella pertussis*.[99] Shaving of the bacterial cell surface followed by identification of the released peptides by mass spectroscopy have allowed the identification of surface-exposed proteins in group A *Streptococcus* (GAS)[95] and in GBS.[100] Furthermore, proteomic technologies have been used to identify biomarkers that distinguish virulent isolates of bacterial pathogens from harmless commensals.[101]

Differently from bioinformatic predictions, proteomic technologies also have the ability to identify posttranslational modifications that change the structure, and therefore potentially the antigenic properties, of the vaccine targets. Multiply charged isoforms that represent posttranslational modification such as phosphorylation, as well as smaller mass variants because of proteolytic cleavage, are commonly found in proteomic screens of outer membrane proteins by 2D-PAGE in *E. coli*.[102,103] On the basis of these data, it has been estimated that the fraction of proteins that undergo posttranslational modifications can represent up to 42% of the *E. coli* proteome.[102]

Prediction of immunogenicity

Of obvious interest for the selection of candidate antigens is the possibility to computationally predict the immunogenicity of the proteins that are on the surface of the bacterial cells. Most vaccines work by inducing serum antibodies, requiring the activation of B cells. Despite numerous efforts using a variety of computational techniques (for a review of available software and online resources, see Ref. 104), an exhaustive assessment of their predictive power has shown that their rate of success is only marginally better than random,[105] possibly because B cell epitopes are often conformational. Although recent approaches based on 3D protein structures have shown encouraging results,[106] their large-scale use is limited by the availability of crystallographic data.

In contrast to the case of B cell epitopes, considerable improvements have been made in T cell epitope prediction methods, thus allowing the inclusion of cellular mediated immunity in the RV framework. A large number of computational algorithms have been proposed,[104,107] and databases of predicted and experimentally determined epitopes are available.[108] In parallel, many technological advancements and experimental studies have allowed the validation of prediction algorithms and the elucidation of the role of cellular immunity in vaccine efficacy (for a recent comprehensive review, see Ref. 107).

Gene expression

It is increasingly appreciated that it is essential for potential vaccine targets to be expressed by pathogens during the infection process, and that in many cases antigens poorly expressed in *in vitro* conditions can be induced *in vivo* by specific signals. One example is the NadA protein, an adhesin present in approximately 50% of the MenB isolates. NadA was found to be protective in an infant rat model of bacteremia[109,110] and was selected as one of the components of the 4CMenB vaccine against MenB.[4] *In vitro*, the expression of NadA depends on the growth phase and is different in different strains of MenB.[33,109] However, the presence of the *nadA* gene associates significantly with hypervirulent strains; in contrast to most meningococcal surface-associated proteins, sera from children recovering from invasive meningococcal disease react specifically to recombinant forms of NadA.[25] Later studies have shown that NadA expression is tightly regulated by a complex combination of genetic and environmental factors involving the binding of a repressor, NadR, to regions flanking the phase variable promoter of the *nadA* gene (Fig. 4).[111] The presence of 4-hydroxyphenylacetic acid (4HPA), a metabolite of aromatic amino acids found in saliva, can induce NadA expression by alleviating the binding activity of NadR, suggesting that *in vivo* NadA expression can be induced by environmental factors present in the oropharynx.[111,112]

Although measuring the expression of large panels of proteins in a large number of strains or experimental conditions is not feasible, the identification of genes differentially transcribed can be a powerful tool to identify proteins that play a role in the infection process. These approaches

A

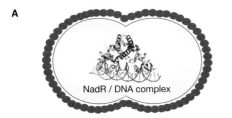

NadR / DNA complex

NadR-metiated *nadA* repression *in vitro*

B

4-HPA / Human Saliva

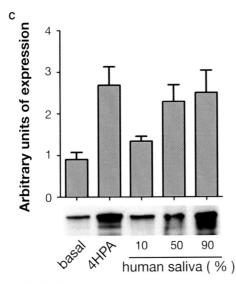

NadR

NadA

NadR-metiated *nadA* induction *in vitro*

C

Figure 4. NadR mediated regulation of NadA expression. (A) The expression of NadA is repressed *in vivo* by the binding of NadR to regions flanking the promoter of NadA. (B) The binding activity of NadR is alleviated by the presence of 4HPA, a metabolite of aromatic amino acids found in saliva. (C) In human saliva NadA is expressed at levels similar to that obtained in the presence of 4HPA, suggesting that environmental factors can trigger the expression of NadA *in vivo*.

use RNA-based techniques—from the conventional expression microarray to the more recent tiling arrays and RNA-Seq technologies—to infer the amount of protein synthesized by bacterial cells at a given time. Soon after the first applications of RV, microarray studies of the differential expression between pathogenic *N. meningitidis* and nonpathogenic *Neisseria lactamica*, upon contact with epithelial cells, was used to identify previously unknown vaccine candidates.[113,114] Overexpression of the *fHbp* protein of *N. meningitidis* has been measured in human blood.[115] Selective enrichment techniques of transcribed sequences[116] have allowed measurement of the level of mRNA transcription *in vivo* in *S. typhi*.[117] An integrated systems biology approach applied to *S. pyogenes* has identified many ways in which this pathogen reacts in a niche-specific manner to the interaction with the human host, identifying new potential vaccine candidates.[118]

New technologies, like RNA-Seq and tiling arrays, that are able to determine the transcriptome independently from genome annotation are increasingly used to validate genome annotation and to elucidate the structure of transcriptional units. In one of the first genome-wide transcriptome determinations using tiling arrays, it was shown that the structure and regulation of the transcriptional units in *L. monocytogenes* are far more intricate than previously known.[119] Strand-specific RNA-Seq has been used to define both the coding and non-coding transcripts in *S. typhi*, identifying many small noncoding RNAs that are likely to be an important regulatory mechanism.[120] Trascriptome analysis through RNA-Seq of several pathogens, such as *H. pylori*,[121] *Campyobacter jejuni*,[122] and *C. trachomatis*,[123] has been performed. The application of these techniques to *in vivo* studies will help to identify genes that are differentially expressed during infection, allowing a more effective selection of target antigens for vaccine formulation.

Discovery of new mechanisms of pathogenesis

The large body of research on previously unknown or poorly characterized surface proteins, initiated by projects based on RV, has substantially increased our knowledge of the mechanisms of interaction between pathogens and the human host, and has led to the discovery of new mechanisms of pathogenesis.

One example is fHbp in *N. meningitidis*. Originally known as GNA1870, fHbp is a surface-exposed lipoprotein that was selected as a vaccine target because of its ability to elicit protective antibodies in an infant rat model of bacteremia. GNA1870 was shown to bind factor H, a component of the alternative complement pathway, and for this reason was renamed fHbp.[36] By inhibiting the activation of the complement cascade, fHbp enhances the ability of bacteria to survive in human serum and might be essential for survival during carriage, when bacteria are often unencapsulated.

Another example is the discovery of pili, long filamentous structures protruding from the surface of cells in Gram-positive organisms. Although it has long been known that Gram-negative bacteria can express pilus-like structures to mediate attachment to host tissues,[124] the presence, structure, and function of pili in Gram-positive bacteria has only recently been characterized, mainly because of their importance as vaccine antigens. Pilus-like structures in a Gram-positive bacterium were first observed in *Corynebacterium renale* using electron microscopy in the late 1960s,[34] and their role in attachment to cells was soon discovered thereafter.[37] However, only recently has the structure and mechanism of assembly of Gram-positive pili been studied in detail.[125] Since then pili have been identified in several species, including *Actinomyces* pp,[126] GAS,[38] GBS,[39,41] and *S. pneumonia*;[127,128] and the way in which they were discovered represents an example of how applied research can produce results of general interest. Gram-positive pili are very different from pili found in Gram-negative bacteria because they are formed by covalent linkage between protein subunits by the action of specialized sortase enzymes and are then anchored to the cell wall. Sortase-mediated attachment to the cell wall is a general mechanism used by Gram-positive bacteria to expose proteins on their surface; and sortase enzymes specifically recognize a conserved carboxy terminal motif (LPXTG). For this reason, proteins containing the LPXTG motif are among those routinely selected in RV projects on Gram-positive bacteria. In most cases, Gram-positive pili are encoded in genomic islands that contain between one and five LPXTG proteins, and between one and three specific sortases. The presence of these genomic structures in many species of *Streptococcus* attracted the attention of researchers looking for vaccine candidates in a specialized variant of RV called *targeted reverse vaccinology*.[129] Components of these genomic structures often prove to be protective in animal models against homologous strains,[38,39,41,130] although their use as vaccine targets is challenging because of their extreme variability[131] and presence only in a subset of virulent strains.[128,132]

Future developments

Integrated approaches

One of the key points in an RV project is that both the bioinformatic analysis and the proteomic analysis identify a large number of candidate vaccines, all of which need to be tested in an animal model to measure their ability to elicit protective antibodies. In an attempt to narrow down the list of potential vaccine targets and to streamline the vaccine development process, the concomitant use of an array of technologies, including bioinformatics, proteomics, screening of human sera using protein arrays, and FACS analysis, has been proposed.[133] By simultaneously predicting/testing the conservation, expression, surface exposure, and immunogenicity of the predicted antigens, this experimental strategy allows an accurate selection of bacterial vaccines without using *in vitro* and/or *in vivo* protection assays, thus dramatically decreasing the costs of vaccine projects and maximizing the chances of success.

Single cell expression

Most of the steps in the RV antigen selection procedure rely on the assumption that genetically homogeneous populations of bacterial cells will display homogeneous phenotype. However, it is well known that marked phenotypic heterogeneities can be identified even in clonal cultures,[134] where individual microbial cells can exhibit variable degrees of resistance to antibiotics, motility, or expression of virulence determinants.

Phenotypic heterogeneity of a population is thought to allow bacteria to adapt to variations in the environment, leveraging on their large population size. The main advantage of these mechanisms is that because they do not involve irreversible genetic modifications the population of bacteria can revert to the original state once the transient stimulus is removed, thus providing an ideal solution to the problem of adapting to short-time environmental fluctuations. Bacterial pathogens have adopted these mechanisms in cases in which the infection process involves selective bottlenecks, and to provide a reservoir of escape mutants that survive the action of the adaptive host immune system. In other cases, structures with high fitness costs are expressed only transiently, as recently shown for the type III secretion system *ttss-1,* the main virulence factor of *S. enteric* serovar Typhimurium that, at any given time, is present only in a fraction of the bacterial population *in vitro.*[135] This phenomenon poses a significant challenge to the use of vaccine targets of antigens that are not consistently expressed by the entire bacterial population, as in the case of the Var antigen in *Plasmodium falciparum.*[136]

Several mechanisms have been identified as the cause of these heterogeneities, including the presence of variations at the genome or epigenetic levels. Hypermutable loci have been recognized as one of the mechanisms that allow the generation of a huge number of genomic variants via the combination of different variants at individual loci. Polymerase slippage on simple sequence repeats is one of the best understood mechanism that generate hypermutability at selected loci, often resulting in inactivation of genes through phase variation.[137] These and other subtle mechanisms have been suggested to be responsible for the observed virulence differences between carriage and disease strains of *N. meningitidis.*[138] The existence of minority sequence heterogeneities in a clonal population of bacteria is very difficult to identify with conventional sequencing technologies that usually determine only a consensus sequence in which low copy number variants are averaged out. NGS technologies, with the high level of coverage that they can attain, will provide the basis for a genome-wide identification of these loci.

Other mechanisms that are likely to be much more widespread than currently thought can produce phenotypic heterogeneities in the absence of genotypic differences, as suggested in the case of the pilus expression in pilus-positive strains of *S. pneumonia.*[139] These mechanisms rely on the intrinsically non-linear nature of many expression regulatory networks.[134] A certain degree of cell-to-cell and time-dependent fluctuations in protein expression is unavoidable, and the relevance of this grows for proteins present in low copy numbers.[140] These fluctuations, when occurring in a molecular circuitry that includes feedback loops, can allow single cells to reversibly switch between mutually exclusive states,[141] effectively turning metabolic pathways into decision-capable circuits.[142] One of the first well-studied examples of a fluctuation-induced switch between two alternative stable states is the lambda switch in bacteriophages;[143] the role of fluctuation-induced switches has also been studied in many other microbial biological processes, from chemotaxis in *E. coli*[144] to viral latency in HIV.[145] Although it is hard to imagine the fitness advantage of these mechanisms in a fixed environment, it is now well understood that these mechanisms can actually confer a selective advantage in fluctuating environments.[146] Moreover, it has been shown that these complex regulatory circuitries can, in turn, modulate host physiology in a nontrivial way.[147]

Technical and methodological advances in experimental techniques and data analysis are boosting interest in cell-to-cell variability.[148–152] Determination of copy number variations in a clonal population of *E. coli* has shown the extent to which such fluctuations are an intrinsic property of single cell measurements of both the transcriptome and the proteome.[149] Large-scale application of single cell expression measurement technologies to populations of bacterial cells grown in infection-mimicking cultures is likely to provide valuable information that can be used in screening libraries of potential vaccine targets, allowing concentration on those that are consistently expressed by all members of the bacterial population or whose expression is essential during the infectious process.

Conclusions

Despite the many difficulties and pitfalls, RV has been a revolution in the field of vaccine discovery for infectious diseases, and has been instrumental in advancing vaccines for bacteria that were thought intractable. At the same time, the introduction into vaccine research of high-throughput technologies, such as NGS and proteomic technologies, has brought new insights into many aspects of the biology of infectious diseases and allowed the use of experimental data in several steps of the RV process that a decade ago were based only on bioinformatic predictions. Since their introduction, these technological advancements have greatly improved the efficiency of the vaccine target identification, selection, and development process. Further improvements are still possible that will widen the scope of

RV. For instance, use of large-scale screening technologies based on sequencing of complete genomes could increase the chances of success and speed the development of some viral vaccines, particularly for complex viruses, such as human cytomegalovirus, that have a coding capacity, the complexity and sophisticated regulation mechanisms of which we are now starting to appreciate.[153]

In this review, we have presented an overview of the aspects of RV that have undergone major changes, with an emphasis on the possibilities, opened by new technologies, to focus the costly testing in animal models on those molecules that have a high chance of success.

Bringing a new vaccine from basic research to a product ready for the market through the many stages of development is a challenging task that sometimes requires formulating completely new scientific paradigms; RV is a good example of such a paradigm. Although many of its original premises have changed, the RV approach, and more generally the use of omics approaches, is, and will continue to be in the future, a fundamental part of vaccine research projects.

Acknowledgments

The authors wish to tank Antonello Covacci and Marirosa Mora for critical reading of the manuscript; Isabel Delany, Luca Fagnocchi, Sébastien Brier, and Nathalie Norais for giving access to unpublished data, and Giorgio Corsi for artwork.

Conflicts of interest

The authors declare no conflicts of interest.

References

1. Fleischmann, R.D., M.D. Adams, O. White, *et al.* 1995. Whole-genome random sequencing and assembly of *Haemophilus influenzae* Rd. *Science* **269:** 496–512.

2. Pizza, M., V. Scarlato, V. Masignani, *et al.* 2000. Identification of vaccine candidates against serogroup B meningococcus by whole-genome sequencing. *Science* **287:** 1816–1820.

3. Tettelin, H., N.J. Saunders, J. Heidelberg, *et al.* 2000. Complete genome sequence of *Neisseria meningitidis* serogroup B strain MC58. *Science* **287:** 1809–1815.

4. Giuliani, M.M., J. Adu-Bobie, M. Comanducci, *et al.* 2006. A universal vaccine for serogroup B meningococcus. *Proc. Natl. Acad. Sci. U.S.A.* **103:** 10834–10839.

5. Git, A., H. Dvinge, M. Salmon-Divon, *et al.* 2010. Systematic comparison of microarray profiling, real-time PCR, and next-generation sequencing technologies for measuring differential microRNA expression. *RNA* **16:** 991–1006.

6. Boerno, S.T., C. Grimm, H. Lehrach & M.R. Schweiger. 2010. Next-generation sequencing technologies for DNA methylation analyses in cancer genomics. *Epigenomics* **2:** 199–207.

7. Nobuta, K., K. McCormick, M. Nakano & B.C. Meyers. 2010. Bioinformatics analysis of small RNAs in plants using next generation sequencing technologies. *Methods Mol. Biol.* **592:** 89–106.

8. Maione, D., I. Margarit, C.D. Rinaudo, *et al.* 2005. Identification of a universal Group B streptococcus vaccine by multiple genome screen. *Science* **309:** 148–150.

9. Cheng, L., W. Lu, B. Kulkarni, *et al.* 2010. Analysis of chemotherapy response programs in ovarian cancers by the next-generation sequencing technologies. *Gynecol Oncol.* **117:** 159–169.

10. Metzker, M.L. 2010. Sequencing technologies – the next generation. *Nat. Rev. Genet.* **11:** 31–46.

11. Hacker, J. & J.B. Kaper. 2000. Pathogenicity islands and the evolution of microbes. *Annu. Rev. Microbiol.* **54:** 641–679.

12. Nakano, M., S. Yamamoto, A. Terai, *et al.* 2001. Structural and sequence diversity of the pathogenicity island of uropathogenic Escherichia coli which encodes the USP protein. *FEMS Microbiol. Lett.* **205:** 71–76.

13. Galan, J.E. 2001. Salmonella interactions with host cells: type III secretion at work. *Annu. Rev. Cell Dev. Biol.* **17:** 53–86.

14. Cornelis, G.R. 2000. Molecular and cell biology aspects of plague. *Proc. Natl. Acad. Sci. U.S.A.* **97:** 8778–8783.

15. Odenbreit, S., J. Puls, B. Sedlmaier, *et al.* 2000. Translocation of Helicobacter pylori CagA into gastric epithelial cells by type IV secretion. *Science* **287:** 1497–1500.

16. Tettelin, H., V. Masignani, M.J. Cieslewicz, *et al.* 2005. Genome analysis of multiple pathogenic isolates of Streptococcus agalactiae: implications for the microbial "pan-genome". *Proc. Natl. Acad. Sci. U.S.A.* **102:** 13950–13955.

17. Tettelin, H., D. Riley, C. Cattuto & D. Medini. 2008. Comparative genomics: the bacterial pan-genome. *Curr. Opin. Microbiol.* **11:** 472–477.

18. Touchon, M., C. Hoede, O. Tenaillon, *et al.* 2009. Organised genome dynamics in the Escherichia coli species results in highly diverse adaptive paths. *PLoS Genet.* **5:** e1000344.

19. Donati, C., N.L. Hiller, H. Tettelin, *et al.* 2010. Structure and dynamics of the pan-genome of Streptococcus pneumoniae and closely related species. *Genome Biol.* **11:** R107.

20. Muzzi, A. & C. Donati. 2011. Population genetics and evolution of the pan-genome of Streptococcus pneumoniae. *Int. J. Med. Microbiol.* **301:** 619–622.

21. Harris, S.R., I.N. Clarke, H.M. Seth-Smith, *et al.* 2012. Whole-genome analysis of diverse Chlamydia trachomatis strains identifies phylogenetic relationships masked by current clinical typing. *Nat. Genet.* **44:** 413–419, S411.

22. Stecher, B., R. Denzler, L. Maier, *et al.* 2012. Gut inflammation can boost horizontal gene transfer between pathogenic and commensal Enterobacteriaceae. *Proc. Natl. Acad. Sci. U.S.A.* **109:** 1269–1274.

23. Croucher, N.J., S.R. Harris, C. Fraser, *et al.* 2011. Rapid pneumococcal evolution in response to clinical interventions. *Science* **331:** 430–434.

24. Smillie, C.S., M.B. Smith, J. Friedman, *et al.* 2011. Ecology drives a global network of gene exchange connecting the human microbiome. *Nature* **480:** 241–244.

25. Litt, D.J., S. Savino, A. Beddek, *et al.* 2004. Putative vaccine antigens from Neisseria meningitidis recognized by serum antibodies of young children convalescing after meningococcal disease. *J. Infect. Dis.* **190:** 1488–1497.

26. Masignani, V., M. Comanducci, M.M. Giuliani, *et al.* 2003. Vaccination against Neisseria meningitidis using three variants of the lipoprotein GNA1870. *J. Exp. Med.* **197:** 789–799.

27. Seib, K.L., B. Brunelli, B. Brogioni, *et al.* 2011. Characterization of diverse subvariants of the meningococcal factor H (fH) binding protein for their ability to bind fH, to mediate serum resistance, and to induce bactericidal antibodies. *Infect. Immun.* **79:** 970–981.

28. Brehony, C., D.J. Wilson & M.C. Maiden. 2009. Variation of the factor H-binding protein of Neisseria meningitidis. *Microbiology* **155:** 4155–4169.

29. Kodama, Y., E. Kaminuma, S. Saruhashi, *et al.* 2010. Biological databases at DNA Data Bank of Japan in the era of next-generation sequencing technologies. *Adv Exp Med. Biol.* **680:** 125–135.

30. Ravn, U., F. Gueneau, L. Baerlocher, *et al.* 2010. By-passing in vitro screening–next generation sequencing technologies applied to antibody display and in silico candidate selection. *Nucleic Acids Res.* **38:** e193.

31. Nagarajan, N. & M. Pop. 2010. Sequencing and genome assembly using next-generation technologies. *Methods Mol. Biol.* **673:** 1–17.

32. Cahill, M.J., C.U. Koser, N.E. Ross & J.A. Archer. 2010. Read length and repeat resolution: exploring prokaryote genomes using next-generation sequencing technologies. *PLoS One* **5:** e11518.

33. Martin, P., T. van de Ven, N. Mouchel, *et al.* 2003. Experimentally revised repertoire of putative contingency loci in Neisseria meningitidis strain MC58: evidence for a novel mechanism of phase variation. *Mol. Microbiol.* **50:** 245–257.

34. Yanagawa, R., K. Otsuki & T. Tokui. 1968. Electron microscopy of fine structure of Corynebacterium renale with special reference to pili. *Jpn. J. Vet. Res.* **16:** 31–37.

35. Donnelly, J., D. Medini, G. Boccadifuoco, *et al.* 2010. Qualitative and quantitative assessment of meningococcal antigens to evaluate the potential strain coverage of protein-based vaccines. *Proc. Natl. Acad. Sci. U.S.A.* **107:** 19490–19495.

36. Madico, G., J.A. Welsch, L.A. Lewis, *et al.* 2006. The meningococcal vaccine candidate GNA1870 binds the complement regulatory protein factor H and enhances serum resistance. *J. Immunol.* **177:** 501–510.

37. Honda, E. & R. Yanagawa. 1975. Attachment of Corynebacterium renale to tissue culture cells by the pili. *Am. J. Vet. Res.* **36:** 1663–1666.

38. Mora, M., G. Bensi, S. Capo, *et al.* 2005. Group A Streptococcus produce pilus-like structures containing protective antigens and Lancefield T antigens. *Proc. Natl. Acad. Sci. U.S.A.* **102:** 15641–15646.

39. Lauer, P., C.D. Rinaudo, M. Soriani, *et al.* 2005. Genome analysis reveals pili in Group B Streptococcus. *Science* **309:** 105.

40. Roh, S.W., G.C. Abell, K.H. Kim, *et al.* 2010. Comparing microarrays and next-generation sequencing technologies for microbial ecology research. *Trends Biotechnol.* **28:** 291–299.

41. Rosini, R., C.D. Rinaudo, M. Soriani, *et al.* 2006. Identification of novel genomic islands coding for antigenic pilus-like structures in Streptococcus agalactiae. *Mol. Microbiol.* **61:** 126–141.

42. Crisafulli, G., S. Guidotti, A. Muzzi, *et al.* 2012. An extended multi-locus molecular typing schema for Streptococcus pneumoniae demonstrates that a limited number of capsular switch events is responsible for serotype heterogeneity of closely related strains from different countries. *Infection Genet. Evol.*

43. Maiden, M.C., J.A. Bygraves, E. Feil, *et al.* 1998. Multilocus sequence typing: a portable approach to the identification of clones within populations of pathogenic microorganisms. *Proc. Natl. Acad. Sci. U.S.A.* **95:** 3140–3145.

44. Enright, M.C. & B.G. Spratt. 1998. A multilocus sequence typing scheme for Streptococcus pneumoniae: identification of clones associated with serious invasive disease. *Microbiology* **144**(Pt 11)**:** 3049–3060.

45. Enright, M.C., N.P. Day, C.E. Davies, *et al.* 2000. Multilocus sequence typing for characterization of methicillin-resistant and methicillin-susceptible clones of Staphylococcus aureus. *J. Clin. Microbiol.* **38:** 1008–1015.

46. Enright, M.C. & B.G. Spratt. 1999. Multilocus sequence typing. *Trends Microbiol.* **7:** 482–487.

47. Enright, M.C., B.G. Spratt, A. Kalia, *et al.* 2001. Multilocus sequence typing of Streptococcus pyogenes and the relationships between emm type and clone. *Infect. Immun.* **69:** 2416–2427.

48. Grundmann, H., S. Hori, M.C. Enright, *et al.* 2002. Determining the genetic structure of the natural population of Staphylococcus aureus: a comparison of multilocus sequence typing with pulsed-field gel electrophoresis, randomly amplified polymorphic DNA analysis, and phage typing. *J. Clin. Microbiol.* **40:** 4544–4546.

49. Chan, M.S., M.C. Maiden & B.G. Spratt. 2001. Database-driven multi locus sequence typing (MLST) of bacterial pathogens. *Bioinformatics* **17:** 1077–1083.

50. Altschul, S.F., W. Gish, W. Miller, *et al.* 1990. Basic local alignment search tool. *J. Mol. Biol.* **215:** 403–410.

51. Pearson, W.R. & D.J. Lipman. 1988. Improved tools for biological sequence comparison. *Proc. Natl. Acad. Sci. U.S.A.* **85:** 2444–2448.

52. Thompson, J.D., T.J. Gibson & D.G. Higgins. 2002. Multiple sequence alignment using ClustalW and ClustalX. In *Current Protocols in Bioinformatics*. Andreas D. Baxevanis, Chapter 2: Unit 2. 3. Wiley. New York.

53. Edgar, R.C. 2004. MUSCLE: multiple sequence alignment with high accuracy and high throughput. *Nucleic Acids Res.* **32:** 1792–1797.

54. Li, H. & R. Durbin. 2010. Fast and accurate long-read alignment with Burrows-Wheeler transform. *Bioinformatics* **26:** 589–595.

55. Li, H., B. Handsaker, A. Wysoker, *et al.* 2009. The Sequence Alignment/Map format and SAMtools. *Bioinformatics* **25:** 2078–2079.

56. Harris, S.R., E.J. Feil, M.T. Holden, *et al.* 2010. Evolution of MRSA during hospital transmission and intercontinental spread. *Science* **327:** 469–474.

57. Marttinen, P., W.P. Hanage, N.J. Croucher, *et al.* 2012. Detection of recombination events in bacterial genomes from large population samples. *Nucleic Acids Res.* **40:** e6.

58. Delcher, A.L., K.A. Bratke, E.C. Powers & S.L. Salzberg. 2007. Identifying bacterial genes and endosymbiont DNA with Glimmer. *Bioinformatics* **23:** 673–679.

59. Delcher, A.L., D. Harmon, S. Kasif, *et al.* 1999. Improved microbial gene identification with GLIMMER. *Nucleic Acids Res.* **27:** 4636–4641.

60. Salzberg, S.L., A.L. Delcher, S. Kasif & O. White. 1998. Microbial gene identification using interpolated Markov models. *Nucleic Acids Res.* **26:** 544–548.

61. Salzberg, S.L., M. Pertea, A.L. Delcher, *et al.* 1999. Interpolated Markov models for eukaryotic gene finding. *Genomics* **59:** 24–31.

62. Lukashin, A.V. & M. Borodovsky. 1998. GeneMark.hmm: new solutions for gene finding. *Nucleic Acids Res.* **26:** 1107–1115.

63. Guo, F.B., H.Y. Ou & C.T. Zhang. 2003. ZCURVE: a new system for recognizing protein-coding genes in bacterial and archaeal genomes. *Nucleic Acids Res.* **31:** 1780–1789.

64. Larsen, T.S. & A. Krogh. 2003. EasyGene–a prokaryotic gene finder that ranks ORFs by statistical significance. *BMC Bioinformatics* **4:** 21.

65. Zhu, H., G.Q. Hu, Y.F. Yang, *et al.* 2007. MED: a new non-supervised gene prediction algorithm for bacterial and archaeal genomes. *BMC Bioinformatics* **8:** 97.

66. Nielsen, P. & A. Krogh. 2005. Large-scale prokaryotic gene prediction and comparison to genome annotation. *Bioinformatics* **21:** 4322–4329.

67. Denoeud, F., J.M. Aury, C. Da Silva, *et al.* 2008. Annotating genomes with massive-scale RNA sequencing. *Genome Biol.* **9:** R175.

68. Martin, J., W. Zhu, K.D. Passalacqua, *et al.* 2010. Bacillus anthracis genome organization in light of whole transcriptome sequencing. *BMC Bioinformatics* **11**(Suppl 3)**:** S10.

69. Mader, U., P. Nicolas, H. Richard, *et al.* 2011. Comprehensive identification and quantification of microbial transcriptomes by genome-wide unbiased methods. *Curr. Opin. Biotechnol.* **22:** 32–41.

70. Li, W., J. Feng & T. Jiang. 2011. IsoLasso: a LASSO regression approach to RNA-Seq based transcriptome assembly. *J. Comput. Biol.* **18:** 1693–1707.

71. Trapnell, C., B.A. Williams, G. Pertea, *et al.* 2010. Transcript assembly and quantification by RNA-Seq reveals unannotated transcripts and isoform switching during cell differentiation. *Nat. Biotechnol.* **28:** 511–515.

72. Guell, M., V. van Noort, E. Yus, *et al.* 2009. Transcriptome complexity in a genome-reduced bacterium. *Science* **326:** 1268–1271.

73. Jaffe, J.D., H.C. Berg & G.M. Church. 2004. Proteogenomic mapping as a complementary method to perform genome annotation. *Proteomics* **4:** 59–77.

74. Ansong, C., N. Tolic, S.O. Purvine, *et al.* 2011. Experimental annotation of post-translational features and translated coding regions in the pathogen Salmonella Typhimurium. *BMC Genomics* **12:** 433.

75. Gardy, J.L. & F.S. Brinkman. 2006. Methods for predicting bacterial protein subcellular localization. *Nat. Rev. Microbiol.* **4:** 741–751.

76. Nair, R. & B. Rost. 2002. Sequence conserved for subcellular localization. *Protein Sci.* **11:** 2836–2847.

77. Yu, C.S., Y.C. Chen, C.H. Lu & J.K. Hwang. 2006. Prediction of protein subcellular localization. *Proteins* **64:** 643–651.

78. Chou, K.C. & H.B. Shen. 2006. Large-scale predictions of gram-negative bacterial protein subcellular locations. *J. Proteome Res.* **5:** 3420–3428.

79. Shen, H.B. & K.C. Chou. 2007. Gpos-PLoc: an ensemble classifier for predicting subcellular localization of Gram-positive bacterial proteins. *Protein Eng. Des. Sel.* **20:** 39–46.

80. Chang, J.M., E.C. Su, A. Lo, *et al.* 2008. PSLDoc: protein subcellular localization prediction based on gapped-dipeptides and probabilistic latent semantic analysis. *Proteins* **72:** 693–710.

81. Su, E.C., H.S. Chiu, A. Lo, *et al.* 2007. Protein subcellular localization prediction based on compartment-specific features and structure conservation. *BMC Bioinformatics* **8:** 330.

82. Matsuda, S., J.P. Vert, H. Saigo, *et al.* 2005. A novel representation of protein sequences for prediction of subcellular location using support vector machines. *Protein Sci.* **14:** 2804–2813.

83. Gardy, J.L., C. Spencer, K. Wang, *et al.* 2003. PSORT-B: Improving protein subcellular localization prediction for Gram-negative bacteria. *Nucleic Acids Res.* **31:** 3613–3617.

84. Gardy, J.L., M.R. Laird, F. Chen, *et al.* 2005. PSORTb v.2.0: expanded prediction of bacterial protein subcellular localization and insights gained from comparative proteome analysis. *Bioinformatics* **21:** 617–623.

85. Yu, N.Y., J.R. Wagner, M.R. Laird, *et al.* 2010. PSORTb 3.0: improved protein subcellular localization prediction with refined localization subcategories and predictive capabilities for all prokaryotes. *Bioinformatics* **26:** 1608–1615.

86. Yu, N.Y., M.R. Laird, C. Spencer & F.S. Brinkman. 2011. PSORTdb–an expanded, auto-updated, user-friendly protein subcellular localization database for Bacteria and Archaea. *Nucleic Acids Res.* **39:** D241–244.

87. Bulashevska, A. & R. Eils. 2006. Predicting protein subcellular locations using hierarchical ensemble of Bayesian classifiers based on Markov chains. *BMC Bioinformatics* **7:** 298.

88. Niu, B., Y.H. Jin, K.Y. Feng, *et al.* 2008. Using AdaBoost for the prediction of subcellular location of prokaryotic and eukaryotic proteins. *Mol. Divers* **12:** 41–45.

89. E-komon, T., R.J. Burchmore, P. Herzyk & R.L. Davies. 2012. Predicting the outer membrane proteome of Pasteurella multocida based on consensus prediction enhanced by results integration and manual confirmation. *BMC Bioinformatics* **13:** 63.

90. Goudenege, D., S. Avner, C. Lucchetti-Miganeh & F. Barloy-Hubler. 2010. CoBaltDB: Complete bacterial and archaeal

orfeomes subcellular localization database and associated resources. *BMC Microbiol.* **10:** 88.

91. Rey, S., J.L. Gardy & F.S. Brinkman. 2005. Assessing the precision of high-throughput computational and laboratory approaches for the genome-wide identification of protein subcellular localization in bacteria. *BMC Genomics* **6:** 162.

92. Shatkay, H., A. Hoglund, S. Brady, *et al.* 2007. SherLoc: high-accuracy prediction of protein subcellular localization by integrating text and protein sequence data. *Bioinformatics* **23:** 1410–1417.

93. Thieu, T., S. Joshi, S. Warren & D. Korkin. 2012. Literature mining of host-pathogen interactions: comparing feature-based supervised learning and language-based approaches. *Bioinformatics* **28:** 867–875.

94. Walters, M.S. & H.L. Mobley. 2010. Bacterial proteomics and identification of potential vaccine targets. *Expert Rev. Proteomics* **7:** 181–184.

95. Rodriguez-Ortega, M.J., N. Norais, G. Bensi, *et al.* 2006. Characterization and identification of vaccine candidate proteins through analysis of the group A Streptococcus surface proteome. *Nat. Biotechnol.* **24:** 191–197.

96. Ferrari, G., I. Garaguso, J. Adu-Bobie, *et al.* 2006. Outer membrane vesicles from group B Neisseria meningitidis delta gna33 mutant: proteomic and immunological comparison with detergent-derived outer membrane vesicles. *Proteomics* **6:** 1856–1866.

97. Berlanda Scorza, F., F. Doro, M.J. Rodriguez-Ortega, *et al.* 2008. Proteomics characterization of outer membrane vesicles from the extraintestinal pathogenic Escherichia coli DeltatolR IHE3034 mutant. *Mol. Cell Proteomics* **7:** 473–485.

98. Wright, A., R. Wait, S. Begum, *et al.* 2005. Proteomic analysis of cell surface proteins from Clostridium difficile. *Proteomics* **5:** 2443–2452.

99. Tefon, B.E., S. Maass, E. Ozcengiz, *et al.* 2011. A comprehensive analysis of Bordetella pertussis surface proteome and identification of new immunogenic proteins. *Vaccine* **29:** 3583–3595.

100. Doro, F., S. Liberatori, M.J. Rodriguez-Ortega, *et al.* 2009. Surfome analysis as a fast track to vaccine discovery: identification of a novel protective antigen for Group B Streptococcus hypervirulent strain COH1. *Mol. Cell Proteomics* **8:** 1728–1737.

101. Cash, P. 2011. Investigating pathogen biology at the level of the proteome. *Proteomics* **11:** 3190–3202.

102. Lopez-Campistrous, A., P. Semchuk, L. Burke, *et al.* 2005. Localization, annotation, and comparison of the Escherichia coli K-12 proteome under two states of growth. *Mol. Cell Proteomics* **4:** 1205–1209.

103. Alteri, C.J. & H.L. Mobley. 2007. Quantitative profile of the uropathogenic Escherichia coli outer membrane proteome during growth in human urine. *Infect. Immun.* **75:** 2679–2688.

104. Korber, B., M. LaBute & K. Yusim. 2006. Immunoinformatics comes of age. *PLoS Computat. Biol.* **2:** e71.

105. Blythe, M.J. & D.R. Flower. 2005. Benchmarking B cell epitope prediction: underperformance of existing methods. *Protein Sci.* **14:** 246–248.

106. Haste Andersen, P., M. Nielsen & O. Lund. 2006. Prediction of residues in discontinuous B-cell epitopes using protein 3D structures. *Protein Sci.* **15:** 2558–2567.

107. Sette, A. & R. Rappuoli. Reverse vaccinology: developing vaccines in the era of genomics. *Immunity* **33:** 530–541.

108. Kim, Y., J. Ponomarenko, Z. Zhu, *et al.* 2012. Immune epitope database analysis resource. *Nucleic acids Res.* **40:** W525–530.

109. Comanducci, M., S. Bambini, B. Brunelli, *et al.* 2002. NadA, a novel vaccine candidate of Neisseria meningitidis. *J. Exp. Med.* **195:** 1445–1454.

110. Capecchi, B., J. Adu-Bobie, F. Di Marcello, *et al.* 2005. Neisseria meningitidis NadA is a new invasin which promotes bacterial adhesion to and penetration into human epithelial cells. *Mol. Microbiol.* **55:** 687–698.

111. Metruccio, M.M., E. Pigozzi, D. Roncarati, *et al.* 2009. A novel phase variation mechanism in the meningococcus driven by a ligand-responsive repressor and differential spacing of distal promoter elements. *PLoS Pathog.* **5:** e1000710.

112. Brier, S., L. Fagnocchi, D. Donnarumma, *et al.* 2012. Structural insight into the mechanism of DNA-binding attenuation of the Neisserial adhesin repressor NadR by the small natural ligand 4-hydroxyphenylacetic acid. *Biochemistry.* **51:** 6738–6752.

113. Grifantini, R., E. Bartolini, A. Muzzi, *et al.* 2002. Previously unrecognized vaccine candidates against group B meningococcus identified by DNA microarrays. *Nat. Biotechnol.* **20:** 914–921.

114. Grifantini, R., E. Bartolini, A. Muzzi, *et al.* 2002. Gene expression profile in Neisseria meningitidis and Neisseria lactamica upon host-cell contact: from basic research to vaccine development. *Ann. N. Y. Acad. Sci.* **975:** 202–216.

115. Echenique-Rivera, H., A. Muzzi, E. Del Tordello, *et al.* 2011. Transcriptome analysis of Neisseria meningitidis in human whole blood and mutagenesis studies identify virulence factors involved in blood survival. *PLoS Pathog.* **7:** e1002027.

116. Daigle, F., J.Y. Hou & J.E. Clark-Curtiss. 2002. Microbial gene expression elucidated by selective capture of transcribed sequences (SCOTS). *Methods Enzymol.* **358:** 108–122.

117. Sheikh, A., R.C. Charles, N. Sharmeen, *et al.* 2011. In vivo expression of Salmonella enterica serotype Typhi genes in the blood of patients with typhoid fever in Bangladesh. *PLoS Negl. Trop. Dis.* **5:** e1419.

118. Musser, J.M. & F.R. DeLeo. 2005. Toward a genome-wide systems biology analysis of host-pathogen interactions in group A Streptococcus. *Am. J. Pathol.* **167:** 1461–1472.

119. Toledo-Arana, A., O. Dussurget, G. Nikitas, *et al.* 2009. The Listeria transcriptional landscape from saprophytism to virulence. *Nature* **459:** 950–956.

120. Perkins, T.T., R.A. Kingsley, M.C. Fookes, *et al.* 2009. A strand-specific RNA-Seq analysis of the transcriptome of the typhoid bacillus Salmonella typhi. *PLoS Genet.* **5:** e1000569.

121. Sharma, C.M., S. Hoffmann, F. Darfeuille, *et al.* 2010. The primary transcriptome of the major human pathogen Helicobacter pylori. *Nature* **464:** 250–255.

122. Chaudhuri, R.R., L. Yu, A. Kanji, *et al*. 2011. Quantitative RNA-seq analysis of the Campylobacter jejuni transcriptome. *Microbiology* **157:** 2922–2932.

123. Albrecht, M., C.M. Sharma, R. Reinhardt, *et al*. 2010. Deep sequencing-based discovery of the Chlamydia trachomatis transcriptome. *Nucleic Acids Res.* **38:** 868–877.

124. Proft, T. & E.N. Baker. 2009. Pili in Gram-negative and Gram-positive bacteria–structure, assembly and their role in disease. *Cell Mol. Life Sci.* **66:** 613–635.

125. Ton-That, H. & O. Schneewind. 2003. Assembly of pili on the surface of Corynebacterium diphtheriae. *Mol. Microbiol.* **50:** 1429–1438.

126. Kelstrup, J., J. Theilade & O. Fejerskov. 1979. Surface ultrastructure of some oral bacteria. *Scand. J. Dent. Res.* **87:** 415–423.

127. Barocchi, M.A., J. Ries, X. Zogaj, *et al*. 2006. A pneumococcal pilus influences virulence and host inflammatory responses. *Proc. Natl. Acad. Sci. U.S.A.* **103:** 2857–2862.

128. F. Bagnoli, M. Moschioni, C. Donati, *et al*. 2008. A second pilus type in Streptococcus pneumoniae is prevalent in emerging serotypes and mediates adhesion to host cells. *J. Bacteriol.* **190:** 5480–5492.

129. Mora, M. & J.L. Telford. 2010. Genome-based approaches to vaccine development. *J. Mol. Med. (Berl).* **88:** 143–147.

130. Gianfaldoni, C., S. Censini, M. Hilleringmann, *et al*. 2007. Streptococcus pneumoniae pilus subunits protect mice against lethal challenge. *Infect. Immun.* **75:** 1059–1062.

131. Falugi, F., C. Zingaretti, V. Pinto, *et al*. 2008. Sequence variation in group A Streptococcus pili and association of pilus backbone types with lancefield T serotypes. *J. Infect. Dis.* **198:** 1834–1841.

132. Moschioni, M., C. Donati, A. Muzzi, *et al*. 2008. Streptococcus pneumoniae contains 3 rlrA pilus variants that are clonally related. *J. Infect. Dis.* **197:** 888–896.

133. Bensi, G., M. Mora, G. Tuscano, *et al*. 2012. Multi High-Throughput Approach for Highly Selective Identification of Vaccine Candidates: the Group A Streptococcus Case. *Mol. Cell Proteomics.* **11:** M111.015693.

134. Avery, S.V. 2006. Microbial cell individuality and the underlying sources of heterogeneity. *Nat. Rev. Microbiol.* **4:** 577–587.

135. Sturm, A., M. Heinemann, M. Arnoldini, *et al*. 2011. The cost of virulence: retarded growth of Salmonella Typhimurium cells expressing type III secretion system 1. *PLoS Pathog.* **7:** e1002143.

136. Ralph, S.A. & A. Scherf. 2005. The epigenetic control of antigenic variation in Plasmodium falciparum. *Curr. Opin. Microbiol.* **8:** 434–440.

137. Moxon, R., C. Bayliss & D. Hood. 2006. Bacterial contingency loci: the role of simple sequence DNA repeats in bacterial adaptation. *Annu. Rev. Genet.* **40:** 307–333.

138. Schoen, C., H. Tettelin, J. Parkhill & M. Frosch. 2009. Genome flexibility in Neisseria meningitidis. *Vaccine* **27**(Suppl 2)**:** B103–111.

139. De Angelis, G., M. Moschioni, A. Muzzi, *et al*. 2011. The Streptococcus pneumoniae pilus-1 displays a biphasic expression pattern. *PLoS One* **6:** e21269.

140. Elowitz, M.B., A.J. Levine, E.D. Siggia & P.S. Swain. 2002. Stochastic gene expression in a single cell. *Science* **297:** 1183–1186.

141. Smits, W.K., O.P. Kuipers & J.W. Veening. 2006. Phenotypic variation in bacteria: the role of feedback regulation. *Nat. Rev. Microbiol.* **4:** 259–271.

142. Balázsi, G., A. van Oudenaarden & J.J. Collins. 2011. Cellular decision making and biological noise: from microbes to mammals. *Cell* **144:** 910–925.

143. Shea, M.A. & G.K. Ackers. 1985. The OR control system of bacteriophage lambda. A physical-chemical model for gene regulation. *J. Mol. Biol.* **181:** 211–230.

144. Korobkova, E., T. Emonet, J.M. Vilar, *et al*. 2004. From molecular noise to behavioural variability in a single bacterium. *Nature* **428:** 574–578.

145. Weinberger, L.S., J.C. Burnett, J.E. Toettcher, *et al*. 2005. Stochastic gene expression in a lentiviral positive-feedback loop: HIV-1 Tat fluctuations drive phenotypic diversity. *Cell* **122:** 169–182.

146. Thattai, M. & A. van Oudenaarden. 2004. Stochastic gene expression in fluctuating environments. *Genetics* **167:** 523–530.

147. Tan, C., P. Marguet & L. You. 2009. Emergent bistability by a growth-modulating positive feedback circuit. *Nat. Chem. Biol.* **5:** 842–848.

148. Brehm-Stecher, B.F. & E.A. Johnson. 2004. Single-cell microbiology: tools, technologies, and applications. *Microbiol. Mol. Biol. Rev* **68:** 538–559.

149. Taniguchi, Y., P.J. Choi, G.W. Li, *et al*. 2010. Quantifying E. coli proteome and transcriptome with single-molecule sensitivity in single cells. *Science* **329:** 533–538.

150. Bandura, D.R., V.I. Baranov, O.I. Ornatsky, *et al*. 2009. Mass cytometry: technique for real time single cell multitarget immunoassay based on inductively coupled plasma time-of-flight mass spectrometry. *Anal. Chem.* **81:** 6813–6822.

151. Qiu, P., E.F. Simonds, S.C. Bendall, *et al*. 2011. Extracting a cellular hierarchy from high-dimensional cytometry data with SPADE. *Nat. Biotechnol.* **29:** 886–891.

152. Kalisky, T. & S.R. Quake. 2011. Single-cell genomics. *Nat. Methods* **8:** 311–314.

153. Stern-Ginossar, N., B. Weisburd, A. Michalski, *et al*. 2012. Decoding human cytomegalovirus. *Science* **338:** 1088–1093.

Ann. N.Y. Acad. Sci. ISSN 0077-8923

The National Institutes of Health Center for Human Immunology, Autoimmunity, and Inflammation: history and progress

Howard B. Dickler,[1] J. Philip McCoy,[1] Robert Nussenblatt,[2] Shira Perl,[1] Pamela A. Schwartzberg,[3] John S. Tsang,[4] Ena Wang,[5] and Neil S. Young[6]

[1]Center for Human Immunology, National Institutes of Health, Bethesda, Maryland. [2]Laboratory of Immunology, National Eye Institute. [3]Genetic Disease Research Branch, National Human Genome Research Institute. [4]Laboratory of Systems Biology, National Institute of Allergy and Infectious Diseases. [5]Laboratory Services Section, Department of Transfusion Medicine, Office of Deputy of Clinical Care, Clinical Center, National Institutes of Health, Bethesda, Maryland. [6]Hematology Branch, National Heart, Lung, and Blood Institute, National Institutes of Health, Bethesda, Maryland

Address for correspondence: Robert Nussenblatt, Chief, Laboratory of Immunology, NIH—National Eye Institute, 10 Center Drive, Bethesda, MD 20892. drbob@nei.nih.gov

The Center for Human Immunology, Autoimmunity, and Inflammation (CHI) is an exciting initiative of the NIH intramural program begun in 2009. It is uniquely trans-NIH in support (multiple institutes) and leadership (senior scientists from several institutes who donate their time). Its goal is an in-depth assessment of the human immune system using high-throughput multiplex technologies for examination of immune cells and their products, the genome, gene expression, and epigenetic modulation obtained from individuals both before and after interventions, adding information from in-depth clinical phenotyping, and then applying advanced biostatistical and computer modeling methods for mining these diverse data. The aim is to develop a comprehensive picture of the human "immunome" in health and disease, elucidate common pathogenic pathways in various diseases, identify and validate biomarkers that predict disease progression and responses to new interventions, and identify potential targets for new therapeutic modalities. Challenges, opportunities, and progress are detailed.

Keywords: human; immunology; autoimmunity; inflammation

The history of the Center for Human Immunology, Autoimmunity, and Inflammation

Planning

In early 2006, Elias Zerhouni, director of the National Institutes of Health (NIH), initiated a process for the development of an intramural roadmap, parallel to the previously established extramural roadmap that focuses on translational research, with the goal of conducting research distinctive from work supported by extramural grants.

A lengthy series of meetings involving intramural scientists at all levels of experience and on all the NIH campuses ensued over the next year. Based on a draft proposal for an initiative for a detailed study of the human immune system in health and disease that was presented to Michael Gottesman and Elias Zerhouni in March 2007, approval was given to proceed with more concrete planning. In early June, Gottesman asked Neil Young to lead this effort as director, focusing on the immediate task of developing a business plan to present at a second retreat in the fall. The Trans-NIH Committee was reconstituted as a steering committee for the center with several additional members. Working with Gorgio Trinchieri and Ronald Germain, and with the help of McKinsey & Company, a business plan was developed and presented by Young at a second NIH Intramural Research Retreat in October 2007.

doi: 10.1111/nyas.12101

The draft proposal and the business plan became the foundation of the Center for Human Immunology (CHI) Charter. The charter was further developed collaboratively with the input of Young, Trinchieri, and Germain, as well as Daniel Kastner (NIAMS), and with the participation of the entire steering committee. This charter was extensively presented to all institute directors, institute scientific directors, and all intramural immunologists over the course of several months and was subsequently approved in September 2008.

The creators of the CHI were motivated by the desire to establish a structure capable of drawing on the strength of the intramural programs in immunology and clinical research to generate critical new knowledge in immunology and inflammation, and especially to solve problems in translating such knowledge into clinical practice. Three aspects of the present difficulty of efficient translation of basic immunologic knowledge into clinical practice provided the impetus for the establishment of the CHI. First, the enormous field of immunology is highly fragmented, both within the basic sciences and in the clinic among medical subspecialists studying many different diseases. This is a particular problem in the NIH intramural program because nearly all the institutes are disease focused, and each receives an independent budget directly from Congress, which makes cooperative research across institutes much more difficult. Second, there is a perception of the difficulty, compounded by a relative lack of success, in translating promising insights from the laboratory and animal models of human disease and from other clinical experiences into patient care, and ultimately into practice. Finally, many new technologies with potential applications in the laboratory and clinic are simply too difficult and/or expensive for individual laboratories to master or utilize effectively.

These difficulties were directly addressed in the CHI mission statement, including the following three statements:

1. The center is envisioned as a cooperative enterprise, with representatives from many NIH institutes working together on focused projects with clearly stated and shared goals.
2. CHI will provide capabilities often unavailable to individual laboratories because of cost, complexity, or novelty in three distinct areas:

(a) assays of immune cells and their products, mainly based on flow cytometry and other emerging multiplexed techniques; (b) high-throughput systems technologies, involving the use of new methods for large-scale examination of the genome, gene expression, epigenetic modulation, as well as the proteome, lipidome, and metabolome, and the application of advanced biostatistical and computer modeling methods for mining these diverse data to aid in understanding immune function and pathology; and (c) protocol development, with staff dedicated to efficient translation of science to the clinic while meeting appropriate ethical and regulatory requirements for human research.

3. The center's focus is human immunology, normal but especially pathologic, with an emphasis on shared pathophysiologic mechanisms that underlie disease. This includes recognized immunologically mediated diseases, organ-specific autoimmunity, and the role of inflammation in a wide variety of common diseases, including cancer, atherosclerosis, and neurologic degeneration.

Budget and refocus

The charter and the business plan (the latter was developed by a respected external consultant) were ambitious, incorporating many high-throughput multiplex platforms and targeting multiple diseases. Thus, the proposal was for a budget of $65 million over 5 years, a staff of 65–70, and laboratory space of 20,000–25,000 ft^2. However, when the institutes began to discuss resources to support the CHI, fiscal and physical constraints resulted in a much more modest budget and more limited laboratory space (5000 ft^2). A memorandum of understanding signed in April 2009 by seven institutes established a budget of $2.55 million/year for 5 years, along with a verbal promise that if the CHI was successful, there would be increased resources in the future. The National Institute of Arthritis and Musculoskeletal and Skin Diseases (NIAMS) was the largest contributor in terms of the percentage of the institute budget (the director, Stephen Katz, was a staunch supporter), with the National Cancer Institute (NCI), the National Institute of Allergy and Infectious Diseases (NIAID), and the National Heart, Lung, and Blood Institute (NHLBI) contributing

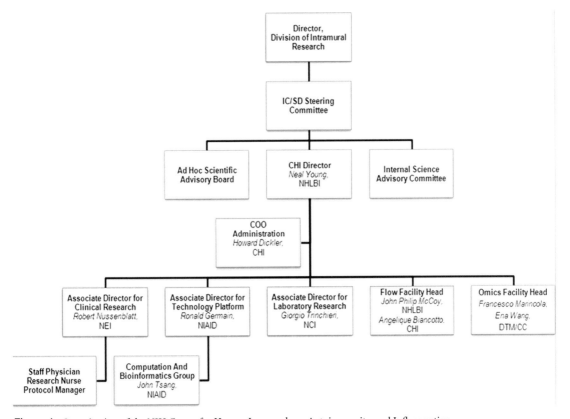

Figure 1. Organization of the NIH Center for Human Immunology, Autoimmunity, and Inflammation.

substantial amounts. Significant support also came from the National Institute of Neurological Disorders and Stroke (NINDS), the National Institute of Child Health and Human Development (NICHD), and the National Institute of Diabetes and Digestive and Kidney Diseases (NIDDK).

This budget reality forced the CHI to limit the number of high-throughput multiplex platforms to single-nucleotide polymorphism (SNP) analysis, RNA and miRNA expression, highly detailed flow cytometric analysis of immune cells, and extensive analysis of serum cytokines. The goal became to use biostatistics and computational modeling to combine these dense data sets to develop new insights into normal human immune function and the pathophysiology of immune-mediated diseases, a novel approach. Studies were limited to one large and a handful of smaller studies per year, and these were carefully chosen to have very clean demarcations between groups that would lend themselves to this approach.

Organization

As noted above, Gottesman had asked Young to serve as director, and Young, in turn, asked those that had helped shape the charter to serve as associate directors: Trinchieri for laboratory research, Kastner for clinical research, and Germain for the technology platforms. Subsequently, when Kastner assumed new responsibilities as scientific director of the National Human Genome Research Institute (NHGRI), Robert Nussenblatt (National Eye Institute, NEI) became associate director for clinical research (Fig. 1). Two platform facilities were established, one for cell preparation and storage, and for omics headed by Franco Marincola and Ena Wang (both part-time from the Department of Transfusion Medicine of the Clinical Center (DTM/CC)), and another for flow and cytokine analyses headed by Phil McCoy (NHLBI, part-time) and Angelique Biancotto. The position of chief operating officer was established to provide day-to-day leadership because of the limitations on the amount of time each of the directors could allocate to the CHI, owing to the responsibilities of their primary appointments; Howard Dickler filled this position. Subsequently, John Tsang (NIAID, part-time) assumed leadership of the bioinformatics group. The CHI leaders meet weekly to make policy, scientific, and strategic decisions.

The CHI receives advice and counsel on both scientific and administrative matters from three committees. The steering committee comprises the directors of the funding institutes or their designees (one deputy director and one scientific director), and convenes at six-month intervals. The ad hoc external advisory board is made up of outside experts, convenes yearly, and is primarily responsible for providing ideas on new platforms and new directions. The internal science advisory committee consists of a senior scientist from each of the NIH institutes, meets every two months, and has responsibility for reviewing and approving all studies that the CHI undertakes.

Start-up (April–December 2009)

The CHI began life in borrowed space while new administrative and laboratory space was under construction. Space for administrative and clinical personnel was lent by the NHLBI, while temporary administrative offices and laboratories were provided by the NHLBI, NIAMS, and DTM/CC. The initial aim was to become functional as quickly as possible. Because the CHI began life in the middle of a fiscal year, the majority of first-year funds were utilized to purchase the high-throughput machines needed for the platforms. Personnel for the administrative and clinical units were recruited efficiently and were in place by the fall. It took considerably longer to recruit the personnel for the laboratories and especially for the bioinformatics unit (Fig. 2). Platforms were established and validated for SNP analysis, dense flow cytometric analysis (up to 10 tubes of 15 colors), 70 serum cytokines, and expression of RNA and miRNA. Standard operating procedures were established for the separation and preservation of peripheral blood mononuclear cells (PBMC) that retained high viability when thawed.

The CHI took advantage of the expected H1N1 pandemic to conduct their first large study, which examined the immune systems in 200 normal NIH employees before, and at various time points after, perturbation with H1N1 and seasonal influenza vaccines. The two goals were to establish a large

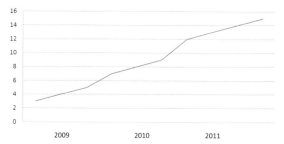

Figure 2. Timeline of hiring of CHI personnel.

database that began to define the parameters of the normal immune system, and to see how it changed after perturbation. The protocol was written and approved by an institutional review board during the summer, the subjects were recruited and screened in the early fall, and the study was conducted as soon as the H1N1 vaccine became available. This study is described in detail in the section that follows. Toward the end of this period, CHI administrative space came online and the CHI had its first home.

Attaining full function and productivity (January 2010–December 2011)

The goal for this period was to attain full function and productivity within the limitation of resources. The CHI embarked on numerous additional protocols during this period, including additional perturbations of the human immune system and studies in several autoimmune and inflammatory conditions. The clinical group was very active in writing protocols, obtaining needed approvals, screening subjects, and enrolling participants. These efforts resulted in significantly increased usage of the NIH Clinical Center and are detailed in a later section. The laboratory cores recruited and trained additional technicians, set up quality control measures, and added additional platforms. Most importantly, the CHI recruited a bioinformatics group under the leadership of John Tsang, a tenure-track investigator at the NIAID and Assistant Director for Informatics at the CHI. This group began the important work of developing approaches to integrate the various dense data sets in order to draw novel and robust biological insights. This was been a laborious effort, as there were no existing applications that could be used for this purpose; these efforts are ongoing. By the end of December 2011, the CHI laboratories were completed and brought online.

Also during this period, the true trans-NIH nature of the effort expanded. Investigators from eight different institutes and the Food and Drug Administration (FDA) were active in CHI studies. Their enthusiasm for the mission of the CHI, and the gratis donation of their time and expertise were key ingredients in propelling the CHI forward. This was fortunate because, given its limited budget, the CHI could not otherwise have obtained the participation of scientists at such high levels. The informal nature of participation also circumvented lengthy approval processes in the various institutes.

External review of the CHI and the future

In the summer of 2011, the CHI was invited to report on its progress to the assembled directors of the NIH and its institutes. There was considerable enthusiasm for what the CHI had accomplished in slightly over two years, and Harold Varmus (NCI) suggested that a review of the CHI by a panel of outside experts would be helpful in the institutes' consideration of future funding. This outside review was held at the end of November 2011. The panel, chosen by senior NIH immunologists, included Raymond N. DuBois (University of Texas MD Anderson Cancer Center), Larry Turka (University of Pennsylvania), Karolina Palucka (Baylor University), and Rafi Ahmed (Emory University School of Medicine). The chairs of the review, Griffith Rodgers (NIDDK) and Michael Gottesman (NIH), prepared a summary of the reviewer's comments that stated, in part:

> Progress in establishing the CHI has been outstanding in the 2.5 years since it was initiated. This is reflected in the recruitment of a talented staff, expert leadership, appropriate investment in instrumentation, and an excellent choice of initial projects. The emphasis on a 'Systems' approach, especially the involvement of Ron Germain and John Tsang, has added an important dimension to the data analysis. Continuing this trajectory is strongly encouraged.

The reviewers recommended an increase in support to $4 million/year for the fiscal years 2014–2018. The NIH institutes are currently considering their levels of support. However, enough commitments have been made that support will be increased above current levels, and the breadth of that support is wider (more supporting institutes). This additional support will be targeted to increasing throughput to allow the CHI to expand its efforts.

It is important to note that the CHI intends to share its data not only through publication but also by placing the data online. Additionally, cooperation with other groups undertaking similar efforts, such as the NIAID-supported Human Immune Project Consortium, are ongoing, as well as are efforts to standardize cell phenotyping (see below), which, if successful, would be a major step in moving this technology into the clinic.

The robust immune platforms developed to date

Clinical sample collection—processing and repository

The CHI has developed standard operating procedures (SOP) for blood and serum collection, PBMC isolation, and control-rate freezing for long-term storage. Human PBMCs isolated using a ficoll gradient are cryopreserved in freezing medium consisting of the intracellular cryoprotecting agent dimethylsulfoxide (DMSO) 10%, plus 90% heat-inactivated fetal bovine serum (HI-FBS). Cells suspended in the freezing medium are cryopreserved at control-rate steps to a temperature of $-120\,°C$ to minimize cell damage, and are then transferred into the vapor phase of a liquid nitrogen (LN_2) tank at $-156\,°C$ ($+/-20\,°C$) until use. The implementation of Leucosep^{TM} tubes (Greiner Bio-One North American Inc, Monroe, North Carolina) for PBMC isolation makes the procedure more robust and reduces laboratory technician handling variation. The control freezing of PBMC appears critical for the maintenance of high viability and function of cells ($>95\%$), including B cells, as verified by B cell ELISPOT assays. Those SOPs have been implemented for all CHI-initiated protocols and have been shared with intra- and extramural collaborators. They are publically available on the CHI website (http://www.nhlbi.nih.gov/resources/chi/sop.htm).

To control for the reliability of storing conditions of frozen cells, the Rees wireless monitor system (Rees Scientific Corp., Easton, Maryland) was implemented to prevent undocumented failures related to power shortage and/or maintenance and instrument malfunction. A web-based automated sample inventory and tracking system (FreezerPro,

RURO, Inc. Frederick, Maryland) has been implemented for efficient sample management and utilization.

To study transcriptional patterns of blood components directly *ex vivo*, the Paxgene blood RNA tube (Becton, Dickinson and Company, San Jose, California) is used for RNA isolation in selected protocols. The integrity and comparability of the isolated RNA is currently being compared with RNA isolated from PBMC samples to address potential biases related to the depletion of granulocytes occurring during PBMC isolation.

PBMCs for gene expression analysis are freshly isolated *ex vivo* and directly lysed in the RNA isolation reagent Qiazol, which protects mRNA from degradation for a minimum of 18 months at $-80\ ^\circ$C to maintain the integrity of the PBMC transcriptome without experiencing freeze and thaw processes. Total RNA isolated from those samples using miRNeasy is used for micro-RNA profiling, gene expression analysis, RNAseq, and real-time PCR.

Flow cytometry and cytokine Luminex platforms

Immunophenotyping of peripheral blood leukocytes is performed for all clinical research protocols. To maximize both the breadth and depth of immunophenotyping, a series of 10 tubes has been developed, each comprising 15 colors.[1] The immunophenotypes examined encompass a wide spectrum of memory and naive T cells, T helper (Th)1, Th2, Th17, regulatory T (T_{reg}), memory and naive B cells, dendritic and natural killer (NK) cell subsets, and monocytes. As all samples for these studies are cryopreserved peripheral blood mononuclear cells (PBMCs), no immunophenotyping of neutrophils is performed. Data are collected on a LSR-Fortessa cytometer (BDIS, San Jose, CA) and analyzed using Flowjo software. Large lots of reagents are purchased for this panel in order to minimize any lot-to-lot variation occurring during a study. As this immunophenotyping panel could theoretically identify over 20,000 subsets of cells, the data are initially analyzed for approximately 150 of the most prominent subsets. The data files are saved for more in-depth analysis, as interest dictates. Some of these data are also provided to collaborators working on automated approaches for data analysis (e.g., FlowCAP),[2] as such efforts would yield more

consistent, in depth, and timely analysis than currently possible.

The flow cytometry platform is also a key participant in the Federation of Clinical Immunology Societies Human Immunophenotyping Consortium (FOCIS-HIPC) and the NIAID U19-HIPC efforts to harmonize immunophenotyping for clinical trial research.[3] To this end, a five-tube panel consisting of eight colors each has been devised. These panels are supplied as lyophilized reagents in 96-well plates (lyoplates) for distribution to immunology centers around the world. Additionally, standard cell sample controls are distributed to each center to assess the degree of harmonization achieved. These data are also provided to the FlowCAP effort in order to assist in the development of automated approaches for data analysis—an effort that will substantially enhance harmonization of these data. Standardization of data and the ultimate replacement of a manual process for reading results with an automated methodology are major goals of clinical immunologists. Reaching these goals will permit studies to be performed at multiple sites, which would increase the robustness of studies enormously.

The levels of cytokines in cryopreserved serum are measured using Luminex multiplex bead array assays (Austin, TX). A total of 69 analytes are measured using five kits from Bio-Rad (Hercules, CA) to provide the most comprehensive and practical assessment of common cytokines and chemokines. These are performed on the Luminex100 instrument, and standard curves are obtained according to the manufacturer's instructions. Data are analyzed using Bio-Plex software (from Bio-Rad). Large lots of these plates are purchased to minimize lot changes within a study, and one bridge control sample is run on all plates to permit normalization of the data.

Omic platforms implemented at the CHI

A whole transcriptome platform from Affymatrix HumanGene 1.0 ST array (Affymatrix, Santa Clara, CA) was selected using a new chip design that covers the full length of each transcript by probing individual exons. The advantage of this design comes from the fact that it targets only functional transcripts with superior accuracy compared to the conventional $3'$-biased design. Each array comprises more than 257,430 unique, 25-mer oligonucleotide probes that interrogate more than 28,000 genes. The data generated from this platform can be used for expression level analysis as well as splicing variants analysis, which have important biologic implications in biologic process in general, and more specifically in immunology. Each transcript value is estimated using the mean of multiple probe sets representing the same transcript, which makes transcript data much more accurate and highly reproducible. The specially designed whole-transcript (WT) RNA amplification method by Ambion replaced the 3′ IVT method, yielding robust amplification of cRNA with one round of amplification using a minimum of 50–100 ng of total RNA. To explore transcript variance, polymorphism, and noncoding RNAs, the CHI has adapted the Genome Analyzer II (Illumina, San Diego, CA) for high-throughput and high-resolution sequence analysis. Functional variants identified by the sequencing approach can be validated in broader study cohorts through targeted resequencing using barcoded amplicons generated by the BioMark System (Fluidigm, San Francisco, CA). The Bio-Marker system can also validate marker transcript expression levels in real time with minimum cost per sample and per reaction.

The influenza vaccination study

As one of the pilot projects for the CHI program, a study was initiated that was designed to evaluate variation in normal responses to vaccination for influenza. Influenza vaccination provides a model perturbation that is routinely used in both healthy and ill adult and pediatric populations. Upon vaccination, there is an early activation of innate cells, along with the subsequent activation of T and B cells, leading to a transient increase in plasmablasts in the blood and the robust production of antibody. Thus, immunization activates multiple arms of the innate and adaptive immune system that allow global evaluation of immune function. Moreover, analysis of antibody titers provides an easily followed assay for examining the generation of protective immunity, which can be compared to multiple immune parameters for evaluation of correlates with protective immunity. In turn, these can be used to build systems biology models for prediction of responses.

Studies on influenza vaccination are of high interest to the infectious disease community, in large part because influenza remains a major worldwide risk that causes significant morbidity and mortality due to the pandemic nature of influenza outbreaks. As a result, vaccination for influenza has been the object of intense study, providing seminal information on immunization responses in humans and correlates with protective immunity. Because influenza vaccination is widely recommended for both adults and children, including subjects with a variety of health problems, responses to the vaccine can potentially provide a way to evaluate immune responses and cellular correlates, in general. Responses to this vaccination, therefore, provide information that can be used for comparison of multiple populations and can provide a potential standard for comparison of multiple subjects. These results also provide the material for evaluating variation in immune responses and their potential influence on disease.

Although several groups have taken a systems approaches to evaluating responses to vaccination with influenza, we used influenza vaccination primarily as a means of perturbing the immune system to evaluate the general status of the immune system. In the CHI study, 140 people were immunized with the 2009 seasonal and pH1N1 nonadjuvanted vaccines in two major cohorts. Blood was drawn both before (days −7 and 0) and after vaccination, including days 1, 7, and 70, a sampling procedure designed to examine innate/immediate, adaptive, and long-term responses, respectively. Samples from 63 of these subjects who completed all time points in one cohort were subjected to a panel of CHI's main analyses, including gene expression analyses by microarray, analyses of cytokines and metabolites by Luminex (Austin, TX), extensive flow cytometric analyses of cell populations, and genotyping by SNP. These assays were combined with study-specific tests for influenza titers and B lymphocyte functional assays to evaluate vaccination outcome.

Using data obtained from these assays, along with a combination of bioinformatic analyses, we found major sets of coherent gene expression and cellular changes in response to vaccination. Notably, many of the major gene expression signatures observed had strong overlaps with gene expression and pathway signatures that have recently been found in other vaccination studies, including two studies of vaccination for yellow fever, a potent vaccination given to naive subjects. By integrating the data sets, we further showed that many of these signature genes are associated with increases in plasmablast frequencies, which can be used to build predictive models, as have been done in other studies. However, most remarkably, the data facilitated the building of accurate predication models using day 0 parameters alone. Intriguingly, these models can be built using cell population frequencies. Such work has obvious implications for predicting responses to vaccines, as well as for extensions to other types of studies involving analyses of the effects of the immune system on outcome, including prospective studies of diverse diseases and drug interventions.

The influenza study has also provided material for setting up and standardizing analyses. For example, evaluation of multiple cell populations by high-density marker flow analysis (as described above) revealed a high degree of variability in the frequency of cell populations among normal donors, particularly the frequencies of cell populations expressing markers of activation or cytokine production. Such populations are likely to reflect variation in the immune activation states of individual subjects, as has been well documented, but care must be taken to evaluate technical variation in the assays. To address this issue, a well-defined apheresed sample was used for comparative purposes, and independent PBMC samples from 24 normal donors from the second cohort of the influenza vaccine study were evaluated over the course of a 2-month period. Notably, a high degree of concordance was observed between runs of the same control apheresed sample, supporting the consistency of the results and highlighting the importance of interexperimental controls. Together, we think the findings of this study will provide important new insight into evaluation of immune responses, as well as insight into improved methods for analyses of the immune system.

Other CHI studies

Despite tremendous progress in the discovery of components of the immune system and understanding of their interactions from *in vitro* and animal experiments, our understanding of the human immunome remains quite limited. This limited knowledge significantly impairs progress in both elucidating the pathophysiology of immune-mediated diseases and the development of new therapies. The traditional bench to bedside approach that utilizes findings from mouse models to human disease is increasingly recognized as flawed, mostly due to the extensive differences between species and, of equal importance, because of the high interindividual variability present in humans

but absent in inbred laboratory animals. The immune system is inherently dynamic, with marked changes in response not only to antigens, immunogens, and pathogens, but also to circadian rhythm, metabolic (food intake) variations, and physical and emotional stress. Some effects are of short duration and rapidly resolve to steady-state conditions; others exert a longer lasting effect. The need to control for many of the factors that affect the immune system, such as diet, environment, and time of day is of special importance in clinical trials (as opposed to mice that live in a highly controlled environment). We can minimize some effects by using measures like admission to inpatient units, but we cannot eliminate them. Many factors are hard or even impossible to control, including unrecognized comorbidities and genetic factors, OTC drug consumption, diet, and psychosocial stress.

The CHI conducts trials (Table 1) in patients with various immune-mediated diseases as well as in healthy volunteers to better characterize the normal immunome. The unique setting of the NIH Clinical Research Center, with 250 inpatient beds, access to highly specialized research nursing staff, and the availability of laboratory technicians around the clock to process samples, facilitates and encourages the conduct of high-quality clinical research. Ten clinical trials have been initiated by the CHI since its founding in 2009, as summarized in Table 1. Below, we describe some of the protocols, and discuss some of the debates and challenges we have encountered during the design and implementation of these trials.

The extensive phenotyping approach developed by the CHI utilizes multiple platforms that require large amounts of blood. Obviously, research subjects' safety limits the amount of blood that can be sampled (per NIH guidelines, up to 550 mL over an 8-week period), so time points for sampling need to be chosen carefully. Sampling can be performed at rest and in presumed steady state in order to measure variations in the immune system among individuals. Alternatively, testing can be performed in disease states, assuming the disease (or its treatment) sufficiently affects the immune system to overcome interindividual variation. Finally, studies can be performed during synchronized perturbation of the immune system of healthy subjects. The choice of intervention must take into account the risk associated with the perturbation, the optimal

Table 1. CHI's studies and collaborations[a]

Study title (short title)	Disease	Number of subjects	Status	Comments	Clinicaltrials. gov
Effects of flu vaccine on the immune system	Healthy volunteers	203	Advanced data analysis		NCT00995527
Effects of systemic steroids on the immune system	Healthy volunteers	20	Data analysis		NCT01281995
Effects of statins on inflammation	Healthy volunteers	20	Sample collection	10 subjects normal CRP; 10 subjects elevated CRP	NCT01200836
Low-dose IL-2	Healthy volunteers	12	Data analysis	6 subjects 100,000/m^2 6 subjects 200,000/m^2	NCT01445561
Innate immune response to HIN1 vaccine	Healthy volunteers	23	Data acquisition		NCT00995527
The immune system during pregnancy	Healthy volunteers	40	Sample collection		NCT01200979
The immune system in Hermansky-Pudlak syndrome	HPS or familial pulmonary fibrosis	11 5	Data acquisition		NCT01200823
Multiple sclerosis	Newly diagnosed high inflammatory MS with flu vaccine perturbation	10 10	Sample collection		NCT01200823
Effects of long-term steroid exposure on the immune system	Cushing's disease	10	Sample collection		NCT01200823
Oral tolerance in uveitis	Uveitis	40	Sample collection		NCT01195948

[a]HPS, Hermansky-Podlak syndrome; MS, multiple sclerosis.

dose, the method of delivery, and effects on absorption and metabolism.

Our choice of perturbation test for the first CHI study was strongly influenced by the emergence of the swine-origin H1N1 flu pandemic in 2009. The fear of a pandemic highlighted our limited understanding of the basic immunologic response to a challenge by a mild antigen, such as the split-inactivated influenza vaccine. H1N1 was a new antigen to which most of the population was then naive, so the primary immune response could be assessed, as opposed to a recall response obtained during the seasonal flu vaccination. Since flu was a weak antigen (compared to yellow fever vaccination), it was a good test for the sensitivity of our various assays and of the computational approach.

In fact, the overarching question of the study at its inception was whether alterations in the immune system would be detectable. The strong clinical indication for vaccination minimized ethical concerns for the study subjects, all of whom were healthcare workers for whom vaccination was mandated.

The use of flu perturbation can be further expanded to disease and unique physiological states. We are currently studying the response to flu vaccination in multiple sclerosis and in healthy pregnant women, the latter a circumstance notable for risk aversion in clinical research.

In the flu study and subsequent protocols, timing of sampling is important and often requires compromises with ideal experiments that can be performed in animal models. The more frequent the

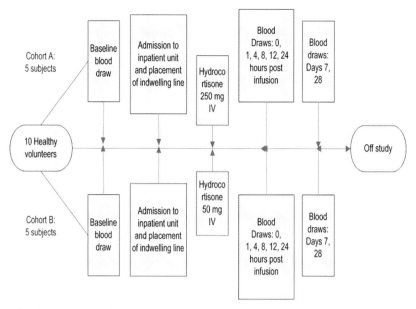

Figure 3. Protocol outline: the effects of systemically administered corticosteroids on the immune system of healthy volunteers.

sampling, the less blood can be obtained at any one time point for more in-depth analysis. Conversely, if sampling frequency is reduced, a critical stage in the development of the immune response might be missed. In contrast to homogeneous mouse populations, humans are likely to develop similar responses but over slightly different time courses. Our approach to capture both critical time points and also allow for deep analysis has been to pilot in a small cohort to establish an approximate secular course for the response. Subsequently, a larger cohort can be assayed at fewer time points. This approach was used in the study of the innate immune response to H1N1 vaccine.

We set out to study the innate immune response to H1N1 vaccine, working under the assumption that most subjects would be naive. The first question we considered was: Is the innate response to a split inactivated vaccine prominent enough to allow detection in peripheral blood, and if so, what would be the time course for such a reaction? Because of the lack of prior relevant information in the literature, we chose to have the first four subjects serve as a pilot for detailed study of the time course of the immune response. The vaccine's brochure reported fever 6–12 h postvaccination in young first-time vaccine recipients, suggesting a higher likelihood for detecting innate immune response in that time window.

We therefore measured gene expression changes by microarray every 2 h for the initial 16 h following administration of the vaccine, and every 6 h up to 36 h postvaccination. Initial analysis of the timeline suggested that the majority of the changes occurred within 8–12 h postvaccination. Based on these data, for the main cohort of the study we collected samples at baseline and at 8, 12, and 24 h. The focus on fewer time points allowed for larger amounts of blood collection at each time point, and hence deeper phenotyping, including comprehensive flow cytometry analysis. We applied this same approach to study the effects of corticosteroids on the immune system of healthy volunteers (Fig. 3).

Corticosteroids were first used in 1948 to treat rheumatoid arthritis[4] and have since become the most commonly prescribed class of immunomodulatory therapeutics. They are used in therapy for an array of medical conditions, including rheumatic, allergic, autoimmune, endocrine, hematologic, dermatologic, pulmonary, neurologic, and oncologic diseases. However, despite their ubiquitous clinical use, there is a paucity of information on the effects of systemically administered corticosteroids in humans, and no previous study has examined their effects on the human immunome.

In designing a study to examine the action of corticosteroids on the human immunome, the first debate was the choice of agent and dose. The corticosteroid family contains multiple compounds that differ in potency and action. They are utilized at different doses and regimens in different conditions. Among the synthetic and naturally occurring corticosteroids, hydrocortisone exhibits the least variation in absorption and metabolism in humans. It is equivalent in potency and anti-inflammatory properties to the naturally occurring steroid hydrocortisone (cortisol), and it has a rapid onset of action, with biologic activity detected within 1 h of administration. An infused dose of hydrocortisone is nearly completely excreted within 12 h. We chose to study a low therapeutic dose of 50 mg and a moderate 250 mg dose (equivalent to 50 mg prednisone).

A two-step trial design was used (similar to the innate response to H1N1 vaccine), wherein the first step informed the time course for sampling of the second step. Each step had two cohorts: one for each dose (50 or 250 mg). To complement the study of the effects of a single dose of steroids, we developed a collaboration to study patients with Cushing's disease, which is characterized by increased secretion of endogenous steroids (cortisol). NIH investigators have been studying this very rare disease (incidence 2–4/million), enabling us to phenotype the immune system under long-term exposure to steroids without an underlying immune-mediated disease.

HMG-CoA reductase inhibitors (statins) represent another commonly used class of medications. Statins are presumed to have significant effects on the immune system that are not well characterized. Statins are potent inhibitors of HMG-CoA reduc-

tase, a key enzyme in cholesterol synthesis, and have been successfully used for primary and secondary prevention of cardiovascular disease. The main action of statins is believed to be reduction in LDL cholesterol synthesis. However, the preventive effects of statins on cardiovascular disease appear to be well beyond their cholesterol-lowering effects. In the JUPITER trial, 17,000 healthy subjects with normal blood cholesterol levels (LDL < 130) and elevated C-reactive protein (CRP > 2 mg/L), a marker of inflammation, were randomized to therapy with statins versus placebo. The study found significant reductions in fatal and nonfatal myocardial infarction, stroke, and death from cardiovascular disease.[4] This study did not establish a mechanism for the effects of statins; however, the concomitant 37% reduction in CRP levels suggests that reduction in inflammation might have been a major contributing mechanism. An understanding of the mechanism (Fig. 4) by which statins affect the immune system may help us to better define the patient population that might benefit from such therapy and potentially develop drugs that act more selectively and potently on the relevant immunologic pathway(s).

Another immune-active medication that has been drawing great interest is interleukin-2 (IL-2). Investigation into the role of T_{reg} and NK cells in immunity led to multiple trials investigating the therapeutic application of IL-2 in different disease states (Fig. 5). These preliminary studies suggest that very low-dose IL-2 therapy (0.5–1 mIU/m^2/day) can induce preferential immune reconstitution by

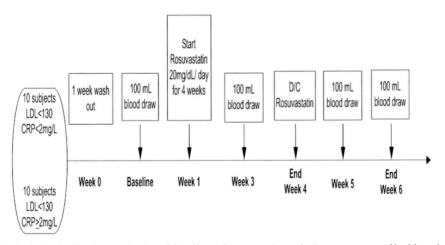

Figure 4. Study design for the characterization of the effects of rosuvastatin on the immune system of healthy volunteers with normal cholesterol with or without elevated C-reactive protein.

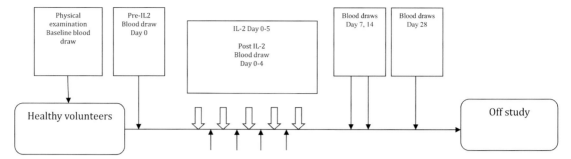

Figure 5. Study outline: ultra-low-dose Il-2 in healthy volunteers; six subjects were treated with 100,000 IU/m^2 followed by a second cohort of six subjects treated with 200,000 IU/m^2.

selective expansion of T_{reg} and NK cells.[5–7] We designed a clinical trial to evaluate the effects of very low-dose interleukin-2 therapy on the immunome. We also aimed to determine the optimal IL-2 dose for preferential expansion of T_{reg} and NK cells in immunocompetent healthy volunteers. The results from this study would be valuable as a control group for studying immunopathology of a broad spectrum of diseases, including cancer, immunodeficiency, autoimmune disease, and hematopoietic stem cell transplantation.

The CHI approach to the study of the human immunome can be further expanded to physiological states such as pregnancy. Traditionally, it has been suggested that pregnancy causes an immunosuppressed state that facilitates fetal tolerance and results in increased susceptibility to infection. Although the suppression has been characterized as a global T cell defect, the observation that the increase in susceptibility is restricted only to specific intracellular bacteria and viruses is consistent with a downregulation of only certain components of the innate immune system. Progress in the treatment and management of infections during pregnancy will require further understanding of the changes to the immune system that occur during pregnancy. It is hypothesized that there is a fundamental downregulation in the innate immune system that occurs during pregnancy and remains until delivery. Pregnancy-induced changes in serum cytokines may influence naive CD4$^+$ differentiation to different subpopulations. We designed a study to evaluate blood samples drawn from pregnant women during early, middle, and late pregnancy, as well as in postpartum women. These samples were compared to those of healthy, nonpregnant women to study changes in the innate and adaptive immune system. The effects of pregnancy on the immune system make pregnant women more vulnerable to influenza, especially H1N1. Therefore, the addition of clinically indicated flu vaccination with postvaccine blood draws is of special importance in this study.

The CHI approach has proven valuable in assessing therapies and their mechanisms of action. In a randomized trial comparing the effects of horse- and rabbit-derived antithymocyte globulin (ATG) in patients with previously untreated severe aplastic anemia, horse ATG was significantly more effective in inducing hematologic remission. Phenotyping of lymphocyte reconstitution posttreatment provided a putative explanation for this clinical effect that was unexpected and contrary to the *in vitro* predictions. While rabbit ATG promoted T_{reg} cells *in vitro*, this effect was overwhelmed by its more severe reduction in all CD4$^+$ cells *in vivo*. T_{reg} cell number was the most dramatic difference among all measurements of lymphocyte subsets and cytokines between horse and rabbit ATG in patients.[8]

CHI education and interactions with the extramural immunologic community

From the very beginning, educational efforts and interactions with the extramural immunologic community have been an important part of the CHI. These efforts fell into three areas, as described below.

NIH symposia and other lecture series
The CHI has organized large yearly one-day symposia, the purpose of which is to bring leaders in human immunology and new immunology technologies to the NIH campus to discuss their work and interact with the leadership and members

of the CHI: "Inaugural CHI Conference—Big Questions in Human Immunology" (2008), "Meeting the Human Immunology Challenge" (2009), "Influenza and the Immune System" (2010), and "High Technology in Clinical Immunology" (2011). Each symposium was well attended (300–450 participants) and produced useful discussions. Two additional lecture series were begun under the auspices of the CHI. The CHI Thursday noon lectures featured visiting professors' presenting novel human translational research and/or novel technologies, which provided a valuable source of ideas that helped shape CHI efforts.

The Novel Experimental Research Developments (NERD) series is an educational activity representing a joint effort among the Infectious Disease and Immunogenetic Section (IDIS), the DTM, and the CHI. Its scope is to reach the intramural community with primary focus on the CHI membership. The NERD series favors the presentation of novel technical and methodological advances relevant to basic and/or clinical research that would not typically fit the broader purposes of most scientific lecture series held at the NIH.

Training program in clinical immunology

The CHI has established a one-week internship for clinical fellows from other disciplines who are interested in conducting research in immune-mediated diseases. The objectives are to increase an understanding of the need to study the human immune system and to define the normal immunome, promote a realization of the limitations and challenges of this study, introduce the relevant methods, and explore immune-mediated diseases outside of the fellow's specific discipline/specialty. Initially, this program was 1 week in length with a planned extension to 2 weeks in the following year. Our long-term target is a formal curriculum for 6 months of fellowship training.

The CHI is a Federation of Clinical Immunology Societies (FOCIS) Center of Excellence

This designation has provided the CHI with the opportunity for both educational and interactive efforts. It provided the opportunity to send young NIH investigators to the FOCIS training programs at a reduced cost. CHI hosted the FOCIS meeting on immunophenotyping standardization in February 2011. It also established the Bedside to Bench

& Back (BB&B) Lecture Series, which is an educational activity supported jointly by the CHI and the FOCIS. Its scope is to serve as a bridge between the intramural and local extramural immunology communities, promoting cultural exchange and collaboration among scientists and clinicians who share common interests in translational studies aimed at unraveling the intricacy of the human immune system. Through thought-provoking lectures, BB&B hopes to deliver innovative science and trigger novel investigations.

The CHI: advantages, challenges, and the future

NIH's CHI is a coordinated effort, in the human sense of multiple agents acting toward a common goal. Broadly, all science can be viewed as a collective striving toward truth, but the details vary depending on the organization. For individual scientific laboratories, there is a clear hierarchy of professor or laboratory chief, junior faculty, fellows, and students, with obvious roles, incentives and expectations, and mechanisms of interaction. The human genome sequencing effort was a massive aggregated effort, but the goal was straightforward; enormous, central, and dedicated funding dictated its organization, benchmarks, and quality control. In comparison, the CHI has had special advantages but also particular challenges.

Adding to the history of CHI described above, there were several inherent problems present at the start. First, CHI was perceived as a top–down initiative, perhaps politically motivated. Second, as the budget of the Intramural Program of NIH is fixed, allocation of funds is viewed as a zero-sum game, in which every winner implies a loser; additionally, there was the usual skepticism that resources would be diverted to the interests of the organizers. Third, many NIH scientists were uncomfortable with the stress of new and unfamiliar technologies, and especially computational approaches to large data sets, and with the contrast to hypothesis-generating rather than classical hypothesis–testing science. Further, the central role of technology platforms as drivers of experiments and the primacy of computational approaches conflicted with the expectations of core facilities for specific assays, and of the statistician who entered the laboratory after the data were generated. Finally, the fact that the CHI was a voluntary and participatory activity—there were no dues or any requirements for membership other than interest in the venture—also puzzled some who viewed the center as a possible source of grant-like support. In retrospect, some of this confusion was secondary to errors made by the CHI. For example, the new center advertised to the NIH community its interest in proposals for appropriate research to take place at the CHI, with the intents of publicizing CHI goals, democratizing its processes, and generating ideas. The CHI was inundated by mini-grant requests; many contained excellent scientific ideas but were inappropriate for the CHI vision. At its inception, the CHI was simply unable to rank, approve, or act on these proposals, which led to much disappointment among the proposers. Similarly, group meetings to discuss the sorts of big questions in immunology, which the CHI might address over the long term, could devolve into heated arguments over the virtues of the CD4$^+$ cell over the macrophage, or the centrality of particular cytokines. This experience made the proposed influenza trial appealing, as it did not belong to any single investigator's domain, it was likely to provide large numbers of healthy volunteers to establish a database containing the outlines of the human immunome, and was a test of the practicality of the CHI's nascent SOP, logistics of sample handling and testing in the platform laboratories, and the quality of newly hired staff. Indeed, the hypothesis of the flu protocol was that a mild perturbation, a single injection of a killed viral vaccine antigen, would lead to consistent detectable alterations in the immune system, and if alterations appeared, that a computational approach combining data from several multiplex platforms would yield interesting results.

The CHI enlisted many generals to serve as its leadership, individuals with vast experience in diverse areas, heads of large NIH laboratories and branches, all of whom had limited extra time and continuing obligations to their main occupations, and to meeting the stringent requirements for success before quadrennial review boards that determine forward funding in the intramural program. That these individuals enthusiastically contributed enormous time and energy to the CHI was strong evidence of the soundness of the center's underlying goals. The CHI benefited from simple techniques like a weekly breakfast with excellent espresso and good pastries. The diversity of interests of the CHI leaders was an enormous plus, as their expertise encompassed the most basic aspects of immunology, animal models, cell biology and imaging, genetics and genomics, as well as clinical trial design and implementation. There may have been advantages to having a director who was not a classical immunologist but rather a clinical researcher. The status and strength of the CHI leadership seemed most compatible with a flat management hierarchy, with big decisions made by consensus, and even small issues settled among the parties rather than by dictate. Disagreement and arguments, sometimes heated, did occur, but in an atmosphere of trust, respect, and a deeply shared vision of the center's value, aims, and likelihood of success.

Moving forward, there are opportunities and challenges. We have the advantage of stable, indeed, increased funding, evidence of the confidence of the institute directors in the CHI's accomplishments, goals, and importance to the NIH's national mission. Nevertheless, there are concerns of scale. Size matters. Leverage and donated time can be exploited, but a sufficient mass of permanent, diversely specialized staff (especially in computational biology) is critical for sustained growth. The CHI has survived the early learning phase, developed its own culture, and solved many daunting logistical, technical, and especially computational problems: the knowledge gained can be immediately applied to new projects. Organizationally, the CHI will be able to undertake at least one large protocol a year, with the ability to also perform six to eight smaller projects with collaborating investigators. The flow of CHI work is complex: clinical protocol development, patient accrual, sample processing and storage, assays, computation, and finally, manuscript preparation. Each part relates to the other, and balancing the components is not trivial. New technologies, often minimally tested, appear, attract, and supplant the familiar platforms; expertise is needed to assess them, and judgment is required to determine whether and when to implement them. The CHI, as part of the NIH, has obligations to make its data publicly available, but the quality of the data to be released (e.g., raw, refined, or processed) and the timing of release are unresolved issues. Finally, the CHI must maintain enthusiasm for the prospect of an understanding of the human immune system that can result in real clinical applications, diagnostics, and therapeutics, with an impact that is as meaningful and broad as possible.

Acknowledgments

Special thanks need to go to Angelique Biancato, Ronald Germain, Francesco Marincola, Matthew Olnes, and Giorgio Trinchieri.

Conflicts of interest

The authors declare no conflicts of interest.

References

1. Biancotto, A., J.C. Fuchs, A. Williams, *et al.* 2011. High dimensional flow cytometry for comprehensive leukocyte immunophenotyping (CLIP) in translational research. *J. Immunol. Methods* **363:** 245–261.

2. Aghaeepour, N., *et al.* 2013. Critical assessment of automated flow cytometry data analysis techniques. *Nat. Methods* **10:** 228–238.

3. Maecker, H.T., J.P. McCoy & R. Nussenblatt. 2012. Standardizing immunophenotyping for the Human Immunology Project. *Nat. Rev. Immunol.* **12:** 191–200.

4. Ridker, P.M., E. Danielson, F.A. Fonseca, *et al.* 2008. Rosuvastatin to prevent vascular events in men and women with elevated C-reactive protein. *N. Engl. J. Med.* **359:** 2195–2207.

5. Shah, M.H., A.G. Freud, D.M. Benson, Jr., *et al.* 2006. A phase I study of ultra low dose interleukin-2 and stem cell factor in patients with HIV infection or HIV and cancer. *Clin. Cancer Res.* **12:** 3993–3996.

6. Lechleider, R.J., P.M. Arlen, K.Y. Tsang, *et al.* 2008. Safety and immunologic response of a viral vaccine to prostate-specific antigen in combination with radiation therapy when metronomic-dose interleukin 2 is used as an adjuvant. *Clin. Cancer Res.* **14:** 5284–5291.

7. Zorn, E., M. Mohseni, H. Kim, *et al.* 2009. Combined CD4+ donor lymphocyte infusion and low-dose recombinant IL-2 expand FOXP3+ regulatory T cells following allogeneic hematopoietic stem cell transplantation. *Biol. Blood Marrow Transplant.* **15:** 382–388.

8. Scheinberg, P., O. Nunez, B. Weinstein, *et al.* 2011. Horse versus rabbit antithymocyte globulin in acquired aplastic anemia. *N. Engl. J. Med.* **365:** 430–438.